# BUILDING A SCIENCE OF NURSING EDUCATION:

## FOUNDATION FOR EVIDENCE-BASED TEACHING-LEARNING

Cathleen M. Shultz, PhD, RN, CNE, FAAN
*Editor*

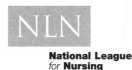

NLN

**National League**
*for* **Nursing**

National League for Nursing
61 Broadway
New York, NY 10006
212-363-5555 or 800-669-1656
www.nln.org


ISBN 1-934758-05-1


The NLN's Priorities for Research in Nursing Education and Science Building Model are included with permission of the National League for Nursing.


All of the photos in this book are included with the permission of the College of Nursing at Harding University (Searcy, AR). Gratitude is expressed to Jeff Montgomery, Eric Swanson and Kyle Vath for taking the photos.


Cover design by Brian Vigorita
Art Director, Laerdal Medical Corporation


Printed in the United States of America

# Building a Science of Nursing Education:

## Foundation for Evidence-based Teaching-Learning

# TABLE OF CONTENTS

# LIST OF TABLES

# LIST OF FIGURES

In the NLN's 2008 Strategic Plan, the fourth goal reads as follows: "Advancement of the Science of Nursing Education: Promote evidence-based nursing education and the scholarship of teaching." This book, *Building a Science of Nursing Education: Foundation for Evidence-Based Teaching–Learning,* is clearly dedicated to the achievement of this goal. The strategic plan cited above is relatively new, having only existed for slightly more than one year. However, the goal of advancing the science of nursing education is not new to the NLN. This book represents a seven-year journey of unblinking determination by the amazing members of the NLN Task Group on Teaching-Learning Paradigms and the contributing authors. Their journey in bringing this work to life is documented in the preface and the first two chapters of the book, where Drs. Shultz, Gresley, and Sullivan speak boldly about the paucity of nursing education search descriptors and actual research findings in existing electronic databases.

Although the task group members were delayed, they were not defeated. In this book they introduce the first model for building a science of nursing education; provide a framework for organizing and reporting research findings in nursing education; describe in depth the essentials of learning; and walk the reader through the domains of teaching and learning in nursing education. Finally, with an eye toward the future, they provide an overall summary of their work and the gaps in nursing education research that stand ready to be filled by nurse educator scholars.

For the seven years of the journey, there are seven chapters in this book. With the clear vision of the academic nurse scholar, the authors sketch in detail the cluttered path that was followed and the opportunity for others to transform that narrow path into an electronic highway of access to nursing education research, and thus build the science of nursing education.

In a position statement from 2002, "The Preparation of Nurse Educators," the NLN issued a major, historical challenge: "The teaching of nursing must be evidence-based with research informing what is taught, how learning is facilitated and evaluated, and how curricula/programs are designed." In order to make the challenge even more controversial, the following was added: "Educators whose area of scholarship is pedagogical, rather than clinical in nature should be encouraged, supported and rewarded for this contribution." In other words, nursing education research is nursing science and should have equal footing with clinical nursing research in our reward and value system. Nursing education research touches the patient, family, community, and the world through the hands of all those students prepared by nurse educators. This book represents a powerful step in disseminating the good news: the science of nursing education is good for patient care.

The NLN is all about nursing education and, yes, the NLN is all about patient care. In the following pages, you will see the task group members and contributing authors unveil the rubrics of the science that is the foundation for nursing education. This is a book whose subject has come of age. *Building the Science of Nursing Education* — the right book, the right time, and the right message.

*Beverly Malone, PhD, RN, FAAN*
*Chief Executive Office*
*National League for Nursing*

# PREFACE

At no other time in the history of nursing has there been such a compelling need to examine our educational practices. Clearly the public and employers desire graduates who can think critically, practice safely and effectively, and relate as caring, compassionate professionals. Although it can be argued that these are not necessarily new expectations of nursing graduates, the dramatic changes in the practice environment have redefined what it means to deliver safe and competent care. Not only are nurse educators challenged to prepare students for the increasing complexities of the practice environment, they are also expected to do so within the time frame of the academic program. Admittedly, the task often seems daunting, calling for nurse educators to reexamine their current pedagogical assumptions and practices, determine which practices are most effective to meet the current and projected needs of the nursing profession, propose new and/or modified strategies, and discard practices that are not evidence-based.

As the first and now enduring leader in nursing education for all program types, the National League for Nursing (NLN) recognized the need to support the scholarship of nursing education. Among other initiatives, the NLN created a task group to synthesize existing nursing education research findings. The purposes were to provide a foundation of research findings for current and aspiring nurse educators and to identify gaps in existing research for nurse educator scholars. We engaged experienced nurse educators in the United States and South and Central America for this challenge; every effort was made to include global nurse educator research findings. This book is the result of that task group's work over a seven-year period. The publication is a resource for graduate students, new nurse educators, new and experienced scholars, and seasoned nurse educators to assist them in understanding the scope and use of existing nursing education science and to create new areas of research. Another audience that this book addresses is those in the publishing business who create and sustain publishing companies, especially those who print nursing education research. The authors have identified strengths and weaknesses of existing publications. A plea is made to fill those gaps, accept quality study designs that are theoretically based, and develop a consistent terminology base that eases the retrieval of studies from electronic databases. We implore you to join nurse educators in creating a strong, useful science of nursing education.

We, the task group members and chapter authors (see Appendix A), initially thought our task could be accomplished within two years, a typical time frame for research and writing activities. Very early, we encountered a major barrier to identifying the research that is discussed in Chapter 2. We discovered that most of the nursing education research is not retrievable in existing electronic databases using existing search descriptors. Further complicating the retrieval was that numerous studies were published in books such as the *Annual Review of Nursing Education*. These were not in electronic databases even though we knew they existed. As a result, we often used time-intensive hand searches. Once that barrier was resolved, categories to collect and describe the research were chosen. These findings are synthesized in Chapters 3 through 6. The combined efforts of the authors inspired the Building a Science of Nursing Education Model presented in Chapter 1. Chapter 7 discusses challenges to current and future nurse educator scholars. Finally, nurse educators are directed to the appendices for compilations of current electronic databases and journals that publish nursing education research for assistance in their scholarship development. Our colleagues in this project summarized nursing education research from the Spanish and Portuguese languages and these are located in the appendices. In essence, Chapters 1 and 2 establish the development and context for this book. Chapters 3 through 6 synthesize published research studies about learning in the cognitive, psychomotor and affective domains of learning. Chapter 7 holistically presents the research literature gaps and future evidence-based teaching-learning needs of nurse educators. A summary of each chapter follows.

### Chapter 1. Building a Science of Nursing Education

This chapter follows the evolutionary development of this book from a conceptual idea to its actual publication. The task group's purposes and the relationship of Ernest Boyer's Scholarship of Engagement to nursing education are discussed. The nature and development of a science are explored, as well as the present nurse educator role and core competencies expected of nurse educators. National nursing education research priorities are presented. Finally, the Building a Science of Nursing Education Model, the very first for nursing education, and created by the task group authors, is discussed.

### Chapter 2. A Framework for Organizing and Reporting Research Findings: Using a Common Language

The development of this chapter was initially hampered by search descriptors in existing literature databases. The task group's efforts to extract, locate, and obtain research findings are summarized so that new nurse educator scholars, those who archive the databases, and librarians have an increased awareness of the existing logistical problems. In an effort to disseminate findings in a logical, relevant manner for readers, the task group selected a well-known and useful model that is explained in this chapter. The task group does not suggest that Bloom's model become the end-all for nursing education. Rather, the major terms of the model are used to organize the meta-analysis of literature. The authors believe that future nurse educators will create an even better organizing framework.

### Chapter 3. Essentials of Learning

A comprehensive, in-depth overview of learning theories, emerging nursing pedagogies, the learner and the teacher are presented. Research about learner characteristics that affect learning are summarized; these include intelligence, motivation level, aptitude, learning style and brain function. The learning environment and technology searches yielded few studies that affect learning. Teacher characteristics, thinking styles, personality, relationships with students, and teaching styles have been studied with limited findings. Nurse educator competencies developed by another NLN task group are discussed. Critical thinking, as an aspect of learning, has been researched with a general focus, as a measurement within a course or program in relationship to other factors such as teaching.

### Chapter 4. Teaching-Learning in the Cognitive Domain

Recognizing Chickering's *Seven Principles for Effective Teaching Practices in Undergraduate Education*, research studies, though few, are summarized. Effective, evidence-based cognitive learning methods are scarce. Most studies were one-time, isolated studies that have not been replicated in the literature. Prominent teaching practices in the cognitive domain that were researched include lecture, discussion, collaborative learning, and critical thinking.

### Chapter 5. Teaching-Learning in the Psychomotor Domain

The psychomotor domain includes development of basic motor skills, coordination and physical movement. Bloom's early research has been developed into a taxonomy of progression by Reilly and Oermann. Stages of psychomotor skill progression are delineated. This domain's research is the most extensive in nursing education and is analyzed into categories of faculty roles when teaching psychomotor skills, instructional strategies, and evaluation. Studies on lecture, work-based learning, simulations/simulators, objective structured clinical examinations, problem-based learning, student-centered approaches to learning skills, use of multimedia, and computer-based learning for teaching psychomotor domain learning are synthesized. In addition, research on evaluating psychomotor skill performance is included. The chapter is rich in research findings and new teaching methods. However, the psychomotor domain research in nursing education remains in its infancy.

### Chapter 6. Teaching-Learning in the Affective Domain

Research in the affective domain remains a challenge to nurse educators as well as related disciplines. The domain is broad, complicated, and abstract, with few measurement tools other than self-reports, perceptions, and attitudinal scales to indicate progress. Using the professional values verified in the American Nurses Association's *Code of Ethics* (2001), professional values, identity, and attitudes were used to organize the chapter. Although research about several professional values is limited, emerging research exists on related professional values such as caring, empathy and civility, and learning while caring for patients who are suffering or experiencing poverty. Nursing student attitudes were studied toward current topics such as nursing research, elders, and mental illnesses. Students' emotional responses to learning in nursing programs were studied, although teaching strategies to address those responses have produced little research. Both instructional and non-instructional strategies that enhance affective learning were identified with no predominant clusters of research; the strategies were diverse and, often, one-time approaches. Studies on faculty behaviors and characteristics that promote affective learning are summarized, as well as research from other professional disciplines. Emerging affective domain national initiatives and product trends are discussed in relation to future nurse educator scholars.

### Chapter 7. Ongoing Development of the Science of Nursing Education

A broad overview of the task group's work is summarized and major gaps in nursing education research findings are discussed. Nurse educator scholars are challenged to continue building the science of nursing education, refining the model in Chapter 1, and building meaningful programs of long-term and multi-site research in nursing education.

This book fills a critical gap in nursing education research and is foundational to nurse educators as they teach, assess learning, strengthen their scholarship, and build the future of nursing education. Evidence generated through research changes education and ultimately, practice. May this book increase nurse educators' awareness of the knowledge and research topics that have been generated and excite nurse educators to further explore and build upon the vast field of nursing education research. Building the science of nursing education is a valuable and necessary undertaking for the challenges ahead.

*Cathleen M. Shultz, PhD, RN, CNE, FAAN*
*Editor*
*President-Elect, National League for Nursing, 2007-2009*
*Chair, NLN Task Group on Teaching-Learning Paradigms, 2001-2006*

# ACKNOWLEDGMENTS

The editor and authors acknowledge the following individuals who volunteered their time and talents to the production of the book. Thank you for your generosity and commitment to nursing education.

## Harding University

Searcy, AR

**Jacqueline Harris, MNSc, RN**
Assistant Professor of Nursing
College of Nursing

**Deanna Nowakowski, BA**
Administrative Assistant
College of Nursing

**Jeff Montgomery, BA**
Director of Photography Services
Public Relations Department

**Eric Swanson, MBA**
Resources Coordinator
College of Nursing

**Jean Waldrop, MS**
Circulation Librarian
Brackett Library

## Janet Martha Phillips, PhDc, RN

Associate Instructor
Project Coordinator, Fairbanks Simulation
  Project, Indiana University School of
  Nursing
Doctoral Candidate, Indiana University
School of Nursing
Indianapolis, IN

## Martha M. Scheckel, PhD, RN

Assistant Professor of Nursing
Winona State University
Winona, MN
2001-2003: Doctoral Student Intern
  at the NLN
Chair, NLN Nursing Education Advisory
  Council, 2003-2005

## Latin American Scientific Nurse Educator Collaborators (see Appendix F)

### Maria da Gloria Miotto Wright, PhD, RN

Inter-American Commission on Drug Abuse
  Control (CICAD)
Organization of American States (OAS)
  Washington, DC

## Federal University of Santa Catarina; Florianopolis/SC, Brazil

**Maria Itayra Coelho de Souza Padilha, PhD, RN**
Professor, Department of Nursing

**Kenya Schmitz Reibnitz**
Nursing Doctoral Student

**Joel Rolim Mancia**
Nursing Masters Student

## University Nuevo Leon; Monterrey, Mexico

**Silvia Espinoza Ortega, MNSc**
Director, Faculty of Nursing

## Brian Vigorita

Art Director
Laerdal Medical Corporation
Wappingers Falls, NY

## Laerdal Medical Corporation

Wappingers Falls, NY

BUILDING A SCIENCE OF NURSING EDUCATION

# DEDICATION

This book is dedicated to...

*... our students, past, present and future, who have inspired and taught us.*

*... nurse educator members of the National League for Nursing, who value their mission to graduate prepared, caring nurses.*

*... the National League for Nursing Board of Governors and staff for creating this Task Group, supporting its work, and being committed to advancing the science of nursing education.*

*... all those who have influenced our development as educators and our thinking about the science of nursing education.*

# CHAPTER 1

## BUILDING A SCIENCE OF NURSING EDUCATION

*Ruth Seris Gresley, PhD, RN, CNE*

"In the university, the tension exists between professing
knowledge as a creative teacher-scholar
and adding to knowledge by scholarly research."

**Armiger, 1974, p. 160**

The tension between adding to knowledge through scholarly research and professing knowledge as a teacher-scholar brought together the critical minds and questioning spirits of a skilled faculty group of teacher-scholars to address the question of the state of the scholarship of teaching and learning in nursing. The work presented in this book focuses on the development of a model for building the science of nursing education and summarizes the extant literature available to support that evolving science.

The expanding body of knowledge developed over the past several decades, starting with the curriculum reform advanced by the National League for Nursing, provides support for evidence-based teaching and learning in nursing (Ironside, 2007). Development of a model for looking at the state of this research and its readiness for use in teaching and learning nursing enhances the science of nursing education. The model depicts a nonlinear, iterative process for building the science of nursing education and the activities involved in such building, and it provides guidance for faculty and students of nursing education to identify ways they can contribute to the science of nursing education.

Tension between the scholarship of teaching and learning the art, science and spirit of nursing is long-standing, as acknowledged by Armiger (1974) almost 35 years ago. Armiger also stated that if nursing does not want to disintegrate as a distinct profession, the uniqueness of nursing science and practice needs to be identified. While the likelihood of nursing disappearing seems somewhat remote, disintegration of the profession is a possibility as measures to contain rising health care costs are sought and some seek to have the work of nurses done more cheaply by others. Defining the sciences of nursing and nursing education, and making scholarship an integral part of nursing must continue so the intellectual work of nurses is seen as a significant contribution to society. This book, developed under the auspices of the National League for Nursing (NLN), reflects the collaborative work of a group of nurse educators to add to the body of knowledge about building a science of nursing education. Its purposes are as follows:

- Describe the concept of scholarship, particularly in connection with the science of nursing education,

- Explore what it means to build a science of nursing education,

- Explore the relationships between the science of nursing education and excellence in nursing education,

- Affirm the significance and uniqueness of the nurse educator role,

- Begin to describe the state of the science of nursing education particularly the teaching and learning aspects, outlining what we know and do not know and what needs to be done to continually build, test and refine the science,

- Review selected research from a variety of fields related to teaching and learning,

- Synthesize relevant research findings about teaching and learning as a way to advance the science of nursing education, and

- Stimulate faculty and those preparing for the faculty role to improve the quality of nursing education through the use of evidence-based teaching practices to enhance learning in the cognitive, affective, and psychomotor domains.

For many nurses coming of age as educated professionals in the last 30 years, concerns about whether nursing is a profession and if it has its own body of knowledge that can be applied in practice took up a great deal of discussion time in graduate school. A decade after Armiger's words, Brown and colleagues (1984) said nursing research was increasing but that a major limitation of the research was its noncumulative nature. Efforts to define nursing as a learned profession were strengthened during this period by work done by nursing scholars on developing and testing theories about the practice of nursing and examining the outcomes of the nursing care provided to clients. This work was crucial to the development of scholarship and a science of nursing practice. However, the noncumulative nature of the research limited changes in practice and education based on the research.

In 1990, Ernest Boyer's book *Scholarship Reconsidered: Priorities of the Professoriate* began a movement in colleges and universities that redefined the nature of scholarship for all faculty. His work, along with others (Rice, 1991), provided a model for defining the scholarship of teacher-scholars from a much broader perspective than funded research. Nursing received validation as a practice profession and the developing science of nursing education received support from the rethinking of scholarship through Boyer's scholarship of engagement. Boyer's work traces the changes in the activities of faculty from teaching to advancing knowledge through service and applied research, as well as through the conduct of original research. He identified four types of scholarship germane to faculty work: the scholarship of discovery, which leads to new knowledge; the scholarship of integration, which brings together knowledge from a variety of disciplines to create new perspectives; the scholarship of application, which demonstrates how knowledge is used to enhance the practice of one's profession; and the scholarship of teaching, which uses the process of inquiry about the practices of teaching to identify strategies that most effectively enhance learning. His conclusion that "what we urgently need today is a more inclusive view of what it means to be a scholar - a recognition that knowledge is acquired through research, through synthesis, through practice, and through teaching" (1990, p. 24) provides a strong rationale for the developing science of nursing education.

Boyer, as Armiger did, spoke of the tension in academe between the meaning of scholarship that adds to knowledge through research and the role of the faculty member as a scholar. Is the role of a faculty scholar primarily to discover new knowledge? What is the value of the scholarship of integration, application and teaching to the world of academe? In many academic institutions, scholarship was and still is synonymous with the research generated in disciplines that focus on discovery of new knowledge. In many institutions, disciplined inquiry about learning and teaching does not have the same value as the research done in a controlled laboratory setting. Boyer's work generated interest and discussion about the subject of academic scholarship and the richness of activities that can be included in it. The ensuing work in the academic community about the scholarship of teaching provides a foundation for this book on developing a science of nursing education.

## SCHOLARSHIP REDEFINED

In his book, Boyer (1990) asserted that "We believe the time has come to move beyond the tired old 'teaching versus research' debate and give the familiar and honorable term 'scholarship' a more capacious meaning, one that brings legitimacy to the full scope of academic work" (p.16). He concluded that scholarship, the work of the professoriate, includes four distinct but interrelated dimensions: discovery, integration, application and teaching. His book provided the foundation for a great deal of work and has spurred discussion about scholarship in academe, particularly as it relates to professional disciplines.

Boyer's scholarship of discovery reflects the traditional definition of scholarship, the discovery of knowledge through original or specialized research. This effort is the pursuit of knowledge for its own sake. This scholarship continues to be important in our current efforts to understand the world around us, discover new treatments and approaches, learn from our past, appreciate the significance of differences, and improve human conditions. However, as Boyer notes, this is not the only type of scholarship.

The scholarship of integration reaches across the many disciplines that have generated knowledge about the nature of life and living. Nursing has been committed to a foundation in the liberal arts and sciences since it moved into the academic setting, and more recent recognition of the value of interdisciplinary collaboration reinforces the need to reach across disciplinary lines, gather a variety of ideas and understandings, and put them together in new and creative ways. The integrative form of scholarship requires exquisite critical thinking skills as it challenges old notions of knowledge as being owned by any one discipline. Integration reframes knowledge and allows it to be applied to new problems or applied to old problems in new ways. Integration involves looking at the knowledge for connections across disciplines and interpreting research in terms of larger patterns. Boyer said that being engaged in integration means asking "What do the findings mean?" (p. 19).

The third form of scholarship described by Boyer, application, is designed to apply knowledge to the needs and problems of society, a form of scholarship that clearly has relevance for nursing and nursing education. Using knowledge for improving the world or for service is one form of scholarship that nursing clearly encompasses. While many in the world of academe provide service to their campuses, nursing faculty and students use knowledge to address health problems and societal needs throughout the curriculum as well as through professional activity. Rigor and accountability are hallmarks of professional activity and the scholarship of application just as they are hallmarks of the scholarship of discovery, partly since integrative scholarly work leads to "new intellectual understandings...as theory and practice interact and one renews the other" (Boyer, 1990, pp. 22-23). This type of scholarship clearly includes evidence-based practice in nursing and nursing education that leads to building science.

The scholarship of teaching, the form most relevant to this book and to the development of the science of nursing education, is "the most difficult of the four forms of scholarship to describe" (Rice, 1991, p.14) since there are at least three elements. The first element is "the synoptic capacity, the ability to draw the strands of a field together in a way that provides coherence and meaning" (p. 14). The second element of the scholarship of teaching is what some refer to as "pedagogical content knowledge," or the capacity to represent a subject. The third element addresses "what we know about learning" (p. 15). Boyer (1990) said "teaching can be well regarded only as professors are widely read and intellectually engaged" (p. 23). "Teaching, at its best, means not only transmitting knowledge, but transforming and extending it as well" (p. 24). Teaching is tied to the other

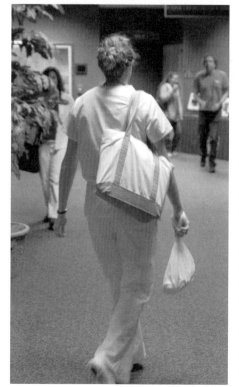

three forms of scholarship outlined by Boyer because it brings together knowledge from a number of fields in a manner that makes connections between disciplines, and transmits information in ways that can be understood by others so that they can make meaning of the information for useful purposes.

It is clear that Boyer's work on scholarship is particularly germane to nursing education. Each form of scholarship is critical to help faculty discover knowledge about how students learn a practice, draw from education and other disciplines to enhance their ability to teach and evaluate learning most effectively, apply knowledge in ways that help them meet the learning needs of diverse student populations, and engage in evidence-based teaching practices. Thus, there are many dimensions to building a science of nursing education, and every faculty member can contribute to that effort in some way.

## THE NATURE AND DEVELOPMENT OF SCIENCE

But what is science? The definition that guided the development of this book defines a science as "a comprehensive, internally consistent body of knowledge about a particular field (e.g., nursing, education) that is built over time by a variety of scholarly endeavors, tested, applied in practice, and continually refined" (T. Valiga, [June 19,] 2003, personal communication). The characteristics of science explicated by McEwen and Wills (2002, p. 6) (see Table 1.1) also was helpful.

| Table 1-1. Characteristics of Science  (McEwen & Wills, 2002, p. 6) |
| --- |
| 1. Science must show [a] certain coherence. |
| 2. Science is concerned with definite fields of knowledge. |
| 3. Science is preferably expressed in universal statements. |
| 4. The statements of science must be true or probably true. |
| 5.The statements of science must be logically ordered. |
| 6. Science must explain its investigations and arguments. |

Discussions about science reflect that it can be considered both a process and a product. That is, science is the act of developing a body of knowledge as well as the actual body of knowledge itself. Science developed through Boyer's four forms of scholarship — discovery, integration, application and teaching — come together in systematic ways that "advance the teaching, research and practice of nursing through rigorous inquiry that 1) is significant to the profession, 2) is creative, 3) can be documented, 4) can be replicated or elaborated, and 5) can be peer-reviewed through various methods" (AACN, 1999, p. 2). The science of nursing education will develop through the Scholarship of Teaching and Learning (SoTL), which "goes beyond being a good teacher (facilitating significant student learning) and beyond being a scholarly teacher (reading the pedagogical literature, attending teaching development activities, etc.). It involves the systematic reflection on teaching and/or learning and the public sharing of the work" (McKinney, 2003, p.1). Thus, the development of a science of nursing education requires a cadre of teacher-scholars who provide leadership regarding the scholarship of teaching and learning the practice of nursing.

## SIGNIFICANCE OF THE NURSE EDUCATOR ROLE

With the current crisis in nursing education, the shortage of nursing faculty, the pressure to produce increasing numbers of students in shorter periods of time, the increasing use of part-time faculty, the aging of the full-time nursing faculty workforce, and the frequent use of non-doctorally prepared faculty, it is even more critical that schools of nursing prepare and support faculty scholars who can help identify effective and efficient ways to facilitate learning and professional growth (NLN, 2002a, 2002b). The concern for nursing education is not whether the part-time and non-doctoral faculty members understand nursing, but whether or not they understand education. Of the 2,837 graduates of master's or doctoral programs in 2001, only 8 % (227) had prepared as educators. Sadly, this number did not even fill the gap left by the 350 resignations from full-time faculty positions that same year (Southern Regional Education Board, 2002), let alone meet new demands.

Concern regarding the educational preparedness of faculty is not unique to nursing. The Association of American College and Universities in conjunction with the Council of Graduate Schools (1997) offers a variety of graduate student programs, one of which is Preparing Future Faculty (PFF). The purpose of the PFF program is to ensure that students preparing to become members of the academic community are conversant in all roles they will be expected to fill as faculty. This includes pedagogical initiatives, research, and service activities. Such an emphasis is particularly relevant in nursing, since many of our faculty come to academe from practice settings and have a limited understanding of the complex role they will assume. Through trial and error or trial by fire, these clinicians came to appreciate that being a faculty member is more than just lecturing or supervising clinical activities. Promotion and tenure requirements may sound like a foreign language to clinical practitioners, and the intricacies of curriculum development also need to be learned. If nursing is to do a better job of preparing the next generation of teachers to also be scholars, the development of the science of nursing education will be a significant step in that process.

One of the core competencies of nurse educators identified by the NLN (Halstead, 2007) is "Engage in Scholarship." This means that faculty "draw on evidence-based literature to improve teaching; exhibit a spirit of inquiry about teaching and learning; design and implement scholarly activities in an established area of expertise; disseminate nursing and teaching expertise through various means and to a variety of audiences; possess skill in grant writing; and demonstrate qualities of a scholar: integrity, courage, perseverance, vitality and creativity" (NLN, 2005, pp. 22-23). Halstead (2007) states that "scholarship is an essential component of the nurse educator role and nurse educators must engage in those professional activities that systematically advance the science of nursing and the science of nursing education" (p. 144).

## THE SCIENCE OF NURSING EDUCATION

The science of nursing education refers to an integrated, comprehensive body of knowledge about how individuals learn to be a nurse or a specialist in some area of nursing, how teachers best enhance that learning, how curriculum design and implementation affect learning, how learning and outcomes of the educational enterprise are managed, and what skills nurse educators need to prepare graduates for the ambiguous, uncertain, unpredictable, constantly changing world in which they will live and practice nursing. At present, this science is in its infancy. Nursing education programs, to a large extent, are traditional, fairly rigid, and inflexible, rather than innovative, as they would be if they were grounded in evidence.

If graduates of basic and advanced nursing programs are to provide the leadership that is needed to provide quality care, promote the health of our nation and create a preferred future for the profession, then educational programs need to be innovative, flexible and responsive to change. To make wholesale change based on "hunches" or "gut feelings" is not defensible. Instead, changes must be made in nursing education that arise from what has been learned through research about teaching and learning.

Such research is referred to as pedagogical research and is conducted by scholars in numerous fields for nursing. Such research identifies the most effective approaches to help students achieve desired learning outcomes for providing quality care to individuals, families, and communities, and for the advancement of the profession itself. With increasing expectations of evidence-based clinical practice, the teaching and learning of that practice also must be evidence-based. It is no longer enough to hope that nursing students learn what they need to know to practice nursing. Instead faculty must use teaching and evaluation strategies that research demonstrates have the most success achieving desired learning outcomes.

## THE SCIENCE OF NURSING EDUCATION MODEL

Building the science of nursing education can be guided by the priorities for research in nursing education formulated by the NLN (2008) (see Table 1.2). (Readers are encouraged to check the NLN website http://www.nln.org/research/priorities.htm for revisions and updates.)

Priority 3, the Development of the Science of Nursing Education: Evidence-Based Reform, stimulated the development of the Science of Nursing Education Model shown in Figure 1.1. The model is a conceptual picture of the multiple processes involved in building the science of nursing education. Building the science of nursing education is a nonlinear, iterative process in which all activities noted in the model need to occur and all can be done simultaneously.

**Table 1.2. NLN's Priorities for Research in Nursing Education**

## Innovations in Nursing Education: Creating Reform

- New pedagogies
- Use of instructional technology, including new approaches to laboratory/simulated learning
- Flexible curriculum designs
- Community-driven models for curriculum development
- Processes for reforming nursing education
- Educational systems and infrastructures
- Student/teacher learning partnerships
- Community-based nursing and service learning strategies
- Clinical teaching models
- Teaching evidence-based practice
- New models for teacher preparation and faculty development, particularly as they relate to minority faculty and preparation for teaching diverse student populations

## Research in Nursing Education: Evaluating Reform

- Economics of and productivity in nursing education
- Quality improvement processes
- Program evaluation models
- Student and teacher experiences in schools of nursing
- Evaluating the success of diverse student populations
- Nursing education innovations, including facilitators and barriers to innovation and reform
- Best practices in schooling, teaching, and learning
- Grading, testing and evaluation of students, faculty and curricula

## Development of the Science of Nursing Education: Evidence-Based Reform

- Best practices in schooling, teaching, and learning
- Nursing education database development
- Strategies supportive of nursing education researchers
- Validation of key concepts and keywords related to evidence-based teaching practices
- Meta-analysis related to innovation or evaluation in nursing education
- Concept analysis related to innovation or evaluation in nursing education

**Figure 1.1.** *Science of Nursing Education Model*

## NATIONAL LEAGUE FOR NURSING
## BUILDING A SCIENCE OF NURSING EDUCATION MODEL*

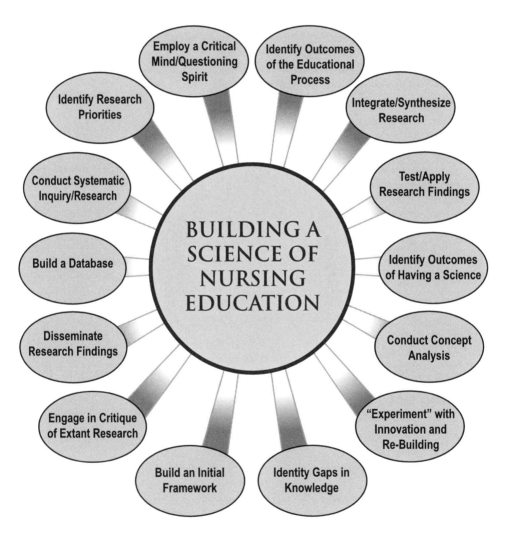

*Developed by NLN Task Group on Teaching Learning, 2003

The authors of this book employed critical minds and questioning spirits to put into words the concepts that would guide building a science of nursing education. They started with the NLN's research priorities for nursing education, which focus on improving teaching and evaluation practices in order to obtain better student learning outcomes for improved quality of care to individuals and communities. Research priorities help members of the discipline/profession clarify the gaps in knowledge that need scholarly attention so those gaps can be filled and the practice of those professionals can be evidence-based.

As gaps are filled by scholars who conduct systematic inquiry/research, test and apply research findings, and integrate and synthesize research findings, databases of information can be built that can be accessed by others interested in adding to the science of nursing education. The availability of databases fosters the dissemination of research findings, which is a critical piece of any process of inquiry. Currently, there are many more avenues of dissemination with the development of additional journals and the advent of the Internet, making scholarly material more accessible. With improved dissemination of available work, faculty scholars can critique extant research, extend investigations, and develop new knowledge based on intradisciplinary, interdisciplinary and global collaboration.

Ultimately, frameworks related to the practice of teaching will evolve, concept analyses of ideas in these frameworks will be conducted, gaps in knowledge will be identified, and ongoing scholarly activities that continually build the science will occur. Research findings will be tested and applied by faculty scholars, and research that reflects measurable outcomes of the educational process will be integrated and synthesized into the evolving science of nursing education. The value of having a science of nursing education will be clearly seen as faculty teacher-scholars with critical minds and questioning spirits continually retrace their steps through the model of building a science of nursing education and add to the knowledge about teaching and learning the art, science and spirit of nursing. The ultimate outcome will be improved patient care.

Subsequent chapters of this book introduce the reader to the framework used to organize and report research findings in teaching and learning in the cognitive, affective, and psychomotor domains. The research of teaching and learning in each of those domains is analyzed and synthesized, and gaps in our current knowledge base are identified. Finally, the reader is invited to reflect on future endeavors for building the science of nursing education and how each of us can contribute to that work.

## REFERENCES

AACN (American Association of Colleges of Nursing). (1999). Position statement on defining scholarship for the discipline of nursing. [Online]. Available: http://www.aacn. nche.edu/Publications/positions/scholar.htm.

Armiger, Sr. B. (1974). Scholarship in nursing. Nursing Outlook, 22(3), 160-164.

Boyer, E. L. (1990). Scholarship reconsidered: Priorities of the professoriate. New York: John Wiley & Sons.

Brown, J. S., Tanner, C. A., & Padrick, J. P. (1984). Nursing's search for scientific knowledge. Nursing Research, 33(1), 22-32.

Council of Graduate Schools. (1997). Preparing future faculty. Faculty roles and responsibilities. [Online]. Available: http://www.preparing-faculty.org/PFFWeb.Roles.htm.

Halstead, J. A. (2007). Nurse educator competencies: Creating an evidence-based practice for nurse educators. New York: National League for Nursing.

Ironside, P. M. (2007). On revolutions and revolutionaries. New York: National League for Nursing.

McKinney, K. (2003). Applying the scholarship of teaching and learning. The Teaching Professor, 17(7), 1, 5, 8.

McEwen, M., & Wills, E. M. (2002). Theoretical basis for nursing. Philadelphia: Lippincott, Williams & Wilkins.

National League for Nursing. (2005). The scope of practice for academic nurse educators. New York: Author.

National League for Nursing. (2008). Priorities for research in nursing education. [Online]. Available: http://www.nln.org/research/priorities.htm.

National League for Nursing. (2002a). Position statement: Funding for nursing education research. [Online]. Available: http://www.nln.org/aboutnln/Position Statements/funding051802.pdf.

National League for Nursing. (2002b). *Nurse educators 2002: Report of the faculty census survey of RN and graduate programs*. New York: Author.

Rice, E. R. (1991, Spring). The new American scholar: Scholarship and the purposes of the university. *Metropolitan Universities*, 7-18.

Southern Regional Education Board, Council on Collegiate Education for Nursing. (2002). Red alert: Nursing faculty shortage worsens in SREB states. [Online]. Available: http://www.sreb.org/programs/nursing/publications/redalert.asp.

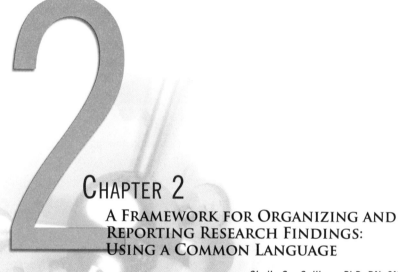

# Chapter 2

## A Framework for Organizing and Reporting Research Findings: Using a Common Language

*Sheila Cox Sullivan, PhD, RN, CNE*

"The years teach much which the days never knew."

**Emerson**

In 2001, the NLN Task Group on Teaching-Learning Paradigms was charged to conduct a meta-analysis of nursing education research in order to summarize the current state of the literature regarding teaching and learning. To fulfill that charge, Task Group members (see Appendix B) reviewed the educational literature from nursing and other health-related disciplines, as well as select disciplines outside the health professions. As the group attempted to collect, organize, and synthesize research findings on teaching and learning, it became clear that there was no common set of search terms to obtain relevant information, nor was there any overarching framework used to link one study to another. Even within nursing itself, there was no common search term language for retrieving the literature, and there was no framework to organize studies. Thus, the authors were challenged to develop a framework to organize the findings in a way that would be meaningful to and usable for faculty and nursing education scholars.

As the authors considered how best to present the results of the extensive literature reviews, one consideration was to present the information by the discipline from which the research originated (i.e., nursing, medicine, respiratory therapy, psychology, etc.). This suggestion was rejected because it did little to clarify the data, and it promoted separation, rather than integration, of research findings. Another consideration was to organize findings into behavioral and humanistic perspectives; however, this approach failed to provide a structure that could capture the comprehensiveness of the literature being reviewed. The group then considered adapting the Synergy Model adopted by the American Association of Critical-Care Nurses (2000), but while this framework showed some promise, it again failed to capture the totality of extant literature. Finally, it became evident that Bloom's Taxonomy (1956) of cognitive, affective, and psychomotor learning would be an excellent way to organize and present findings. Developed by Benjamin Bloom, a master educator, this framework was prominent in the literature as a conceptual model, it provided a broad framework capable of capturing all the concepts in the interdisciplinary teaching and learning literature, and it is familiar to most nurse educators.

## BLOOM'S TAXONOMY

Learning, teaching, and assessment/evaluation have been framed historically within a behavioral approach influenced by behavioral psychology. With this approach, planned learning outcomes frequently consist of lists of specific tasks that are sequenced, hierarchically, from simple to complex. Mastery of lower level knowledge and skills is assumed to be necessary before one can progress to more difficult tasks, and teachers often focus on student performance of isolated tasks rather than on the integration of learning and performance of tasks in combination. Such a perspective contributes to a focus on teaching rather than learning and the testing of less complex knowledge and skills, primarily because these are relatively easy to identify, teach, and evaluate. The behavioral approach may continue to be most useful for individualized instruction, training programs and simple tasks, but its relevance to helping students learn to function effectively in a complex world has been called into question.

Since the mid-1980s, through the influence of cognitive psychology, higher education has placed an increased emphasis on outcomes, or what learners actually know and can do upon completion of a course of study. This approach encourages the learning of more complex concepts since it supports the belief that students are capable of thinking and reasoning, and learning is not reduced to performance of a list of simple tasks: learning, instead, is acknowledged to be a complex, holistic, integrative, and contextual (i.e., influenced by real-world situations) process.

Clearly, learning in one domain affects learning in other domains. In order for one to engage in professional practice, one must be able to integrate learning in all three domains. For example, while one may have mastered the psychomotor skill of using a stethoscope, absence of the theoretical understanding (cognitive) of what one is hearing renders the activity meaningless. Further, if the understanding of the assessment does not produce a plan of care reflective of the client's worldview or personal priorities (affective), the patient receives suboptimal care.

While research and contemporary perspectives on teaching and learning have moved education beyond Bloom's thinking, the framework outlined over 50 years ago remains relevant. Teachers still are concerned with what students know and how they think, representative of the cognitive domain. They increasingly focus on helping students become aware of their own values while accepting that others' values may be different, appreciate how values drive actions, and (in fields like nursing) internalize the values of one's profession, all of which are reflective of the affective domain. And, in practice fields like nursing, teachers are still concerned that students are capable of performing certain skills safely, efficiently, and effectively, illustrative of the psychomotor domain. Thus, this framework continues to have value for today's educators.

The notions of detailed, teacher-directed objectives and rigid hierarchies of learning, all of which are evident in Bloom's original work, are incongruent with today's ideas of student-centered, flexible education. However, the basic concepts of cognitive, psychomotor, and affective learning continue to have merit, particularly in nursing education.

## DOMAINS OF LEARNING: COGNITIVE, PSYCHOMOTOR, AND AFFECTIVE

Nursing faculty design educational experiences to help students build their knowledge base, perform a variety of clinical skills, work comfortably with technology, develop values that are congruent with those of the profession, and think critically and make sound decisions, among other things. All of these intended outcomes can be classified into Bloom's (1956) domains of learning: cognitive, psychomotor, or affective, which are further explained in Table 2.1.

**Table 2.1. Bloom's Taxonomy of Domains of Learning**

| Learning Domain | Area of Focus | Sample Nursing Outcome |
|---|---|---|
| Cognitive | Intellectual outcomes | Learner will describe pathophysiology of peripheral vascular disease. |
| Psychomotor | Motor skills | Learner will demonstrate subcutaneous injection of insulin. |
| Affective | Interests, values, attitudes, appreciation | Learner will recognize how personal values influence one's perspective on end-of-life issues. |

### Cognitive Domain

Cognitive learning progresses from simple fact recall to judging new concepts and principles (Jefferies & Norton, 2005). Cognitive learning theory is rooted in Gestalt psychology, with its focus on how individuals solve problems and achieve insight (Garrison & Archer, 2000). It is commonly assessed by testing methods designed to evaluate understanding. These ideas are summarized in Table 2.2.

**Table 2.2. Bloom's Taxonomy of Cognitive Domain Learning**

| Level of Understanding | Learner demonstrates by: |
|---|---|
| Knowledge | Recalling previously understood facts |
| Comprehension | Explaining or restating concepts |
| Application | Connecting previously understood material to a new context |
| Analysis | Discriminating differing ideas within a concept and explaining relationships between these ideas |
| Synthesis | Constructing new relationships between ideas or forming new ideas |
| Evaluation | Assessing against a known standard |

### Psychomotor Domain

Although much of nursing practice is intellectual or cognitive in nature, nurses also must be comfortable performing a wide range of skills in order to provide care to diverse populations in varied settings. In addition, they must be able to appropriately adapt the ways in which many skills are performed in light of an individual patient's situation or circumstance. Thus, learning in the psychomotor domain also is important in nursing education.

Psychomotor domain learning refers to the use of basic motor skills, coordination, and physical movement. Simpson (1972) and Harrow (1972) developed popular taxonomies for this domain, both of which suggest that it is through repetitive practice that individuals learn psychomotor skills and are able to perform them with increasing precision, speed, technique (Menix, 2003), and naturalness. However, it is the less-well-known taxonomy developed by Dave (in Armstrong, 1975, pp. 33 - 34) that provides a pragmatic description of learning in the psychomotor domain as shown in Table 2.3. The levels of learning are juxtaposed against the parameters of skill performance for evaluative purposes.

| Table 2.3. Dave's Taxonomy of Psychomotor Domain Learning* | | | |
|---|---|---|---|
| **Level** | **Learner demonstrates by:** | **Parameters of Skill Performance** | **Range of Student Behaviors** |
| **Imitation** | Attempting to replicate an observed task | Coordination | No deviation from what was shown by the expert; copying |
| **Manipulation** | Performing a skill based on instructional criteria rather than visualized perceptions of the task | Control | Lacking to proficient; motions halting to fluid |
| **Precision** | Performing a skill with accuracy and exactness | Time and speed | Slow/Deliberate to quick/fast |
| **Articulation** | Being able to perform multiple skills sequentially and fluidly | Lack of error | Coordinates a series of actions to logical sequencing |
| **Naturalization** | Performing skills with minimal physical or mental effort | Use of judgment | Judgment not exercised to attain accurate application |

* Adapted from R. H. Dave, as reported in Armstrong, R. J. (Ed.). (1975). *Developing and writing behavioural objectives.* Tucson, AZ: Educational Innovators Press.

Psychomotor learning is demonstrated by performance of physical or technological skills, using coordination, dexterity, manipulation, grace, strength, and speed. Fine-motor skills (e.g., suturing, inserting a Foley catheter) involve the use of precision instruments or tools, while gross motor skills (e.g., transferring a patient from bed to chair or performing cardiopulmonary resuscitation) are demonstrated by broader movements or even the use of the entire body. In educational arenas, the behaviors often associated with psychomotor domain learning include bending, grasping, operating, handling, or performing skillfully.

The literature (http://utut.essortment.com/psychomotordeve_pqs.htm) suggests there are three stages through which an individual progresses when learning psychomotor skills: cognitive, associative, and autonomous. In the cognitive stage, learners are consciously trying to "control" psychomotor movements that are, initially, awkward, slow, and deliberate because the learner is imitating the movements observed in another's performance. The learner's execution, even during imitation, often is poor, and learners frequently make errors during this "choppy," slow performance. Frustration levels frequently are high, but diligent practice allows individuals to develop the ability to manipulate the steps of the task, and move onto the next stage.

In the associative stage of psychomotor development, individuals spend less time thinking about every detail of the skill and begin to associate the movements they are learning with other movements already known. For now, the movements are not "hard-wired" into the brain and are not automatic, so learners still must think about every

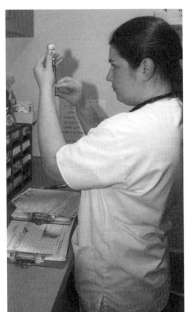

movement. However, performance of the skill begins to be smoother, or more precise, and learners feel less awkward.

The highest stage of psychomotor development is the autonomous stage, when learning is almost complete, although learners can continue to refine the skill through practice. No longer do learners need guidance when performing the skill because the movements have become spontaneous, smooth, and efficient. The learner is able to articulate the movements with other variables that may arise during task performance, and eventually the task becomes like a natural behavior, no longer requiring conscious thought.

### Affective Domain

There is no question that nurses must have a sound knowledge base, be able to make decisions and judgments, think critically, and be at more advanced stages of cognitive development. There also is no doubt nurses must be able to perform many technical skills in a safe, efficient way. However, success in cognitive and psychomotor learning alone is insufficient preparation for a nurse. Such individuals also must internalize a value system that is congruent with nursing's notions of quality patient care (i.e., culturally sensitive, individualized, caring, compassionate, and respectful) and the expectations of a professional (i.e., engage in lifelong learning, exhibit a spirit of inquiry and a questioning mind, and be involved in professional associations). Thus, learning in the affective domain must be attended to along with the cognitive and psychomotor domains.

Affective learning reflects changes in attitude (Clark, 2007). Examples of affective learning in nursing include involving clients in making decisions about their health and revising plans of care based on the client's preferences. Expanding on the concepts of hierarchies and taxonomies originally developed by Bloom in the 1950s, Krathwohl, Bloom, and Masia (1964) identified five categories of affective processes: attending, responding, valuing, organizing, and characterizing values. Table 2.4 expounds upon these categories.

| Table 2.4. Krathwohl, Bloom, & Masia's Taxonomy of Affective Domain Learning | |
|---|---|
| Level | Learner demonstrates by: |
| Attending | Being exposed to an idea |
| Responding | Modifying behaviors in response to exposure to an idea |
| Valuing | Becoming involved with or committed to an idea |
| Organizing | Enmeshing new idea with current value system |
| Characterizing Values | Consistently behaving in ways that are congruent with the embodied value |

Affective competencies are those, "which emphasize a feeling tone, an emotion, or a degree of acceptance or rejection ... as well as interests, attitudes, appreciations and values" (Krathwohl et al., 1964, p. 7). The ultimate goal for learners is internalization, where carefully considered values become a "natural" part of their functioning and influence their thinking and their actions. Indeed, as Krathwohl et al. (1964) stressed, learning in this domain is best demonstrated by changes in learners' actions that are constant despite changing conditions or circumstances. Affective learning has been noted to address "the forces that determine the nature of an individual's life and ultimately the life of an entire people" (Krathwohl et al., 1964, p. 91). It, therefore, is a highly significant aspect of higher education that demands serious attention by faculty.

## SUMMARY

While the three domains of learning — cognitive, psychomotor, and affective — often are discussed and addressed separately, it is understood that learning outcomes typically consist of two or all three domains. For example, cognitive outcomes often have some affective components, and the performance of motor skills typically includes both cognitive and affective elements. While this overlap is essential for educational purposes, it presents challenges when one wishes to examine research on cognitive, affective, or psychomotor learning. Thus, the synthesis of research on teaching and learning in the cognitive, affective and psychomotor domains presented in this book is organized into discrete categories to organize and facilitate discussion. The emphasis on one domain or another is not intended to suggest that faculty should isolate the domains of learning in their design of curricula or selection of teaching/learning and assessment/evaluation strategies.

Having adopted an organizing framework for a meta-analysis of extant literature on teaching and learning, the authors next turned to the topic of learning. The available evidence about this incredibly complex process and its multiple influences is discussed in Chapter 3.

## REFERENCES

American Association of Critical-Care Nurses (2000). *The AACN synergy model for patient care.* [Online]. Available: http://www.aacn.org/WD/Certifications/content/synmodel. pcms?pid=1&&menu=.

Armstrong, R. J. (Ed). (1975). *Developing and writing behavioral objectives.* Tucson, AZ: Educational Innovators Press.

Bloom, B. S., Englehard, M., Furst, E., Hill, W., & Krathwohl, D. (1956). *Taxonomy of educational objectives: The classification of educational goals. Handbook I: Cognitive domain.* London: Longman.

Clark, D. (2007). *Learning domains or Bloom's taxonomy.* [Online]. Available: http://www. nwlink.com/~donclark/hrd/bloom.html.

Garrison, D. R., & Archer, W. (2000). *A transactional perspective on teaching and learning: A framework for adult and higher education.* Oxford, UK: Elsevier Science.

Harrow, A. J. (1972). *A taxonomy of the psychomotor domain: A guide for developing behavioral objectives.* New York: Longman.

Jefferies, P., & Norton, B. (2005). Selecting learning experiences to achieve curriculum outcomes. In D. M. Billings, & J.A. Halstead, *Teaching in nursing: A guide for faculty* (2nd ed., pp. 187-212). Philadelphia: W. B. Saunders.

Krathwohl, D. R., Bloom , B. S., & Masia, B. B. (1964). *Taxonomy of educational objectives: The classification of educational goals. Handbook II: Affective domain.* New York: David McKay.

Menix , K. (2003). Domains of learning: Interdependent components of achievable learning outcomes. *Journal of Continuing Education in Nursing,* 27, 200-208.

Simpson, E. J. (1972). The classification of education objectives in the psychomotor domain. In *Contributions of behavioral science to instructional technology: The psychomotor domain* (pp. 43-56). Washington, DC: Gryphon Press.

BUILDING A SCIENCE OF NURSING EDUCATION

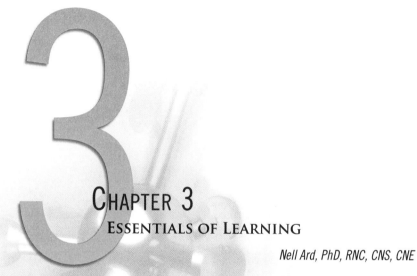

# Chapter 3
## Essentials of Learning

*Nell Ard, PhD, RNC, CNS, CNE*

"Education is not the filling of a pail, but the lighting of a fire."

**William Butler Yeats**

The ultimate goal of nurse educators is to promote student learning. What is learning? How does the learning process occur? How do educators know when learning has occurred? Learning is a complex process that is influenced by factors such as learner characteristics, the learning environment, teacher characteristics, and the teaching methods used. Nurse educators must consider the significance and impact of these factors as they design learning activities in nursing education.

## Definitions of Learning

Learning is a change in the mental processing, emotional functioning, and/or behavior that results from experience. It is the lifelong, dynamic process by which individuals acquire new knowledge or skills and alter their thoughts, feelings, attitudes, and actions. In 1998, a Joint Task Group on Student Learning was created to address principles of learning. The ten

| Table 3-1. Ten Principles of Learning |
| --- |
| "Learning is making and maintaining connections –biologically, mentally, and experientially" (p. 3). |
| "Learning is enhanced by the importance of the context" (p. 4). |
| "Learning is an active search for meaning by the learner — constructing knowledge rather than passively receiving it" (p. 5). |
| "Learning is a developmental, cumulative process involving the whole person, relating past and present, integrating the new with the old, starting from but transcending personal concerns and interests" (p. 6). |
| "Learning is accomplished by individuals who are intrinsically tied to others as social beings, interacting as competitors or collaborators, constraining or supporting the learning process, and able to enhance learning through cooperation and sharing" (p. 8). |
| "Learning is strongly affected by the education climate in which it takes place" (p. 9). |
| "Learning is dependent upon frequent feedback if it is to be sustained, practice if it is to be nourished, and opportunities to use what has been learned" (p. 10). |
| "Learning is formal but also can be informal and incidental" (p. 11). |
| "Learning is grounded in particular contexts and individual experiences, requiring effort to transfer specific knowledge and skills to other circumstances or to more general understandings" (p. 12). |
| "Learning is the ability of individuals to monitor their own learning, to understand how knowledge is acquired, to develop strategies for learning based on discerning their capacities and limitations, and to be aware of their own ways of knowing in approaching new bodies of knowledge and disciplinary frameworks" (p. 14). |

American Association for Higher Education, American College Personnel Association, and National Association of Student Personnel Administration (1998). Powerful partnerships: A shared responsibility for learning, [Online]. Available: http://www.myacpa.org/pub/documents/taskforce.pdf.

principles of learning developed by this coalition have relevance to nursing education and could assist faculty to design more effective learning experiences (American Association of Higher Education [AAHE], American College Personnel Association [ACPA], & National Association of Student Personnel Administrators [NASPA], 1998). Those principles, which are still pertinent a decade later, are listed in Table 3.1.

While none of these principles seems particularly revolutionary, the importance of each of them cannot be underestimated. Educators therefore should consider these principles seriously when designing curricula, teaching strategies, and evaluation methods that will facilitate student learning.

# THEORIES OF LEARNING

Educators have long pondered many questions about learning: how it occurs, what facilitates or hinders the process, what ensures that learning becomes relatively permanent, and other ideas. As a result of these explorations, a number of learning theories have been developed and tested, thereby helping educators understand how individuals acquire knowledge and change their ways of thinking, feeling, and behaving. There are essentially three broad learning categories: behavioral, cognitive, and humanistic. Several of the most significant learning theories are presented here to highlight what is known about the complex process of learning, and a summary of the theories discussed here, along with examples about their use in nursing education, is provided in Table 3.2.

## *Behavioral Learning Theory*

The essential underlying principle in behavioral learning theory is that learning is a response to a stimulus. Skinner (1974) introduced the concept of *operant conditioning*, and he and other behaviorists demonstrated how individuals changed their behavior in response to environmental manipulation. Depending on how an individual is rewarded or "punished" for a particular behavior, he or she will continue to engage in an action or extinguish previously learned responses.

Nursing education utilizes some of the principles of behavioral learning theory in the design and implementation of courses. For example, when students demonstrate they have met the teacher-formulated objectives, they are rewarded with a grade. Operant conditioning, also is the basis for many self-regulated learning experiences, such as computer study modules and linear programs (McKenna, 1995a) used by nurse educators.

## *Cognitive Learning Theory*

Cognitive learning stresses the importance of what goes on "inside" the learner. Additional underlying principles of cognitive learning are (1) rewards are not necessary for learning;

### Table 3.2. Learning Theories and Examples of Their Use in Nursing Education

| Theory | Broad Learning Category | Theorist | Examples of Use in Nursing Education/Activities |
|---|---|---|---|
| Behavioral Learning Theory | Behavioral | Skinner (1974) | Behavioral objectives; self-directed learning programs |
| Cognitive Learning Theory | Cognitive | Gagne (1965) | Course development — simple to complex; mastery learning |
| Cooperative Learning Theory | Cognitive | Johnson & Johnson (1975) | Learning of skills; group projects |
| Social Learning Theory | Behavioral and Cognitive | Bandura (1977) | Role modeling; preceptorships |
| Humanistic Learning Theory | Humanistic | Maslow (1954) | Case studies, role playing, simulations, self-evaluations |
| Adult Learning Theory | Humanistic | Cross (1981), Knowles (1978), Kolb (1984) | Case studies, role playing, simulations, self-evaluations |
| Experiential Learning Theory | Humanistic | Rogers (1969), Kolb (1984) | Dependent upon style:<br>• Concrete experiences — laboratories, clinical experiences<br>• Reflective observer — logs, journals, brainstorming<br>• Abstract conceptualizer — lectures, papers, analogies<br>• Active experimenter — simulations, case studies |

(2) the learners' goals and expectations, which create disequilibrium, imbalance and tension, are most important in motivating the learner to learn; and (3) past experiences, perceptions, ways of incorporating and thinking about information as well as diverse aspirations, expectations, and social influences affect any learning situation.

Gagne, a cognitive learning theorist, defined learning as "a change in human disposition or capability, which can be retained, and which is not simply ascribed to the process of growth. This learning exhibits itself as a change in behavior" (1965, p. 5). Gagne stated that learning is largely dependent on events in the environment with which the individual interacts. It is not simply an event that happens naturally; instead, learning is an event occurring under certain conditions that can be altered and controlled. The factors that influence learning are mainly determined by the individual's living environment.

Gagne integrated three basic elements: the learner, the stimulus situation, and the response. The learner is any human being who brings past experiences and learning, as well as his/her individual set of learning capabilities, into a new situation. A learning event takes place when the stimulus affects the learner in such a way that his/her performance changes and results in what is called learning.

Gagne also emphasized five different domains of learning, each of which requires a different set of teaching approaches. Those domains of learning are: verbal information, intellectual skills, psychomotor skills, attitudes, and cognitive strategies. Finally, this scholar proposed a hierarchy of learning from simple to complex, where each higher order of learning depends upon the mastery of the one that precedes it.

Nursing education incorporates cognitive learning theory quite extensively. The design of curricula and the organization of content within courses generally are presented from simple concepts to complex concepts, where new material is linked to material previously learned (McKenna, 1995b).

**Cooperative Learning Theory.** Cooperative learning extends cognitive learning theory by incorporating the concept of social constructivism or social cognition (Bastable, 2003; Johnson & Johnson, 1975). The central tenets of cooperative learning are that (a) the learning process is strongly influenced by culture and (b) effective learning occurs through social interaction, collaboration, and negotiation. Many nursing programs have cooperative learning experiences built into skills courses or upper level courses that focus on change, leadership, and the professional role (Baumberger-Henry, 2003; Copp, 2002).

**Social Learning Theory.** Social learning theory is a combination of behaviorist and cognitivist principles of learning. Bandura (1977; 1986) outlined the behaviorist, cognitive, and social cognition dimensions of social life theory, the underlying principle of which is that individuals learn from observation of others. In other words, individuals watch other people, discern what happens to them, and learn from it.

Using role models to enhance learning is grounded in this theory. The role model demonstrates the desirable behavior, which is observed by the learner. The learner then processes this information to memory (retention), calls on that memory in the future to guide his/her performance of the role model's actions (reproduction), and is rewarded or punished (motivation) for that performance.

In more recent studies, Bandura (2001) studied the sociocultural influences on learning and viewed the learner as an agent through which learning experiences are filtered. Social learning theory thereby extends the learning process beyond the educator-learner relationship and the learner's direct experiences to involve the influence of the larger social world.

In nursing education, students often model themselves after teachers and clinicians. Frequently, faculty purposefully use role modeling as a teaching technique (e.g., clinical preceptors), and many nursing textbooks encourage students to find role models who can help them transition from student to graduate nurse roles. However, faculty often may fail to recognize and use many opportunities where they can role model desirable behaviors (e.g., attending professional conferences, expressing excitement about expanding their networks at such meetings, and sharing what was learned from the experience).

### Humanistic Learning Theory

The humanistic theory of learning is concerned with feelings and experiences that lead to personal growth and individual fulfillment. To a great extent, then, humanistic learning theory is motivational theory based on the assumption that all individuals have a desire to grow in positive ways, and is congruent with Maslow's (1954, 1987) hierarchy of needs.

Humanistic learning theory describes the educator as a facilitator of learning rather than an all-knowing authority who conveys information. The central purpose of teaching is to foster curiosity, enthusiasm, initiative, and responsibility rather than the mastery of facts. Thus, the learner is a key player in the teaching/learning process.

In nursing education, humanistic principles are used extensively in the psychiatric components of the curriculum. They also are evident when faculty use reflective practice groups, experiential learning, role-play, case studies, journaling, and dialogues (Ferrari, 2006; Scanlon. 2006).

**Adult Learning Theory.** Knowles' (1978) theory of adult learning, "andragogy," is based upon humanistic principles. The underlying assumptions of Knowles' theory are that adults are (1) autonomous and self-directed, (2) goal oriented, (3) relevancy- and problem-oriented, and (4) practical problem-solvers. In addition, adults have accumulated life experiences that must be built on during the learning process. In essence, Knowles' theory directs teachers of adults to focus more on the process of learning and less on the content being taught.

Cross (1981) developed a model that addresses characteristics of adults as learners. This model attempts to integrate other theoretical frameworks for adult learning such as Knowles' theory, experiential learning, and lifespan psychology. The model consists of two classes of variables associated with learning: personal and situational characteristics.

Nurse educators incorporate components of humanistic learning theory (McKenna, 1995c) when they use case studies, role-playing, simulations, or self-evaluations. However, while many nursing programs state they have adult learners and utilize Knowles' theory, one must question whether principles of adult learning truly are used to design learning experiences for those students. For example, do nurse educators allow students to be autonomous and self-directed? Can students be allowed to pursue their own learning goals? Are faculty certain that every learning experience is relevant?

*Experiential Learning Theory.* Rogers (1969), whose theory evolved as part of the humanistic education movement, delineated two types of learning — cognitive and experiential. He believed that experiential learning was "significant" learning as it addresses the needs and wants of the learner. According to Rogers, learning is facilitated when (a) the learner participates completely in the learning process and has control over its nature and direction, (b) learners are helped to directly confront practical, social, personal or research problems, and (c) self-evaluation is the principal method used to assess progress or success. According to Rogers, an openness to change and valuing learning also are significant factors.

In nursing education, experiential teaching strategies are utilized in a variety of ways. In many regards, clinical education is experiential learning. Additional teaching strategies include role-play, cultural gaming, ethical scenarios, and return demonstrations (Beckman, Boxley-Harges, Bruick-Sorge, & Salmon, 2007; Graham & Richardson, 2008; Sofaer, 1995; Thomas, Clarke, Pollard, & Miers, 2007). Service learning is also a method of experiential learning through which faculty and students meet community needs while developing students' critical thinking and group problem-solving skills and understanding of the sociopolitical processes shaping health (Cohen & Milone-Nuzzo, 2001; Drevdahl, Dorcy, & Grevstad, 2001; Sternas, O'Hare, Lehman, & Milligan, 1999).

## Brain-Based Learning Model

In 1983, a new model of the connections between brain functions and education was introduced (Hart, 1983). Across the years, many individuals have referred to right-brain versus left-brain learning. The right side of the brain deals with feelings and experiences, and is present-oriented with a concrete experiential approach, while the left side of the brain deals with language and is future-oriented with an abstract cognitive approach (Gulpinar, 2005; Kolb, 1984).

In recent years there has been a resurgence of interest in neuroscience and its relationship to education. Brain-based learning is based upon twelve principles (Caine & Caine, 1990; Caine Learning Institute, 2005; Gulpinar, 2005; Jensen, 2000; Roberts, 2002; Weiss, 2000):

- All learning engages the entire physiology;
- Brain/mind is social;
- The search for meaning is innate;
- The search for meaning occurs through "patterning";
- Emotions are critical to patterning;

- Every brain simultaneously perceives and creates parts and wholes;
- Learning involves both focused attention and peripheral perception;
- Learning always involves conscious and unconscious processes;
- There are at least two types to memory — spatial and a set of systems for rote learning;
- Learning is developmental;
- Complex learning is enhanced by challenge and inhibited by threat associated with helplessness and fatigue; and
- Each brain is unique.

Based upon these twelve principles, three elements of optimal teaching have been identified: relaxed alertness, orchestrated immersion in complex experience, and active processing of experience (Caine Learning Institute, 2005; Gulpinar, 2005; Jensen, 2008). *Relaxed alertness* is creating the optimal emotional climate for learning, *orchestrated immersion* is creating optimal opportunities for learning, and *active processing* means creating optimal ways to consolidate learning. Proponents of the model (Caine Learning Institute; Jensen, 2008; Shapiro, 2006) have begun to address instructional approaches and applications to education, and additional work is expected to evolve.

As with any relatively "new" model or theory, brain-based learning has its advocates and others who are challenging at least some underlying aspects of the model (Sternberg, 2008; Willingham, 2008; Willis, 2008). The research in higher education and nursing about this model is absent. (See Chapter 6 for information about its use in the affective domain.)

## Emerging Nursing Pedagogies

New phenomenological pedagogies that are specific to nursing education have been developed by Diekelmann (2000, 2001) and are being refined by Ironside (2001) and others. These pedagogies challenge teachers to question the assumptions of conventional pedagogies such as competency-based education, which is directed toward achieving proficiency in a given role, or problem-based learning, which is directed at resolving or understanding a problem and thinking critically (Diekelmann & Diekelmann, 2000). They also challenge teachers to reform nursing education so that nursing's approaches to teaching and learning are site specific (i.e., they reflect the uniqueness of learners, faculty, institution, and surrounding community) (Andrews et al., 2001).

One of these new approaches — *narrative pedagogy* — evolved from a twelve-year study of the common lived experiences of students, teachers, and clinicians in nursing education (Diekelmann, 2001), and experiences that have been documented in the literature (Diekelmann, 2002a, 2002b, 2002c, 2003; Diekelmannn & Mikol, 2003; Diekelmann & Scheckel, 2003; Diekelmann, Swenson, & Sims, 2003).

Through the original research that led to the formulation of narrative pedagogy, Diekelmann (2001) identified Concernful Practices of Schooling Learning Teaching (p. 57). These nine patterns that describe the common, shared experiences of nursing students and educators and provide a new language for nursing education, are as follows:

- Gathering: bringing in and calling forth;
- Creating places: keeping open a future of possibilities;
- Assembling: constructing and cultivating;
- Staying: knowing and connecting;
- Caring: engendering community;
- Interpreting: unlearning and becoming;
- Presencing: attending and being open;
- Preserving: reading, writing, thinking, and dialogue; and
- Questioning: meaning and making visible.

The nursing literature is now showing examples of how narrative pedagogy has been used in various settings (Bankert & Kozel, 2005; Diekelmann, Ironside, & Gunn, 2005; Kawashima, 2005; Kirkpatrick & Brown, 2004), and research-based literature (Evans & Bendel, 2004; Ironside, 2003, 2006; Young, 2004) now documents its value. According to Diekelmann (2000), "reforming nursing education substantively will require risk and challenging many of the tried-and-true, taken-for-granted assumptions of contemporary teaching and learning" (p. 293). The use of narrative pedagogy in nursing education provides an opportunity for such subtantial reform to begin.

## SUMMARY OF LEARNING THEORIES AND EMERGING PEDAGOGIES

The learning theories and emerging pedagogies described here do much to inform educators, but they are useful only if they are applied as faculty plan experiences to facilitate learning. Since it is the role of the educator to draw on learning theories to design educational experiences that enhance learning, one might ask how this is done. Vandeveer (2005) reviews several of these learning theories and their application to nursing education in terms of the role of faculty, role of student, advantages, disadvantages, and application. Many educators resist selecting a single learning theory and prefer, instead, to draw from several of them simultaneously. This practice is quite acceptable, provided the concepts being blended are consistent with one another. The analysis by Hilgard (1956) illustrates commonalities and shows how one can use several theories simultaneously (see Table 3.3.) Although this analysis is fifty years old, it is still highly relevant and challenges educators to think about their views on and approaches to teaching and learning.

Utilization of a single learning theory or combination of theories is only one aspect of the learning process, however. Figure 3.1 depicts the concept of learning as involving three primary components — the learner, the learning environment, and the teacher — each of which is explored in greater depth and in relation to one another.

## THE LEARNER

The diversity of students in classrooms and clinical groups present a challenge to nurse educators who attempt to address individual learner needs. Although several students in any given class may share certain characteristics such as age, gender or ethnic background, students also are different from one another in many ways, and any of these can affect an individual's ability, capacity, and motivation to learn. Knowing what these factors are will help both learners and teachers create a more positive and effective learning experience.

Some factors known to influence learning are the learners' (1) developmental stage, (2) intelligence, (3) aptitude, (4) motivation level, and (5) learning style. Although one assumes learning is influenced by perceptual, physical and reading abilities, and although these factors are addressed extensively for K-12 learners, review of the literature in higher education and nursing education did not reveal research-based articles pertaining to these factors. Thus they are not addressed here. Also not addressed are a number of other learner characteristics that have received some attention in the nursing and higher education literature, but have not been studied extensively, such as gender, disability, or cultural diversity.

### Developmental Stage

Not surprisingly, developmental psychologists have demonstrated that people of different ages tend to have different preoccupations and focus on different things throughout their lives. Scholars who studied and theorized about such things once thought that individuals moved systematically, task by task, through each stage, and that a person could not progress to the work of a "higher," more advanced, stage until the work of the previous stage was complete. Today's research suggests that progression through various developmental stages is less rigid. It is now accepted that while the idea of progression has significance, there is a great unevenness in growth, and developmental progression is not necessarily orderly or smooth. In addition, regression to an earlier stage is possible. Nearly forty years ago, Chickering (1969) formulated a list of developmental tasks for traditional-age college students that primarily addresses social and emotional development. His theory proposed seven "vectors" of development (see Table 3.4), each of which continues to have relevance for traditional-age and nontraditional students alike.

## Table 3.3. Principles of Teaching from Broad Learning Categories

| | Behavioral | Cognitive | Humanistic |
|---|---|---|---|
| **The Learner** | The learner should be active. Generalization and discrimination suggest the importance of practice in varied contexts so that learning will become appropriate to a wider range of stimuli. | *The perceptual features* of the problem given to the learner are important conditions of learning. *Cognitive feedback* confirms correct knowledge and corrects faulty learning. | The learner's *abilities* are important *Anxiety level* of the individual learner may determine the beneficial or detrimental effects of certain kinds of encouragement. |
| **Process of Learning** | *Repetition* is important to acquire and retain skills and information. | The *organization of knowledge* should be an essential concern of the teacher or educational planner so that the direction from simple to complex is not arbitrary. | *Postnatal development* is as important as hereditary and congenital determiners of ability and interest. |
| **Context of Learning** | *Reinforcement* is important. Desirable or correct responses should be rewarded. | Learning is *internal* based upon goals, past experiences, and ways of thinking. | Learning is *culturally relative* and both the wider culture and the subculture to which the learner belongs may affect learning. |
| **Motivation** | *Novelty in behavior* can be enhanced through imitation of models, cueing or shaping. *Drive* is important in learning. | *Goal setting* by the learner is important as motivation for learning and success and failures determine how future goals are set. *Divergent thinking,* which leads to inventive problem solving or the creation of novel and valued products, is to be nurtured along with convergent thinking, which leads to logically correct answers. | The same objective situation may tap *appropriate* motives for one learner and not for another. The *organization of motives and values* within the individual is relevant. Some long-range goals affect short-range activities. |
| **Learning Environment** | *Conflicts and frustrations* arise inevitably in the process of learning. Recognize and provide for resolution or accommodation. | Environment lends itself to presenting knowledge from *simple to complex and mastery of information. Past experiences and stimuli* affect learning and change in behavior. | The *group atmosphere* of learning (competition vs. cooperation, authority vs. democracy, individual isolation vs. group identification) will affect satisfaction in learning as well as the products of learning. |

*Adapted from Hilgard, E. R. (1956). Theories of learning (2nd ed.). New York: Appleton-Century-Crofts*

## Figure 3.1. Ard's Conceptual Model of Learning

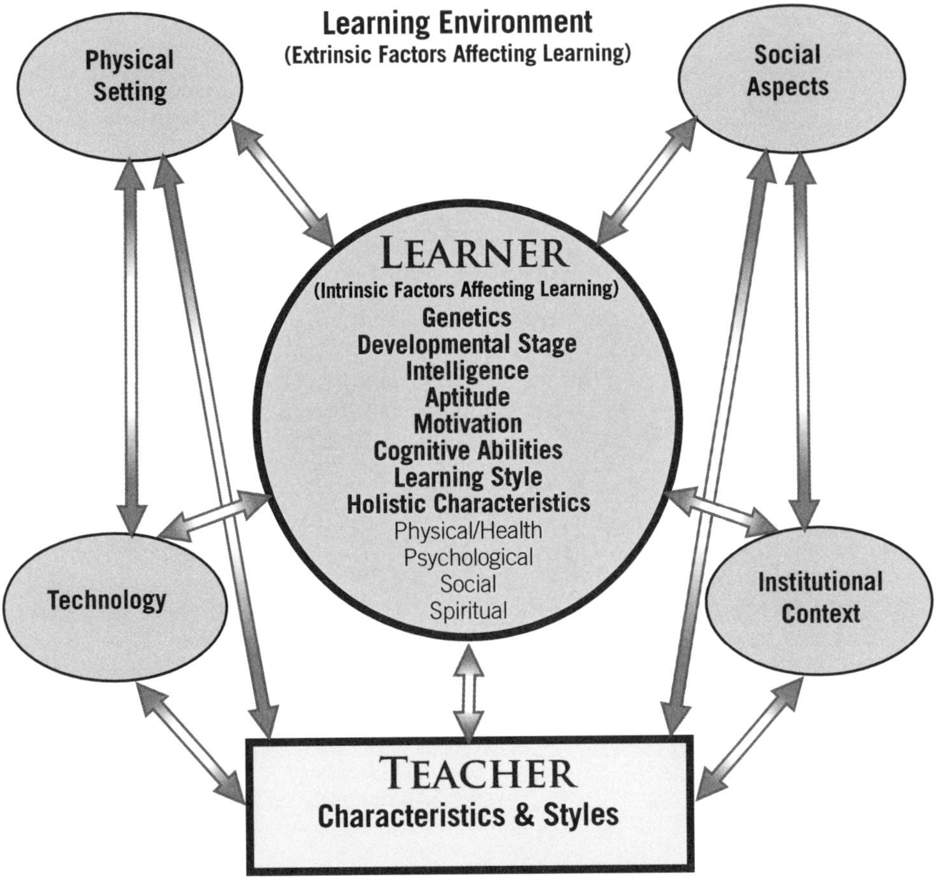

© 2007 by Nell Ard.

Permission to reproduce granted by copyright owner.

| Table 3.4. Chickering's Vectors of Development |
|---|
| • Achieving Competence |
| • Managing Emotions |
| • Becoming Autonomous |
| • Establishing Identity |
| • Freeing Interpersonal Relationships |
| • Clarifying Purposes |
| • Developing Integrity |

The first of Chickering's "vectors" of development is "achieving competence." During this phase, an individual develops basic abilities — intellectual, physical, manual, social, and interpersonal — as well as the confidence to achieve what one sets out to do. A second vector is "managing emotions," where the individual learns how to become more aware of feelings, to trust them more, and to manage them more effectively. Another vector along which an individual develops is "becoming autonomous," where one learns how to live away from parents, becomes emotionally independent, and is freed of continual and pressing needs for reassurance, affection, and approval.

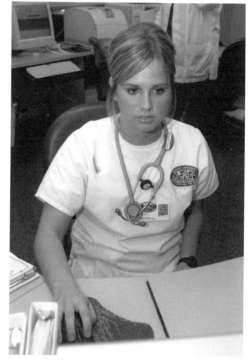

Chickering's (1969) fourth vector of development is "establishing identity," during which individuals further clarify a sense of their own characteristics, physical needs, personal appearance, and sexual identification. The fifth vector, "freeing interpersonal relationships," is where the individual learns to become less anxious, less defensive, less burdened by inappropriate past reactions, and more spontaneous, friendly, warm, and trusting. The next vector Chickering describes is "clarifying purposes," where the individual develops a clearer sense of vocational plans and aspirations, vocational and recreational interests, and lifestyle goals. The final vector identified by Chickering is "developing integrity." The challenge to the individual at this point is to develop a personally valid set of beliefs and values that have some internal consistency and serve as a tentative guide for behavior. (See Chapter 6 for a discussion of the affective domain.) By understanding these vectors of development, teachers can better appreciate how a student's stage of social and emotional development can have a direct impact on his/her ability to learn effectively and affectively.

Cognitive development — the way students think, view knowledge, view their roles as learners, view the role of the teacher, and process information — also plays an important role in an individual's ability to learn. In 1970, Perry outlined a continuum, based on extensive research findings, of progression from dualistic, black/white, right/wrong thinking to a more relativistic perspective, where there is comfort with uncertainty and ambiguity and where the context of a situation is seen as significant in determining "rightness," "wrongness," or the best course of action. Perry described individuals at the upper end of the continuum to be more mature thinkers who carefully consider options, see viable alternatives, and make decisions that are congruent with their own carefully considered values.

Kitchener and King (1990) expanded upon Perry's work and developed The Reflective Judgment Model, which views the reflective thinker as someone who is aware that a problematic situation exists and is able to bring critical judgment to bear on that problem. These researchers found that people vary significantly in the way they think about thinking, and they described a clear pattern of progression, or stages, people go through on their journeys to becoming more complex thinkers.

Understanding how a student's stage of cognitive and affective development can have a direct impact on his/her approach to learning helps faculty design curricula and learning experiences that support students in their current stage of development while simultaneously challenging them to progress to higher levels. Unfortunately, very little of this is done in nursing education, based on the research reviewed (see Chapters 4 and 6).

## Intelligence

Intelligence usually refers to the raw material of thinking power brought to bear on intellectual operations. Intelligence and its measurement are sensitive issues in a pluralistic society, often because significant decisions are made based on results of tests that evolve from a less-than-exact science and that some claim are culturally biased. However, despite this sensitivity, any discussion of learning must address the issue of intelligence.

According to Sternberg (1985), intelligence involves purposive adapting to, selection of, and shaping of real-world environments relevant to one's life. It is the ability to deal with novel situations and unfamiliar tasks, often cutting through to the best solutions by using "automatic" systems for processing information. Finally, it involves a set of governance and coordination mechanisms through which intelligent behavior is accomplished.

Taking a broader perspective, Gardner (1983) offered the Theory of Multiple Intelligences in which he makes two claims. First, Gardner asserts that intelligence involves the ability to manipulate symbol systems, which are associated with each type of intelligence and which involve perception, memory and learning within a specific area. Second, he claims that each individual has seven types of intelligence: linguistic, musical, logical-mathematical, visual-spatial, bodily-kinesthetic, interpersonal and intrapersonal. Since his original formulations, Gardner has identified an eighth intelligence called naturalist, which is an individual's ability to distinguish and categorize objects or phenomena in nature, and he has worked on a ninth area that deals with spiritual intelligence (Klindworth, 1998). According to Gardner's theory, each of the intelligences is present to differing degrees within each person, with some intelligences being better developed than others. Students need to experience learning that allows them to engage and develop all of their intelligences, explore their own intelligences and how they can impact their learning, and have choice in how they learn and are assessed. Therefore, faculty need to attend to students' multiple intelligences and design learning experiences that "tap into" and build each one.

A review of the literature in nursing did not reveal any research-based articles dealing with intelligence, and only three research articles were found in the general higher education literature (Diseth, 2002; Jaeger, 2003; Lassiter, Matthews, Bell, & Maher, 2002). Diseth studied the relationship between intelligence, approaches to learning, and academic achievement in Norwegian undergraduate psychology students using three measures of intelligence; he found no significant relationship between intelligence and academic achievement or approach to learning. Lassiter et al. compared two instruments measuring "intelligence" using a sample of 94 college students and found that the General Ability Measure for Adults (GAMA) and the Kaufman Adolescent and Adult Intelligence Test (KAAIT) accurately estimate overall intellectual functioning. Jaeger explored the theory of emotional intelligence and its affect on graduate students' learning and found that there was a strong relationship between emotional intelligence and academic performance.

Two articles in nursing dealt with the concept of intelligence, but were not research-based (Akerjordet & Severinsson, 2007; Amerson, 2006). Amerson addressed how nursing lectures could apply the theory of multiple intelligence learning, and Akerjordet and Severinsson presented a literature review on the concept of emotional intelligence.

Intelligence has traditionally been considered an important predictor of academic achievement, yet the current research-based literature on this student characteristic is quite limited. Additional research needs to be done in both higher education and nursing to establish the significance of various types of intelligence to each of the domains of learning, academic success, and other outcomes.

## Aptitude

Aptitude is the specific skills and abilities brought to intellectual tasks, and it may be affected by intelligence and motivation. Aptitude is closely related to the concept of achievement, but the two are different: *achievement* is learning one has previously accomplished; *aptitude* is the capacity of an individual for learning at some time in the future. Aptitude of post-secondary students, for example, may refer to their capacity to succeed in college (i.e., general aptitude), as well as their capacity to learn in a specific field of study or be successful in a particular professional field (i.e., specific aptitude).

The two most widely used measures of general aptitude for college are the Scholastic Aptitude Test (SAT) and the American College Test (ACT), which are limited to assessment of precollege students. Prenursing entrance exams that measure specific aptitudes of a candidate's capacity to succeed in a nursing program (e.g., the NLN's Pre-Admission Examination-RN [PAX-RN], Nurse Entrance Test [NET], Health Education System Incorporated Admission Test [HESI], or Psychological Service Bureau Registered Nursing School Aptitude Examination [PSB-RN]) are a growing trend.

A review of the literature in higher education revealed only one research-based article on aptitude. Mau (2001) tested gender differences on the SAT, the ACT, and college grades. In a sample of 10,080 college graduates, he found that males obtained significantly higher scores on the aptitude tests while females had a significantly higher grade point average in their college courses. The basic conclusion was that the more assessments are based on cognitive tests, the greater the male advantage, while the more assessments are based on written work, the greater the female advantage.

A review of the literature in nursing revealed only one research-based article dealing with professional aptitude (Takase, Maude, & Manias, 2006). The study had 346 Australian nurses and compared the nurses' perception of the public's image with self-image of their leadership aptitude. The findings indicated that nurses rated their leadership aptitude more positively than they believed the public viewed them.

There were no nursing articles dealing with general aptitude. Nursing education research could examine aptitudes as a potential variable affecting teaching and learning in all domains.

## Motivation Level

Motivation has to do with the will or desire to put forth effort to learn. It appears simple on the surface, but becomes more complex upon further examination. Wlodkowski (1978) suggests that motivation is "those processes that can (a) arouse and instigate behavior, (b) give direction and purpose to behavior, (c) continue to allow behavior to persist, and (d) lead to choosing or professing a particular behavior" (p. 12).

Motivation is not simply something students have or lack. Instead, motivation is a complex interaction of what students bring to a learning situation and what the learning situation evokes from students. Wlodkowski described six specific components of motivation: attitudes, needs, stimulation, affect (feelings), competence, and reinforcement. Motivation is affected by the learner's *attitudes* about the teacher, the subject, and the setting, all of which are brought to the learning situation. The nature and strength of the student's physical and psychological *needs* also influence motivation, especially regarding a sense of belonging, self-respect, and growth toward one's full potential. The type and degree of *stimulation* provided in the environment — how the classes are organized and the extent of variety, interest, involvement, provocation, and novelty involved — influences student's motivation. The *feelings* the student has about the learning situation — what is being learned, the climate of learning, and the relevance of material to daily life — influence the individual's affect and consequently his/her motivation. Motivation is influenced by the type and degree of *competence* the student expects to develop as a result of the learning experience and by the student's ability to foresee opportunities for applying the information in new environments. Finally, motivation is influenced by the *concrete rewards* that follow learning.

Motivation also can be viewed as both intrinsic and extrinsic. Intrinsic motivation comes from within the person and is considered to be the most effective type of motivation for significant learning and retention. An example of intrinsic motivation is one's desire to be the best at whatever job one undertakes and wanting to learn merely for the satisfaction of learning. Extrinsic motivation comes from outside the individual. Positive feedback from someone who is admired and respected can be a great extrinsic motivator, as can grades. Even though educators may prefer that students be motivated to learn merely from intrinsic factors, the reality is that most students need some extrinsic rewards if their level of motivation is to be heightened. Research regarding motivation — whether intrinsic or extrinsic factors — is limited, especially in nursing education, and needs to be studied, perhaps using the Motivated Strategies for Learning Questionnaire (MSLQ) and conceptual framework for assessing motivation and self-regulated learning developed by Pintrich (2004).

A review of the literature yielded three research-based studies on motivation for learning in higher education (Fritz, Speth, Barbuto, & Boren, 2004; Seale, Chapman, & Davey, 2000; Valle et al., 2003). Additional articles were found that dealt with the motivation of cheating, which will not be discussed here. See Chapter 6 for further findings related to attitude within the affective domain.

In studying 103 undergraduate and graduate college students, Fritz et al. (2004) explored the relationship between learning styles and motivation, using the Approaches to Learning Inventory and the Motivation Sources Inventory to collect data. The results indicated a small significant positive correlation between surface apathetic approach and self-concept internal motivation subscales, a negative correlation between surface apathetic approach and self-concept external motivation subscales, and a negative correlation between strategic approach and self-concept internal motivation subscales. Additional research is needed addressing motivation and learning styles.

Using 98 third-year occupational therapy and physiotherapy students in England, Seale et al. (2000) attempted to discover which type of assessment students found most motivating to their learning. Using an author-developed questionnaire, four factors associated with assessment were found to influence student motivation: perceived relevance of the assessment, perceived content of the assessment, perception of having enthusiastic lecturers, and the group's influence on motivation, which can change as the group matures and shared experiences affect the group's history together. Educators may do well to keep these factors in mind when designing learning activities.

Using 614 university students, Valle et al. (2003) reviewed a learning model that had motivation as an underpinning. They concluded that students' predispositions to feel responsible for their academic behavior is related to a positive self-image, which is an important condition for developing learning-oriented motivation (learning goals). The model supported the use of a combination of learning strategies, which led to students assuming responsibility with a higher level of persistence, perseverance, and tenacity to achieve their goals.

The literature review further revealed only five studies on motivation in nursing. Joshua-Amadi (2003a, 2003b) reviewed motivation regarding recruitment and retention of nurses in the National Health Programs in England. Ten nurses who were interviewed over a six-month period reported leaving the profession because of the motivating factors of low and inequitable pay, lack of appreciation, and lack of growth. Vanhanen and Janhonen (2000) studied factors associated with students' view about nursing when considering whether to pursue it as a profession. Based on findings from 184 Finnish nursing students in three different nursing programs, these researchers concluded that contradictions between students' view of nursing and the philosophy of nursing underlying the study program were a source of motivational problems that resulted in students' dissatisfaction with nursing education. Chan and Wai-Tong (2000) studied student nurses in Hong Kong in their third year of a bachelor of science degree program and found an increase in students' perceived autonomy and motivation for learning in a clinical course when learning contracts were used. Chiu (2005) studied the motivating factors for Malaysian nurses to continue their nursing education and found four interrelated reasons: work-related stimulation or self-growth, compliance with management requirements, professional advancement and keeping up with the profession, and the availability and accessibility of the courses. Braten and Olaussen (2007) studied how enthusiasm and motivation are lost over time during a Norwegian nursing program. The study indicated that changes in motivation could be related to several factors: "disappointments" experienced during training (e.g., nursing work is found to be less glamorous than anticipated); competition between students; strains experienced during nursing practice; and a natural ebbing of one's initial motivation and enthusiasm for something new. The authors encourage faculty to develop interventions to maintain the initial enthusiasm students frequently have upon entering a profession.

Additional research on motivation specific to nursing education needs to be conducted. What motivates individuals to choose a career in nursing? What motivates nursing students to study and to learn? How can nurse educators positively influence student motivation? What behaviors of nurse educators serve to negatively influence student motivation? What effects do admission, retention, progression, and graduation rates have? What impact do program outcomes fostered by external stakeholders (e.g., the state and national Departments of Education, a state board of nursing. and nursing accrediting bodies) have on motivation in nursing education?

## Learning Styles

The final learner characteristic to be discussed here is the student's learning style. Merritt (1989) reviewed the concept of learning styles in nursing education research and found the following: most studies were descriptive, ex post facto investigations; no single model was utilized consistently in the studies; and psychometric properties of the instruments used had not been consistently examined. She stated "more definitive knowledge about learning styles is needed so that the impact of such knowledge in helping people learn can be determined" (p. 17). In order to fully understand the significance of learning styles, educators must know how each component influences a student's desire to learn and her/his ability to learn effectively.

The way an individual processes or learns information describes his/her learning style (Guild & Ganger, 1998). Each person develops a learning style based upon biological, sociological, and environmental life influences, and no learning style is better or worse than another, since learning can occur regardless of the learning style used. Knowing about various learning styles, however, helps teachers make decisions on how to construct learning activities and learning contracts. If a variety of teaching/learning approaches are used, the learning styles of all students will be accommodated, and more students are likely to be satisfied with their learning experiences.

In 1984, Friedman and Alley conducted a comprehensive review of research about learning styles and their measurement. Based on this analysis, these authors formulated six principles on learning style:

- The teacher's preferred style of teaching as well as the student's preferred learning style can be determined.

- Teachers need to recognize that they will have a tendency to teach in a way that is consistent with how they learn.

- Teachers are most helpful when they help learners identify and use their own preferred learning style.

- Learners should be provided with opportunities to learn through their own preferred style.

- Learners should be encouraged and taught ways to diversify their learning styles and preferences.

- Teachers should develop specific learning strategies that support a wide range of learning styles.

Assessing learners' preferred learning styles is an important task of teachers that can be done by asking how they prefer to learn and what enhances their learning, or by observing them in problem-solving situations to determine how they reach conclusions. The learning style also can be assessed through various instruments.

In recent years, the concept of "learning styles" has become a center of attention for many educators, since individuals learn in different ways and each individual may use different learning methods depending upon the situation and the information to be learned. Educators therefore, are urged to discover their students' individual learning styles. But how do educators obtain this information? And what theories underlie the idea of meeting individual students' learning needs?

Learning style theories can be grouped into three basic categories: those that deal with brain functions, those based on personality differences, and those addressing differences in sensory modalities. Many learning-style instruments have been developed based on these categories.

***Brain Function Theories and Instruments.*** In 1972, Ornstein noted that there were differences in left-brain and right-brain functions, but it was not until 1977 that Sperry helped educators understand that the left hemisphere of the brain is predominantly involved with analytical and logical thinking, especially verbal and mathematical functions, while the right hemisphere is specialized for orientation in space, artistic endeavor, body image, recognition of faces, and holistic and rational thinking. Individuals who exhibit pronounced differences in their preferences for linear (analytic) thinking as opposed to holistic (artistic) thinking are said to have a linear (left brain) versus a holistic (right brain) learning style preference.

The Brain Preference Indicator (BPI) is one instrument used to measure brain hemispherical preference (Wonder & Donovan, 1984). Using a carefully developed and theoretically congruent set of questions, it reveals hemispheric dominance and the resultant general style of thought.

***Personality Theories.*** Several learning style theories have their basis in personality differences. Most prominent are those developed by Myers (1980), Gregorc (1982), and Kolb (1984).

Myers developed a personality/learning style theory and the resultant Myers-Briggs Type Indicator (MBTI), based upon Carl Jung's personality theory, which explains personality similarities and differences by identifying the ways people prefer to take in and make use of data from the world around them. The MBTI is not a learning style instrument per se. Instead, it measures differences in personality types that affect how individuals behave and how people tend to interact with one another. The MBTI has four dichotomous preferences — extraversion-introversion, sensing-intuition, thinking-feeling, and judgment-perception; when these preferences are combined with one another, sixteen personality types emerge.

The learning theory, based on the MBTI, postulates that certain personality characteristics have specific learning orientations. Jensen (1987) explained these learning orientations as follows:

- **Extroverts** learn best in situations filled with movement, action, and talk. They enjoy discussion groups, and cooperative projects, but may have trouble sitting still, reading books, and writing.

- **Introverts** learn best alone in periods of concentrated study. They enjoy teacher-centered lectures and may not like discussion. They think before speaking.

- **Sensing** individuals like to focus on the concrete here-and-now as well as on facts and details. They want to put knowledge to use and are quite precise and accurate.

- **Intuitive** individuals like to gain general impressions. They dislike structured and mechanical approaches to learning and prefer open-ended assignments and opportunities for imagination. They may be careless about details.

- **Thinking** individuals prefer performance criteria and want to know how learning will lead to a deeper understanding of how things work. They like rule-based reasoning.

- **Feeling** individuals want to know how learning will affect people, and they are interested in the process of learning. They are motivated by learning that touches convictions and values.

- **Judgment** individuals prefer a structured learning environment with clear goals and deadlines. They enjoy accomplishment, getting assignments done, and achievement.

- **Perception** individuals prefer free-wheeling learning environments, can work on several things at once, and delay closure until the deadline. They may feel imprisoned in a highly structured classroom.

Another theory about learning styles was proposed by Gregorc (1982), who identified four sets of dualities: perception, ordering, processing, and relating. Gregorc's learning styles are based upon the interrelationships of perception and ordering abilities. The perceptual plane has two dimensions, concrete and abstract, and the ordering plane is bi-dimensional: sequential and random. When combined, the two sets characterize four types of learning styles: concrete sequential, abstract sequential, concrete random, and abstract random. In each of these learning styles, learners demonstrate perceived attitudes, motivations, and reasoned thought toward the learning environment. Gregorc believes that most people have the ability to operate to some extent in all four styles. The Gregorc Style Delineator (GSD) is designed to measure the extent to which a learner's pattern of thinking reflects the four modes. A higher score in a mode indicates stronger orientation to that mode.

- **Concrete-sequential** learners tend to operate in a highly structured, conservative manner in which specific details and time schedules are critical. They do not tolerate being interrupted during the performance of a skill and learn best in a quiet environment. Consistency is important to these learners, and they like recognition or a compliment for a job well done. Learning can be enhanced by handouts, demonstrations, hands-on opportunities with guided practice, lectures with visual aids, and computer-aided instruction.

- **Abstract-sequential** learners are global thinkers and surround themselves with language and other symbols of knowledge. They do not learn well when sequence is interrupted, and they need facts and written documentation for reference, as well as a quiet environment in which to concentrate and learn. Their learning can be enhanced by audiotapes, lectures, and supplemental reading.

- **Abstract-random** learners are global thinkers who value relationships and their thinking processes are anchored in feelings. They will ask questions randomly and like a busy environment for learning. Learning is best achieved in groups with the opportunity for discussion and question-and-answer sessions. Learning can be enhanced with color, music, pictures, drawings, symbols, poetry, and humor.

- **Concrete-random** learners tend to seek alternatives and create choices where none existed before. They are very inquisitive, will question motives, focus on the process, and make intuitive leaps or insights. For this type of learner, the "why" is more important than the "how." They do not like detail and have difficulty learning step-by-step. Learning can be enhanced by simulations, computer and board games, case studies, and brainstorming sessions.

The final learning style theory based on personality types is Kolb's Experiential Learning Theory (Kolb, 1984). Kolb believed that learning is a continuous process grounded in the reality that the learner is not a blank slate; instead, every learner approaches a learning situation with preconceived ideas. Kolb believed that learning is a cumulative result of past experiences, heredity, and the demands of the present environment, all of which combine to produce an individualized orientation to learning for each person.

Kolb believed that understanding a person's learning style, including its strengths and weaknesses, represents a major step toward increasing learning power and helping learners get the most from their learning experiences. Kolb's theory states two major principles: (1) most people differ along four modes of learning preferences, Abstract to Concrete, and Reflective Observation to Active Experimentation, and (2) learning style is a combination of these four modes, each of which reflects the dimensions of perception and processing. Kolb used these two sets of polarities to develop the Learning Style Inventory (LSI).

- **Convergent** learners prefer abstract conceptualization and active experimentation. They enjoy problem-solving, decision making, practical application of ideas, finding a single correct answer or solution, and working on technical tasks. They are "thinkers" and "doers."

- **Divergent** learners prefer concrete experience and reflective observation as learning traits. They enjoy organizing many specific relationships into a meaningful gestalt, generating alternative ideas and implications, brainstorming, and imagining. They are "feelers" and "watchers."

- **Assimilative** learners combine the learning modes of reflective observation and abstract conceptualization. They prefer reasoning, creating theoretical models, integrated explanations, and working with ideas, concepts and sound, precise theories. They are "watchers" and "thinkers."

- **Accommodative** learners prefer active experimentation and concrete experiences. They enjoy doing things, carrying out plans, seeking opportunity and risk-taking action, fitting the theory to the facts, and relying on other people for information. They are "doers" and "feelers."

The approach to "learning style" most widely used in the United Kingdom, and often used as an alternative to Kolb's LSI is one that was developed by Honey and Mumford (1986). These researchers used the Kolb model as the basis for their own Learning Styles Questionnaire (LSQ), a tool designed to identify an individual's relative strengths in each of four learning styles: activist, reflector, theorist, and pragmatist (Allinson & Hayes, 1988, 1990).

*Sensory Modalities Theories.* In addition to brain function and personality theories, the concept of learning styles has been addressed in terms of sensory modalities, or one's preferred senses for learning. Of the five senses — taste, smell, touch, sight, and sound — the last two, sight and sound, are very important in most postsecondary settings. It is important to remember, however, that students vary significantly in their capacity for input and output in their "sensory modalities."

Barbe and Swassing (1979) used this idea of sensory modalities to develop a learning style theory that states that all learners have differences in their ability to use sensory modalities. These differences can be expressed as *preferred styles of learning* and are categorized as auditory, visual, and tactile-kinesthetic.

*Auditory* learners like to use their voices and ears, and they learn best by talking and listening. They like to "talk it through" and enjoy lectures and class discussion. Silence can be very disturbing to them. *Visual* learners like to see the words written down. They like pictures, charts, diagrams, graphs, and time lines. They like to have written guidance for their assignment, and they enjoy doing written assignments more than verbal ones. *Tactile-kinesthetic* learners like to be "up and doing." They like to build projects, handle materials, and act out. When they *do* it, they learn it and remember it. They hate sitting still.

Effective teachers are sensitive to the strengths and weaknesses in the sensory modalities that students bring to learning situations. An example of an instrument to measure sensory modalities is the VARK (visual, aural, read/write, and kinesthetic) Inventory (Marcy, 2001).

*Other Measurement Instruments.* In addition to the instruments mentioned, each of which grew from a specific theory, several other instruments exist that are not specific to brain function, personality, or sensory modalities theories. Since these instruments are being used in learning theory research, it is important that they be discussed.

Dunn and Dunn (1978) developed the Learning Style Inventory. This is a self-reporting instrument that is widely used to identify how individuals prefer to function, learn, concentrate, and perform in educational activities. It examines the five basic stimuli that affect a person's ability to learn (environmental elements, emotional elements, sociological patterns, physical elements, and psychological elements) and uses that information to define an individual's learning style. The Learning Style Inventory, which is used primarily in K-12 education, has been modified to create an adult version, the Productivity Environmental Preference Survey (PEPS) (Dunn, Dunn, & Price, 1991).

Riechmann and Grasha (1974) identified three learning preference styles or types: dependent learners, collaborative learners, and independent learners. Dependent learners prefer teacher-directed, highly structured learning experiences, where assignments are explicit and assessed by the teacher. Collaborative learners prefer discussion and favor group projects, collaborative assignments, and social interaction. Independent learners prefer to exercise an influence on the content and structure of learning, and they view the teacher or instructor as a resource. Sadler-Smith (1997) developed the Learning Preferences Inventory (LPI) based upon Riechmann's and Grasha's work.

A final instrument to be discussed is the Revised Approaches to Studying Inventory (RASI) developed by Entwistle and Tait (1994). This instrument is designed to measure an individual's approach to studying in a higher education context in terms of five "*orientations*": deep approach, surface approach, strategic approach, lack of direction, and academic self-confidence. Individuals preferring a *deep approach* to learning try to work out the meaning of information for themselves, do not accept ideas without critical examination, relate ideas to a wider context, and look for the reasoning, justification, and logic behind ideas. Those preferring a *surface approach* to learning rely on rote-learning of material, accept ideas without necessarily understanding them, emphasize acquiring factual information in isolation of a wider picture, and express anxiety about organization and volume of material to be covered. The third approach to learning — the *strategic approach* — incorporates individuals who perceive themselves as having clear goals for studying and are hard workers. These individuals ensure they have the appropriate resources and conditions for successful studying and feel they are generally well organized. Those with a *lack of direction approach* typically have no clear academic or career direction. They just "drift" around in higher education fields. Finally, individuals whose approach is one of *academic self-confidence* perceive themselves as able, intelligent, and competent to cope with the intellectual and academic demands.

***Research-Based Literature on Learning Styles.*** Using ERIC, CINAHL, and Ovid databases, a literature search was conducted in both the nursing and higher education literature. The search revealed several research-based articles on teaching and learning published since 1998, and these are summarized in Table 3.5, which begins on page 65 at the end of the chapter.

The research literature revealed a variety of ways learning styles can be defined: (a) as study preferences (Carnwell, 2000; Fritz et al., 2004; Howard, Hayes, Solomonides, & Swannell, 2001; Lindblom-Ylanne, 2004; Martin, Stark, & Jolly, 2000), (b) as environmental preferences (Andrusyszyn, Cragg, & Humbert, 2001; Diaz & Cartnal, 1999; Harrelson, Leaver-Dunn, & Wright, 1998; Heath, 2000; Hoisington, 2000; Miller, 1998), and (c) as overall learning preferences (Abu-Moghli, Khalaf, Halabi, & Wardam, 2005; Anderson, 1998; Campeau, 1998; Carpio et al., 1999; Chen & Lee, 2000; Coker, 2000; Colucciello, 1999; Cope & Staehr, 2005; DiBartola, Miller, & Turley, 2001; Evans & Waring, 2006; Freeman, Fell, & Muellenberg, 1998; Freeman & Titjerina, 2000; Hativa & Birenbaum, 2000; Hendry et al., 2005; Honigsfeld & Schiering, 2004; Jie & Xiaoqing, 2006; Linares, 1999; May, 2000; McColgin, 2000; McDade, 1999; McLaughlin, 2001;

Morton-Rias et al., 2007; Mupinga, Nora, & Yaw, 2006; Olson & Scanlan, 2002; Reese & Dunn, 2007; Ross, Drysdale & Schulz, 1999; Sandmire, Vromna, & Sanders, 2000; Slater, 2003; Thompson & Bing-You, 1998; Titiloye & Scott, 2001; Vincent & Ross, 2001; Ward, 2003; Wessel et al., 1999). The primary instrument used in all this research about learning styles was Kolb's Learning Style Inventory (Campeau; Carpio et al.; Chen & Lee; Coker; Colucciello, 1999; DiBartola et al.; Freeman et al.; Freeman & Tijerina; Sandmire et al.; Titiloye & Scott; Wessel et al.).

Several studies were also conducted using subjects and educational systems outside the United States (Abu-Moghli et al.; Andrusyszyn et al.; Campeau; Carpio et al.; Chen & Lee; Hativa & Birenbaum; Howard et al.; Jie & Xiaoqing; Lindblom-Ylanne; Martin et al.; Ross et al.; Wessel et al.). While the findings of these investigations are most informative, some may need to be replicated in the United States to determine the applicability of findings to U.S. environments.

Despite the large number of studies about learning styles reported in the literature, most had several of the following limitations: convenience samples, lack of replication, use of multiple "learning style" instruments, and limited underlying theoretical frameworks. The only common themes in learning styles that emerged from this review of the nursing and higher education research literature were the different types of learning styles (Carpio et al.; Chen & Lee; Linares) and efforts to match learning styles with the teacher's style, preceptor's style, or teaching methods (Anderson; Carpio et al.; Chen & Lee; Honigsfeld & Schiering; Linares; McColgin).

Richardson (2005) reviewed the research in teaching and learning over the past 25 years. He believed the research had revealed relationships in students' approaches to learning. From his review, he developed an integrated teaching-learning model that needs to be further tested.

## The Learning Environment

In addition to learner characteristics, including learning style, the learning process is influenced by the environment or setting in which learning takes place. Components of the learning environment include the physical setting itself (e.g., classroom, lab, hospital, or online), as well as the larger institutional context and the social aspects of the setting (e.g., cultural groups represented, gender and age distribution, or the amount of interaction among participants).

### Physical Setting

The physical setting of the learning environment includes the size and arrangement of the classroom or lab, as well as materials available. Arrangement of the classroom can facilitate or stifle communication and interaction. Other influences are comfort, temperature, noise level, lighting, space conducive to the learning, working equipment, colors, accessibility, etc. Where is the teacher located in relation to the students? Are students territorial? Is there enough space to adequately accommodate the number of students? Is there a sufficient amount of equipment to learn a skill in a lab setting, or do students always need to share? How is the teacher viewed by the students — as an expert, formal authority, socializing agent, facilitator, or colleague? Does the classroom have sufficient light? Is it too cold or too hot? Are there distractions? Does the student even see the teacher or other students in person, or is the entire learning experience completed in an online environment?

## Institutional Context

The institutional context is the overall organization's mission/philosophy, culture and climate, as well as the variety of academic disciplines represented. Most institutions have some distinctive mission or purpose that is unique to that institution, serves as the "glue" holding everything together, and incorporates the purposes and the intended outcomes of the educational enterprise.

The culture of an institution is grounded in the shared assumptions of the individuals who participate in that organization. According to Chafee and Tierney (1988), a quick way to focus on the culture of a college or university is to ask what gets done, how it gets done, and who does it. Culture stresses deeply embedded patterns of shared values, assumptions, and beliefs, all of which influence administrative policies, curriculum, schedules, and priorities related to research or instruction.

Climate is the way people in the institution feel about the organization and about one another. The climate can be characterized by satisfaction or dissatisfaction, high morale or low morale, anxiety and stress or excitement/motivation (Tierney, 1990). Climate is current perceptions and attitudes and what it is like to be at the institution at any given point in time. It therefore has more of a psychological basis and is dynamic rather than stagnant.

Part of the institutional context is the variety of academic disciplines represented and how diverse or closely aligned they are. Faculty in different disciplines think differently, approach teaching differently, place different emphases on content to be covered and thinking skills or habits of mind to be developed in their students, and have different attitudes toward their subject matter. All of these factors can affect the learning environment in which students are involved and, ultimately, their learning.

## Social Setting

The social setting in any given learning environment also may have an impact upon learning. The social setting includes gender, ethnicity, age, cultural make-up, amount and extent of interaction, and number of participants. Each learning environment, therefore, is a unique setting in which both teachers and learners need to be flexible and open to various perspectives.

## Research on Learning Environments

The majority of the research reported has been conducted in K-12 settings, which may be reflective of understanding the importance of the learning environment in earlier developmental stages. Several recent research articles (summarized in Table 3.6 which begins on page 80 at the end of this chapter) were found on learning environments in higher education and nursing.

Wanstreet (2006) reviewed 125 non-researched-based articles dealing with learning environments. Several "topics" were identified: (1) learner-learner interactions; (2) learner-instructor interactions; (3) learner-content interactions; (4) learner-interface interactions; (5) computer-mediated communication; and (6) social/psychological connections. Mayer (2003) reviewed the current trends in educational research, as well as the role of computer-based simulations in education and made recommendations regarding future research on learning environments.

Thirteen studies were found in the higher education literature, from which two primary themes emerged: (1) design elements of courses contributing to the learning environment (Ausburn, 2004; Cope & Staehr, 2005; Masui & De Corte, 2005; Schelfhout, Dochy, & Janssens, 2004; Vaatstra & Vries, 2007) and (2) comparison of teaching in an online environment versus traditional or hybrid settings (Barker & Garvin-Doxas, 2004; Bruyn, 2004; Lightfoot, 2006; Romano et al., 2005; Rovai, Ponton, Derrick, & Davis, 2006; Shea, Li, & Pickett, 2006). Two additional studies did not address these two central themes. Nijhuis, Segers, & Gijselaers (2007) studied the relationship between perceptions of the learning environment, personality, and learning strategies used with international business students. They developed four path analyses: (1) personality traits, conscientiousness, and openness and how that relates to learning strategies; (2) students' perceptions of the learning environment and how that influences learning strategies; (3) personality traits and how that influences perceptions of the learning environment; and (4) relationships between conscientiousness, openness to experience, and learning strategies. Scheyvens, Wild, and Overton (2003) assessed how the learning environment supported the academic success of international postgraduate students and how that affected their personal well-being.

Five research-based studies were found in the nursing literature (France, Fields, & Garth, 2004; Nganasurian, 1999; Snelgrove & Slater, 2003; Speziale & Jacobson, 2005; Wong & Chung, 2002). France et al (2004). explored the lived experience of Black nursing students in a predominantly White university setting. The study had four subjects who were interviewed regarding their experiences. The results revealed an environment not conducive to learning due to a perceived lack of relationships, collegiality, and support among classmates. The students also had a poor understanding of how to navigate the educational system.

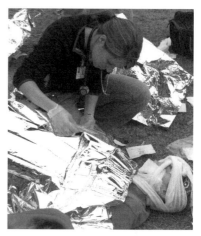

The 1999 study by Nganasurian sought to identify the factors making a positive contribution to learning within mental health care settings. The first phase of the study asked 146 nursing students, staff, and faculty to validate a list of factors thought to be conducive to learning. This information was then used to develop a Likert-type scale to measure the extent to which those factors existed in the student learning environment. In the second phase, 51 mental health nursing student respondents indicated the following factors contribute to learning: (1) practice; (2) 1:1 activity with staff in clinical settings; (3) feedback with activity; (4) good teamwork and integration of the learner into the overall team; (5) wide variety of client problems from which to learn; and (6) a clear link between theory and practice.

Snelgrove and Slater (2003) analyzed the use of the Approaches to Learning Questionnaire with 300 nursing students. The study established the validity of using the tool with this population to gain knowledge about student nurses' approaches to learning and the impact on academic performance.

The fourth study identified how the practices, methodologies, and strategies in RN nurse education have changed in the last five years (Speziale & Jacobson, 2005). They concluded that nursing education needs to develop a high-quality, diverse nursing workforce for the future, where technology will be a recurring theme. They also believe that nursing faculty will need to develop more active learning environments that involve "active" student participation.

Finally, Wong and Chung (2002) explored the diagnostic reasoning process among Hong Kong nursing students who learned in different institutional contexts (a university and a hospital-based school of nursing) to determine whether differences existed. The study had 20 subjects, 10 from each environment. Data were collected using Bigg's Study Process Questionnaire and an exercise in which each subject was asked to identify a differential diagnosis for three simulated scenarios. The results showed no significant difference between the two groups regarding their ability to formulate diagnoses. The study did reveal a difference between the two groups' reasoning patterns. The university-based students used data-driven strategies for decision making, while the hospital-based students used hypothesis-driven strategies for decision making.

The social setting could also include the instructional strategy used — lecture, discussion, online format, demonstration, and so on. Several studies are discussed in later chapters (4-6) dealing with the effectiveness of various teaching strategies in nursing education.

## Technology and Learning

Today's technology affords phenomenal access to knowledge and has had a profound effect on the way teaching and learning occur (Heller, Ortos, & Crowley, 2000). In fact, in many ways it has created new strategies that have transformed teaching and learning. But what evidence exists to document the impact of technology on student learning?

When information is widely available, teachers may no longer be seen as the source of answers, nor may they be the only individuals responsible for imparting knowledge. Instead, they become facilitators of learning. Teachers, therefore, need to understand how technology can be used most effectively to enhance student learning. There are those who believe that technology, in present learning situations, is the overhead projector and blackboard of the past learning environment. In other words, a teaching tool, not a new learning strategy.

Using PubMed and Ovid, an extensive literature search was done using the key terms: learning, technology, education, and nursing. Once again the literature is plentiful, but research-based articles are lacking.

Jones and Paolucci (1999) proposed a framework for selecting technology, using it in educational settings, and evaluating the effectiveness of educational technology in enhancing student learning and achievement. This framework was designed to interrelate instructional objectives, delivery systems and learning outcomes, and it lays a foundation for experimental or quasi-experimental studies, which may contribute meaningful information regarding the effect of technology on learning outcomes.

Billings (2000) also developed a framework to assess the dynamic interaction of technology with other aspects of nursing courses. This framework includes the concepts of outcomes, educational practices, faculty support, learner support, and use of technology. Again, it could serve as a foundation for many research studies.

Premkumar, Hunter, Davison, and Jennett (1998) described the development of a tool to evaluate multimedia resources in health education. This tool could be used to evaluate resources being considered for use in a nursing program. The tool was developed and tested with experts in both technology and education.

An integrative review of the literature on the use of computer-based simulation in the education process was completed by Ravert (2002). She reviewed several studies done between 1980 and 2000, most of which were completed in either a medical school or a nursing program. Ravert concluded that: (1) more research needs to be conducted on the best use of computer-based simulation, and (2) more research needs to be done on the effective use of simulation in basic education as well as in continuing education.

The use of computers in nursing was the focus of Ribbons' (1998) comprehensive literature review. He reported that studies conducted in the 1990s focused primarily on the intricacies of the technology, computer literacy, nurses' attitudes toward computers and information systems, the implementation of computerized systems and the application of nursing information in a computerized environment. Ribbons concluded that very little attention has been given to the cognitive processes required to use information technologies effectively, and formulated five research questions that he believes need to be addressed in nursing: (1) What instructional frameworks underpin the use of computers as cognitive tools? (2) What is the impact of the use of such tools on learners' problem-solving and clinical decision-making abilities? (3) Does the use of generic cognitive tools in nurse education support the concept of cognitive residues — such as skills, understanding, and attitudes acquired during interaction with the computer that remain when the computer is turned off — that are cognitive templates transferable and applicable to a number of contexts? (4) How might contemporary information technologies such as the World Wide Web best be used in the construction of learning environments? (5) What is the best way to manage and evaluate these environments once they are established?

Additional reports discussed the use of technology in a variety of courses and student perceptions regarding technology as a teaching tool (Cartwright & Menkens, 2002; Clark, 1998; Halstead & Coudret, 2000; Kim, 2003; MacDonald & Mason, 1999; Mastrian & McGonigle, 1999; Zalon, 2000). Others reviewed the concept of technology in continuing education for nurses (Billings & Rowles, 2001), as a communication learning tool (Brown, 1999), in distance education (Kuramoto, 1999), and in computer networking use in nursing and health care education (Ward, 1997).

A limited number of studies addressed the effect of technology on learning in nursing and higher education in general and those studies are summarized in Table 3.7, which begins on page 86 at the end of the chapter. The primary themes evident in this literature are determining the effect of different types of technology on learning (Elfrink et al., 2000; Jeffries, Woolf, & Linde, 2003; Klaassens, 1992; MacIntosh, 2001; Weston, 2005) and examining the effect of web-based courses on learning (Atack & Rankin, 2002; Edwards, 2005; Kenny, 2002; Leasure, Davis, & Thievon, 2000). Only one research study addressed the effect of technology on the caring attributes of nurses (Arthur, Pang, & Wong, 2001). Additional studies on caring are summarized in Chapter 6.

In essence, research on the effects of technology on learning in nursing is lacking. The majority of studies suffer from a number of limitations, including the following: researcher-developed questionnaires that are not shown to be valid or reliable, a lack of repetition or duplication of studies, small sample sizes, and a failure to identify an underlying theoretical framework. Additional research is needed on all aspects of technology and its effect on learning in nursing education — basic as well as continuing education.

The use of technology in nursing education is beginning to expand beyond the basic use of computers, including nonresearch articles that explain how technology is being utilized in a variety of settings and ways (Rempher, Lasome, & Lasome, 2003; Simpson, 1997; Skiba, 2005; 2006; 2007a, 2007b, 2007c) and how to adapt teaching to accommodate the net generation of learners that now make up nursing programs (Skiba & Barton, 2006).

## THE TEACHER

The final aspect of the learning model presented at the beginning of this chapter involves the teacher or educator. Just as there is diversity among students, there is diversity among teachers/educators. Essentially, there are two overriding components to the teacher — characteristics and styles — both of which contribute elements to the overall learning process in both the classroom and clinical settings. In nursing education, competencies are also a very important aspect of the teacher (see Chapter 1).

### *Teacher Characteristics*

Each teacher is unique in terms of age, gender, educational preparation, and overall experience, whether in academic or clinical settings, and these characteristics influence the learning environment. In addition, each teacher brings unique cognitive dimensions, personality dimensions, and perceptions of self and others to the learning situation. Each of these latter dimensions is described here.

The cognitive dimension of teachers covers both their personal learning styles and their thinking styles. The same instruments used to assess the learning style of students discussed earlier in this chapter can be used to assess the teacher. It is also believed that teachers tend to teach in a manner consistent with how they learn (Friedman & Alley, 1984). Teachers/educators should, therefore, know their preferred learning style, which will enable them to expand their teaching abilities beyond their "favorite" method. (See Chapters 4 through 6 concerning a variety of teaching methods that address all domains of learning. Chapter 4 also expands upon the cognitive dimension for students.)

Thinking style is how a person prefers to think about material as one is learning about it or after one has already learned it. Thinking styles are emerging from the underlying theory of mental self-government, which is relatively new (Sternberg, 1988, 1997). Sternberg uses the analogy of governing a society to help us understand thinking styles. He says that people use their abilities in many ways to complete daily activities and management tasks, and the preferred ways in which ones does these things is one's thinking style.

Sternberg identified thirteen thinking styles — legislative, executive, judicial, monarchic, heirarchical, oligarchic, anarchic, global, local, internal, external, liberal, and conservative — all of which fall along five dimensions: function (legislative, executive, and judicial), form (monarchic, hierarchical, oligarchic, and anarchic), level (global and local), scope (internal and external), and leaning (liberal and conservative). Thinking styles are posited to fall along a continuum (rather than being dichotomous), and they are not seen as either good or bad. The task a person is performing and the situation in which it is being performed determine the style(s) utilized. Several inventories have been developed that assess Sternberg's theory of mental self-government and thinking styles: Thinking Styles Inventory, Set of Thinking Styles for Students, Students' Thinking Styles Evaluated by Teachers, and the Thinking Styles in Teaching Inventory (Sternberg, 1997).

Four studies in higher education have been done looking specifically at the thinking styles of faculty or students going into education (Evans & Waring, 2006; Zhang, 2001, 2004; Zhang & Sternberg, 2002) (see Table 3.8, which can be found on page 89 at the end of this chapter). Evans and Waring was the only one of these studies done in the United States, but it did not use mental self-government as its underlying framework. The remaining studies had mental self-government as their underlying framework and used a variety of the instruments. Additional research needs to be done on the cognitive dimension of educators in the United States, especially nurse educators.

The personality dimension of teachers is their personal qualities and behaviors. Personality includes how individuals interact with others, what their typical problem-solving methods are, and how they react in difficult or unusual situations. Is the teacher outgoing and engaging? Does the teacher demonstrate enthusiasm and passion for the subject? Is the person conscientious, patient, cheerful, considerate? Personal qualities can also mean the person's physical appearance and dress. The personality theories and instruments discussed earlier in the chapter about the student could be utilized to better understand the teacher as well.

The combination of the cognitive and personality dimension results in how teachers perceive themselves and how they are perceived by others. Is the teacher approachable? Does the teacher demonstrate confidence in the classroom and/or clinical setting? Does the teacher "connect" with the students? Does the teacher demonstrate professional boundaries with students? What type of interpersonal skills does the teacher have with students or professional peers? Only three research-based articles were found in the recent nursing and higher education literature dealing with the personality dimension and/or teacher perception (Gillespie, 2002; Pozo-Munoz, Rebolloso-Pacheco, & Fernandez-Ramirez, 2000; Zhang & Sternberg, 2002).

Gillespie (2002) described experiences of "connection" in the student-teacher relationship and its effect on learning experiences. The study involved eight nursing students who were enrolled in a baccalaureate nursing program, each of whom was interviewed regarding her/his perceived "connection" or lack of "connection" with the clinical instructor. The findings indicated: (1) there are personal and professional components of the connected student-teacher relationship; (2) connection emerged from highly interactive, evolving relationships; (3) the "connected" teacher was characterized by competence, compassion, and commitment; (4) the "fit" of the relationship was dependent upon both teacher-related factors and student-related factors; and (5) the student-teacher connection emerged as a strongly positive influence on the clinical learning experiences. Since this study, Gillespie (2005) has completed an extensive review of the literature using the concept "connection."

Pozo-Munoz et al. (2000) utilized university students' opinions to define the "ideal" teacher. More than 2,000 university students completed a Semantic Differential Scale, which is composed of thirty-nine bipolar adjectives about the teaching staff. The findings revealed four principal attributes of the "ideal" teacher: (1) teaching competency, (2) teaching qualities, (3) teacher's appearance, and (4) directiveness.

The final study investigated the relationship between thinking styles and teacher characteristics (Zhang & Sternberg, 2002). One hundred ninety-three in-service teachers in Hong Kong completed the Thinking Styles Questionnaire for Teachers and an informal demographic questionnaire. The findings indicated there were six teacher characteristics to particular thinking styles, but a causal relationship between thinking styles and teacher characteristics was not found.

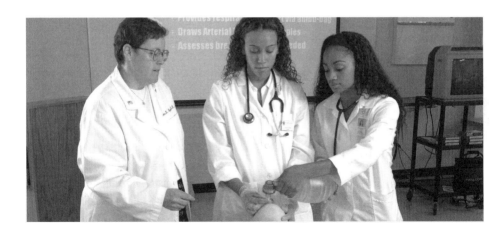

## *Teacher Styles*

Teaching style refers to the characteristic way a teacher goes about his/her work. It consists of natural tendencies as well as consciously developed attitudes, actions, skills, and behavior (Eble, 1980). A teaching style is an outgrowth of the teacher's personality and character, in which a distinctive style or approach emerges. It has also been used as a "catch-all" to encompass whatever the teacher is doing. Eble believes that one's teaching style emerges over time and is a response to positive and negative feedback received from students as well as professional peers.

Richardson (2005) reviewed the research in teaching and learning over the past 25 years. He concluded that the research revealed relationships in teachers' approaches to teaching, and he used this insight to develop an integrated model, which needs to be further tested.

Grasha (2000) provided a review of teaching styles in relationship to instructional technology. He also made recommendations regarding the teaching styles to use with various learning styles.

A review of the literature yielded eight research-based articles on teaching styles since 2000 in higher education (Evans, 2004; Hativa & Birenbaum, 2000; Kreber, 2005; Lindblom-Ylanne, Trigwell, Nevgi, & Ashwin, 2006; Miley & Gonsalves, 2003, 2005; Schaefer & Zygmont, 2003; Stes, Gijbels, & Petegem, 2008; Yacapsin & Stick, 2007) and one in nursing (Schaefer & Zygmont). (See Table 3.9 which begins on page 90 at the end of this chapter for a summary of these studies.)

Each of these studies utilized one of four instruments to measure teaching styles, the primary one being the Approaches to Teaching Inventory (ATI) (Kreber, 2005; Lindblom-Ylanne et al., 2006; Stes et al., 2008). Additional information on the development of this instrument and its validity/reliability is also available in the literature (Meyer & Eley, 2006; Prosser & Trigwell, 2006; Trigwell & Prosser, 2004; Trigwell, Prosser, & Ginns, 2005).

The research specifically on teaching styles is limited. Additional research studies need to be done looking at teaching styles in relation to teaching methodologies, students' learning styles, and the learning environment. Since the teacher's style may influence the learning that takes place more than the teaching method used, this area needs to be studied carefully. The literature supports the concept that knowing something well is simply not enough to teach it effectively. Thus, how one teaches and how one relates to students is a critical piece in achieving positive educational outcomes. (See Chapters 4 through 6 for additional information on teaching methodologies.)

### Nurse Educator Competencies

Understanding the teacher component of the overall complex learning process would not be complete without addressing the competencies of educators. Teaching is a complex process that involves classroom, clinical, and laboratory aspects. The nurse teacher/educator not only brings his/her teaching characteristics and styles to the learning process, but also the academic and nursing professional competencies that have been acquired.

Thought leaders in education and other NLN members began work in 2002 — through a think tank on the educational preparation of nurse educators and a task group on nurse educator competencies — to develop a list of core competencies for nurse educators (NLN, 2005a). After extensively reviewing the literature and seeking feedback from the nursing education community (Halstead, 2007), eight competencies for nurse educators were identified:

- Facilitate Learning
- Facilitate Learner Development and Socialization
- Use Assessment and Evaluation Strategies
- Participate in Curriculum Design and Evaluation of Program Outcomes
- Function as a Change Agent and Leader
- Develop in the Educator Role
- Engage in Scholarship
- Function within the Educational Environment

It is not within the scope of this book to review these competencies in detail, but it is important to consider them as part of the learning "process." Also, these competencies are thoroughly addressed in *The Scope of Practice for Academic Nurse Educators* (NLN, 2005b).

## CRITICAL THINKING: AN ASPECT OF LEARNING

One specific aspect of learning is critical thinking. In nursing, critical thinking has been defined as a logical, context-sensitive, reflective, reasoning process that guides the generation, implementation and evaluation of effective approaches to client care and professional concerns (NLN, 2000). Since critical thinking is so essential to nursing practice, it is necessary that faculty help students develop their critical thinking abilities.

Critical thinking is not a new concept. It has been in the general educational literature since the early 1980s when the essence of the concept was debated and characteristics of critical thinkers were established. Chaffee (1985) identified four characteristics of a critical thinker: (1) being open to new and diverse viewpoints; (2) being able to express and present ideas in an organized manner; (3) having evidence and logical reasoning to support ideas and views; and (4) listening to others but thinking for one's self. Beyer (1987) noted that critical thinkers separate relevant from irrelevant information, spot inconsistencies in a line of reasoning, identify and challenge assumptions, separate verifiable facts from value claims, and identify doubtful or unclear claims and arguments. Brookfield (1987) further asserted that critical thinkers recognize and challenge statements or ideas that may be accepted as true but have no supporting data, identify and explore as many alternatives as possible when analyzing a situation, and utilize logical reasoning skills.

The number of articles on critical thinking in the nursing literature has exploded since the beginning of the 1990s. Using PubMed, ERIC, CINAHL, and Ovid, a literature search generated a long list of references, the majority of which were not research based. Instead, the literature revealed reports of various strategies to teach and learn critical thinking (Elliott, 1996; Hansten & Washburn, 2000; Oermann, 1997; Vanetzian & Corrigan, 1996). Strategies reported in the literature as being used to prompt critical thinking include the following:

- reflective learning (Baker, 1996; Carkhuff, 1996; Forneis & Peden-McAlpine, 2007; Gray, 2003; Lauterbach & Becker, 1996);
- clinical journals or narrative writing (Brown & Sorell, 1993; Chen & Lin, 2003; Cooper, 2000; Degazon & Lunney, 1995; Fang-Chiao & Ming-Chen, 2003; Heinrich, 1992; Kuiper, 2005; Niedringhaus, 2001; Patton et al., 1997; Sorrell, Brown, Silva, & Kohlenberg, 1997; Wong, Kember, Chung, & Yan, 1995);
- ethical debates (Candela, Michael, & Mitchell, 2003; Garrett, Schoener, & Hood, 1996);
- concept maps (Clayton, 2006; Daley, Shaw, Balistrieri, Glasenapp, & Piacentine, 1999; Roberts, Sucher, Perrin, & Rodriguez, 1995);
- learning circles (Heibert, 1996) or tutorial support (Clarke & Lane, 2005) or peer coaching (Ladyshewsky, 2006);
- simulation (Johannsson & Wertenberger, 1996; Rauen, 2001);
- gaming (Kuhn, 1995);
- "think aloud" seminars (Lee & Ryan-Wenger, 1997);
- collaborative testing (Lusk, 2003; Rao & DiCarlo, 2000);
- technology-based assignments (Mastrian & McGonigle, 1999);
- case studies (Mogale & Botes, 2001; Neill, Lachat, & Taylor-Panek, 1997);
- mind mapping (Rooda, 1994); and
- narrative pedagogy (Evans & Bendel, 2004).

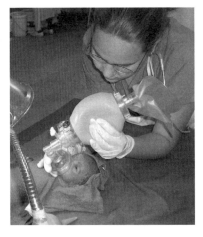

In addition to these reports of teaching strategies used to promote students' critical thinking, the nursing literature presents numerous discussions of the general concept of critical thinking and how it relates to nursing (Brown & Sorrell, 1999; Chenoweth, 1998; Dobrzykowski, 1994; Gendrop & Eisenhauer, 1996; Gordon, 2000; Higuchi & Donald, 2002; Kintgen-Andrews, 1993; Kuiper, 2000; Locsin, 2001; Miller & Malcolm, 1990; Pless & Clayton, 1993; Rane-Szostak & Robertson, 1996; Scheffer & Rubenfeld, 2000; Seymour, Kinn, & Sutherland, 2003; Tanner, 1999; Videbeck, 1997b). Some reviews of the literature or research on critical thinking have been published (Adams, 1999; Beck, Bennett, McLeod, & Molyneaux, 1992; Cody, 2002; Facione & Facione, 1996b; Hickman, 1993; Hicks, 2001; Jones, 1991; Oermann, 1990; Simpson & Courtney, 2002), as have a more limited number of discussions of critical thinking instruments and their use (Adams, 1996; Bondy, Koenigseder, Ishee, & Williams, 2001; Colucciello, 1997; Facione & Facione, 1994; Frye, Alfred, & Campbell, 1999; Smith-Blair & Neighbors, 2000; Stone, Davidson, Evans, & Hansen, 2001; Yeh, 2002).

Some authors have proposed models of critical thinking (Brock & Butts, 1998; Edwards, 1998; Kataoka-Yahiro & Saylor, 1994; Martin, 1996; Redding, 2001; Ulsenheimer et al., 1997; Videbeck, 1997a), but most of these have not been validated. Some publications address critical thinking generally and describe how it was measured throughout a program or an individual course (Alexander & Giguere, 1996; Beckie, Lowry, & Barnett, 2001; Beeken, Dale, Enos, & Yarbrough, 1997; Brown, Alverson, & Pepa, 2001; Carter, 2000; Celia & Gordon, 2001; Chubinski, 1996; Daly, 2001; Dexter et al., 1997; Facione & Facione, 1996a; Gottlieb, 2002; Loving & Wilson, 2000; Miller, 1992; Myrick & Yonge, 2004; Niedringhaus, 2001; Oermann, Truesdell, & Ziolkowski, 2000; O'Sullivan, Blevins-Stephens, Smith, & Vaughan-Wrobel, 1997; Profetto-McGrath, 2003; Saucier, 1995; Sedlak, 1999; Shin, Lee, Ha, & Kim, 2006; Spelic et al., 2001; Thompson & Rebeschi, 1999; Vaughan-Wrobel, O'Sullivan, & Smith, 1997).

As stated, the literature revealed a limited number of research-based articles in nursing. Those that were found are summarized in Table 3.10 which begins on page 93 at the end of this chapter. The primary purpose of these studies is to explore relationships between critical thinking and other factors such as

- bilingualism (Albert, Albert, & Radsma, 2002),
- self-concept (Beeken, 1997; Laird, 2005),

- professionalism (Brooks & Shepherd, 1992),
- learning styles (Colucciello, 1999),
- moral judgment (Ketefian, 1981),
- cognitive development (Rapps, Riegel, & Glaser, 2001),
- research utilization (Profetto-McGrath, Hesketh, Lang, & Estabrooks, 2003), and
- student engagement (Carini, Kuh, & Klein, 2006; Kuh & Klein, 2006).

Additional foci for these studies on critical thinking were (a) the relationship between teaching methods and critical thinking (Chau et al., 2001; Chen & Lin, 2003; Clarke & Lane, 2005; Clayton, 2006; Evans & Bendel, 2004; Forneis & Peden-McAlpine, 2007; Kuiper, 2005; Magnussen, Ishida, & Itano, 2000; Perciful & Nester, 1996; Phillips & Bond, 2004; Profetto-McGrath, 2003; Thompson & Rebeschi, 1999) and (b) the relationship between critical thinking and demographic variables such as age, number of years in nursing practice, level of education and grade point average (Howenstein, Bilodeau, Brogna, & Good, 1996; Ip et al., 2000; Martin, 2002; Maynard, 1996; Saarmann, Freitas, Rapps, & Reigel, 1992; Saint Clair, 1994). One study compared critical thinking between nursing students from two countries (Yeh & Chen, 2003), and several qualitative studies focusing on the development of critical thinking have been conducted (Bethune & Jackling, 1997; DiVito, 2000; Duchscher, 2003; Jones, 2004; Ladyshewsky, 2006; Myrick & Yonge, 2004; Nelms & Lane, 1999; Phillips & Bond; Sedlak, 1997; Tapper, 2004; Wallace, 1996).

A review and analysis of existing research indicates that there is no widely accepted definition of the concept of critical thinking in nursing, there has been minimal replication of studies that would allow nurse educators to generalize findings, and samples are typically small and convenient, which further limits generalization of the findings. In addition, although many methods to teach critical thinking have been proposed, sufficient research has not been conducted to support the validity of these methods in increasing critical thinking abilities/skills. In essence, research studies on teaching/learning strategies to enhance the critical thinking of nursing students are not extensive enough to provide an evidence base for nursing education practices, and more scholarly work is needed. Refer to Chapter 4 for additional discussion of critical thinking findings and the cognitive domain.

## CONCLUSION

The concept of learning has been addressed extensively over the years, but research-based literature concerning learning is lacking, especially in higher education and nursing. A number of the research-based studies that have been reported in nursing and higher education were conducted with students and contexts outside the United States, had small sample sizes, did not specify an underlying theoretical framework, and used instruments whose reliability and validity were questionable or not even reported.

Colleges and universities are increasingly investing attention and energy on issues of teaching and learning. Schools that are learner-centered focus their energies on helping all students be successful learners. Effective learners learn in very different ways, and each individual may use different learning methods depending upon the situation and the information to be learned. Research is increasingly focused on the complexity of the learning process.

Nursing education research about learning has a number of gaps. There is a lack of research studies using a holistic approach inclusive of physical, psychological, social, and spiritual aspects. There is minimal information on what the learner brings to the nursing program — knowledge base, work experience, developmental stage — and how these factors may change teaching practices. And there is very little research involving graduate nursing students, both master's and doctoral.

Several questions about nursing education and its relationship to learning need to be researched. What are the advantages and disadvantages when faculty learning styles are similar to student learning styles? What is the relationship among nursing students, learning environment, and the nursing educator? What factors constitute the "ideal" learning environment in the nursing classroom or clinical area? What kind of environment is most conducive to learning? How does technology influence the learning process?

Nursing also needs to focus attention and energy on issues of teaching and learning. In order to appropriately apply concepts from teaching and learning theories, nurse educators need to understand the theories, continue to study them, reflect upon them, and make appropriate applications in nursing education. Research needs to be conducted on learner characteristics, learning styles, learning environments, teacher/student interactions, the effect of technology on learning, and many other areas.

Research on these and other topics has the potential to improve student learning experiences and enhance students' learning. In addition, it will provide the foundation for evidence-based teaching practices that are needed to develop the science of nursing education. The future of nursing education and the overall profession of nursing depend upon the educational research conducted today and tomorrow. Learning is a complex process. Acknowledging this and responding to the need to expand the research on the overall process can help nurse educators achieve their ultimate goal: facilitating the learning success of students who are exquisitely well prepared to provide safe, quality care to diverse populations.

**Table 3.5. Summary of Research-Based Literature on Learning Styles in Nursing and Higher Education**

| Author(s) | Purpose | Sample | Measurement | Findings |
|---|---|---|---|---|
| Abu-Moghli, Khalaf, Halabi, & Wardam (2005) | To determine Jordanian nursing students' perception of their learning styles. | N=420 Jordanian nursing students | Autonomous Learner Index (ALI) | Majority perceived themselves as independent learners; low percentage indicated good study skills, ability to concentrate while studying, and using time effectively. No statistical significance between learning styles and demographic variables. |
| Anderson (1998) | To determine whether there was a difference in an orientee's perceived satisfaction with orientation, based on whether teaching style of the preceptor and the learning style of the orientee were matched. | Not reported | Myers-Briggs Type Indicator | Those orientees matched with preceptor on personality preferences of introversion or extraversion reported higher levels of satisfaction with orientation that were statistically significant. |
| Andrusyszyn, Cragg, & Humbert (2001) | To study the relationship between multiple distance delivery methods, preferred learning style, content, and achievement. | N=86 nurse practitioners | Researcher-developed questionnaire | Convenience, self-direction, and timing of the learning were more important than delivery method or learning style. Preferred order of learning was reading, discussing, observing, doing, and reflecting. |

**Table 3.5. Summary of Research-Based Literature on Learning Styles in Nursing and Higher Education (continued)**

| Author(s) | Purpose | Sample | Measurement | Findings |
|---|---|---|---|---|
| Campeau (1998) | To explore the distribution of learning styles and preferences for major learning environment characteristics in Emergency Medical Care Assistant (EMCA) students. | N=75 EMCA students | Learning Style Inventory (LSI), researcher-developed questionnaire | Accommodators liked courses with strong emphasis on practical applications and working in groups; Assimilators felt lectures and courses with strong emphasis on theory very useful; Divergers felt a lot of verbal explanation was useful; Convergers desired working with teachers who act as coaches and preferred a strong emphasis on practical applications. |
| Carnwell (2000) | To develop relationships between the need for guidance, materials design and learning styles and strategies. | N=20 "purposively selected" community nurses | Interview | Identified three approaches to studying: systematic waders, speedy focusers, and global dippers. |
| Carpio et al. (1999) | To identify and compare the learning styles of nursing faculty and entry students in two self-directed, problem-based nursing programs. | N=94 generic students, N= 63 post-RN students, and N=22 faculty at a Canadian university; and N=37 incoming nursing students and N=13 faculty at a Chilean university | LSI – English and Spanish versions | Significant difference between the three student groups in active experimentation learning mode; Chilean students were less likely to be active learners; Canadian faculty had higher abstract conceptualization scores than Chilean faculty. |

**Table 3.5. Summary of Research-Based Literature on Learning Styles in Nursing and Higher Education (continued)**

| Author(s) | Purpose | Sample | Measurement | Findings |
|---|---|---|---|---|
| Chen & Lee (2000) | To explore the effects of learning style of students and their faculty on students' academic achievement and teaching satisfaction. | N=201 nursing students and N=24 faculty | LSI and researcher-developed questionnaire | Majority of students were Concrete styles while faculty were Abstract styles; instructors who were Convergers gave significantly higher grades to students than Assimilators; instructors who were Accommodators were much better appreciated by students; no significant difference in academic achievement when the learning styles of students and teachers were matched. |
| Coker (2000) | To examine learning styles of undergraduate athletic training students to determine their consistency in traditional classroom versus clinical settings. | N=26 undergraduate athletic students | LSI | Significant difference between Reflective Observation and Active Experimentation modes across the settings. Fifty-eight percent of the respondents' learning styles changed according to the learning setting. |

**Table 3.5. Summary of Research-Based Literature on Learning Styles in Nursing and Higher Education (continued)**

| Author(s) | Purpose | Sample | Measurement | Findings |
|---|---|---|---|---|
| Cope & Staehr (2005) | To investigate the impact of interventions on student learning approaches. | N=59 students in higher education | Approaches to Studying Questionnaire | Gradual increase in the workload on the subjects annually allowed students to apply deep learning approaches. |
| Diaz & Cartnal (1999) | To compare social learning styles of distance education students with on-campus students. | N=40 distance and N=63 on-campus students in health education classes | Grasha-Reichmann Student Learning Style Scales | Distant students favor independent study while on-campus students were slightly more dependent and collaborative in learning style. |
| DiBartola, Miller, & Turley (2001) | To compare learning outcomes of students with different learning styles in traditional classrooms versus distance education. | Two classes taking same course – one traditional and one distance | LSI and grades | Students in Diverger group demonstrated above average scores in the distance group; learning environment did not influence learning outcome; learning style did not influence learning outcome. |
| Evans & Waring (2006) | To examine the relationship between cognitive style, learning preference, and perceived impact on teaching practices. | N=80 undergraduate education students | Cognitive Styles Analysis; Approaches and Study Skills Inventory for Students (ASSIST); Approaches to Learning; and Preferred Mode of Delivery | Significant difference between three cognitive styles and learning preferences, Wholists being most concerned with speed of delivery and least liking of computer assisted learning. Wholists also preferred less structure and claimed to use more images. |

**Table 3.5. Summary of Research-Based Literature on Learning Styles in Nursing and Higher Education (continued)**

| Author(s) | Purpose | Sample | Measurement | Findings |
|---|---|---|---|---|
| Freeman, Fell, & Muellenberg (1998) | To compare two learning styles — reflective observations versus active experimentation — in terms of learning outcomes. | N=40 clinical laboratory science students | LSI, exam scores | No significant difference between students' examination scores based on learning style; no significant difference in the pattern of exam scores over the semester of learners who were Active Experimentators versus Reflective Observers. |
| Freeman & Tijerina (2000) | To determine allied health students' learning outcomes based upon learner characteristics. | Two classes of physician assistant students | LSI and grades | No relationship between students' learning style and the method of delivery on learning outcomes in the traditional versus online environment. |
| Fritz, Speth, Barbuto, & Boren (2004) | To explore the relationship between learning styles and motivation. | N=103 undergraduate and graduate students | Approaches to Studying Inventory and Motivation Sources Inventory | Significant positive relationship between Surface apathetic approach and Self-concept internal motivation; negative relationship between Surface apathetic approach and Self-concept external motivation; negative relationship between Strategic approach and Self-concept internal motivation. |

**Table 3.5. Summary of Research-Based Literature on Learning Styles in Nursing and Higher Education (continued)**

| Author(s) | Purpose | Sample | Measurement | Findings |
|---|---|---|---|---|
| Harrelson, Leaver-Dunn, & Wright (1998) | To assess the learning styles of undergraduate athletic training students. | N=27 first-year and second-year students | Productivity Environmental Preference Survey | Significant differences in learning preferences between males and females; significant differences between first- and second-year students in their preferences for afternoon learning activities. |
| Hativa & Birenbaum (2000) | To examine the relationship between students' approaches to learning with teaching approaches and discipline. | N=175 engineering and education students in Israel | Motivated Learning Strategies Questionnaire (MLSQ) | Most favored teaching approach was the lecturer who is organized, clear, and interesting. Students preferred teaching approaches that served their learning approaches. No statistically significant differences between disciplines. |
| Heath (2000) | To examine critical thinking abilities, critical thinking dispositions, and preferred learning styles of nursing students throughout a program. | N=71 BSN nursing students | California Critical Thinking Skills Test (CCTST), CCTDI, Watson-Glaser Critical Thinking Appraisal (WGCTA), and Productivity Environmental Preference Survey (PEPS) | No significant growth in CT from entry to exit in program; learning style preferences were most important when learning new or difficult information; as students developed organizational abilities, the need for structure within the learning setting diminished. |
| Hendry et al. (2005) | To investigate the effects of learning styles on self-efficacy, group work, group climate, and assessment performance. | N=24 medical students and N=3 dental students | Learning Style Questionnaire (LSQ) | Workshop training on learning styles had no effect. Students did report greater self-awareness of their own learning and acceptance of others' styles. |

**Table 3.5. Summary of Research-Based Literature on Learning Styles in Nursing and Higher Education (continued)**

| Author(s) | Purpose | Sample | Measurement | Findings |
|---|---|---|---|---|
| Hoisington (2000) | To determine whether there is a relationship between learning styles, computer/Internet experience, age, and comfort using the Internet/WWW. | N=41 ADN students | Quantitative and qualitative: Canfield Learning Style Inventory, Gregorc Style Delineation, researcher-developed comfort scale | No statistical significance between comfort level and learning style; statistically significant relationship between comfort and experience using the Internet and computers; no statistical relationship between students' comfort and age. |
| Honigsfeld & Schiering (2004) | To determine the relationship between learning style preference and implications for teaching style. | N=123 education students | Productivity Environmental Preference Survey (PEPS), Building Excellence Survey and open-ended questionnaire | Majority of participants preferred Verbal kinesthetic learning style with Auditory as the least preferred; late afternoon least preferred time to learn; results indicated a need for guidance, mentoring, and frequent feedback during the learning process that also allows creativity and individual problem-solving opportunities; teaching style was related to the preferred learning style. |

**Table 3.5. Summary of Research-Based Literature on Learning Styles in Nursing and Higher Education (continued)**

| Author(s) | Purpose | Sample | Measurement | Findings |
|---|---|---|---|---|
| Howard, Hayes, Solomonides, & Swannell (2001) | To identify the approaches to studying preferred by nursing students and whether these changed during their education. | N=40 Cohort 1; N=76 Cohort 2 – United Kingdom nursing students | Revised Approaches to Studying Inventory (RASI) | Correlation between age and the deep approach to studying; student nurses changed their approach to studying to favor the deep approach; students who favored deep approach attained higher assessment grades. |
| Jie & Xiaoqing (2006) | To assess the relationship between learning styles and language learning strategies. | N=187 second year students | Myers-Briggs Type Indicator (Chinese); author-developed questionnaire | Significant influence of learning styles on learning strategy choices. High achievers more capable of exercising strategies that are associated with their nonpreferred learning strategies. |
| Linares (1999) | To determine if students and faculty in nursing and allied health demonstrate a predominant learning style and if there is an association between a specific learning style and self-directed learning readiness or prediction of academic success; also to determine whether a discipline-specific learning style could be identified. | N=301 generic BSN students, N=188 RN-BSN students; N=110 allied health students; and N=10 nursing faculty | Self-Directed Learning Readiness Scale; Learning Style Questionnaire (LSQ) | No significant difference in learning styles between students and faculty; Converger style was the predominant style for all subjects; Convergers were significantly more self-directed than either the Accommodators, Assimilators, or Divergers; academic success could not be predicted on the basis of learning style or self-direction. |

**Table 3.5. Summary of Research-Based Literature on Learning Styles in Nursing and Higher Education (continued)**

| Author(s) | Purpose | Sample | Measurement | Findings |
|---|---|---|---|---|
| Lindblom-Ylanne (2004) | To explore students' approaches to learning. | N=11 law students | Reflections on Learning Inventory (RoLI) | RoLI functioned very well as a diagnostic tool in studying counseling; assisted students in becoming aware of approaches to studying, and enabled students to develop more efficient and functional study practices. |
| Martin, Stark, & Jolly (2000) | To assess the relationship between clinical experience, learning style, and performance in an objective structured clinical examination (OSCE) in medical students at the end of their first clinical year. | N=194 medical students | OSCE, Entwhistle Learning Style Inventory, self-reported score of clinical activity | Performance on OSCE was related to well-organized study methods but not to clinical experience; significant relationship between clinical experience and organized deep-learning styles. |
| May (2000) | To explore the relationships among basic empathy, self-awareness, and learning styles of BSN pre-nursing students. | N=380 BSN pre-nursing students | Hogan Empathy Scale (HES), Emotional Empathic Tendency Scale (EETS), revised Private Self-Consciousness subscale, the revised Public Self-Consciousness subscale, LSQ | Students who were less theoretical and pragmatic in their learning styles had higher levels of basic empathy. |

**Table 3.5. Summary of Research-Based Literature on Learning Styles in Nursing and Higher Education (continued)**

| Author(s) | Purpose | Sample | Measurement | Findings |
|---|---|---|---|---|
| McColgin (2000) | To examine the effects of matching learning styles to teaching methods on students' academic performance, amount of perceived learning, and course evaluations. | N=77 first-year nursing students | Grasha-Reichmann Student Learning Style Scale, GPA, final course grade, and Student Instructional Report II | Best predictors of student's final course grade were previous academic performance and type of teaching methodology; the best predictor of perceived learning was the perceived degree of student effort put into the coursework; best predictors of the course evaluation were the degree of student effort, the type of teaching methodology and the match between learning styles and teaching methods. |
| McDade (1999) | To determine the relationship of critical thinking to learning styles. | Nursing, veterinary medicine and dental students | CCTDI; Hanson-Silver Learning Style Inventory for Adults | Positive correlation between intuition-thinking learning style and the total critical thinking disposition score for the entire sample; positive correlation between inquisitiveness and truth-seeking disposition and the intuition-thinking learning style in entire sample; no correlations between demographic variables of age, gender, GPA, previous work experience, learning style, or critical thinking ability. |

**Table 3.5. Summary of Research-Based Literature on Learning Styles in Nursing and Higher Education (continued)**

| Author(s) | Purpose | Sample | Measurement | Findings |
|---|---|---|---|---|
| McLaughlin (2001) | To identify the learning styles of nursing students taking web-based courses and to determine the relationship between perceived course delivery satisfaction and learning style | N=21 graduate nursing students, convenience sample | McCarthy's Learning Type Measure, Course Delivery Satisfaction Questionnaire | No statistically significant correlations between learning style and course delivery satisfaction |
| Miller (1998) | To investigate the effects of the instructional resource Programmed Learning Sequence (PLS) on the achievement and attitudes of college students and their learning styles | Two classes | Semantic Differential Scale; Productivity Environmental Preference Survey; class exams | Exam scores were significantly higher using the PLS rather than traditional method of teaching; significant correlations between learning-style elements and achievement: more quiet environment for book learning, more light for the computer PLS and traditional teaching versus the book PLS; preferred learning with an authority figure who favored the traditional method. |
| Morton-Rias et al. (2007) | To compare student learning styles using two different assessments addressing demographic variables. | N=154 graduate and undergraduate allied health students | Building Excellence (BE); Productivity Environmental Preference Survey (PEPS) | Significant relationship between students' learning style elements — sound, light, temperature, seating design, intake, time-of-day — and mobility, auditory, tactile, and kinesthetic preferences. Gender specific and age-related differences noted in preferences. |

**Table 3.5. Summary of Research-Based Literature on Learning Styles in Nursing and Higher Education (continued)**

| Author(s) | Purpose | Sample | Measurement | Findings |
|---|---|---|---|---|
| Mupinga, Nora, & Yaw (2006) | To determine the learning styles, expectations, and needs of online students. | N=131 industrial education on-line students | Myers-Briggs Cognitive Style Inventory; author-developed questionnaire | Most prominent learning style — introvert, senser, thinker, judger (ISTJ). Three primary expectations — communication with the professor, instructor feedback, and challenging online course. Primary needs were technical support, guidance with sample assignments, similarity in platforms used, and additional reference material. |
| Olson & Scanlan (2002) | To test the relationship between learning style and preference for teaching methods. | N=190 physical therapy students in master's programs | Gregorc Style Delineator, Teaching Methods Scale and Instructional Activities Scale | Weak positive correlations between concrete-sequential learning styles and media-based learning; weak correlation between concrete-random learning style and traditional learning; concrete-random learners had higher self-directed scores while concrete-sequential learners had higher structured teaching scores; high proportion of dual style learners. |

**Table 3.5. Summary of Research-Based Literature on Learning Styles in Nursing and Higher Education (continued)**

| Author(s) | Purpose | Sample | Measurement | Findings |
|---|---|---|---|---|
| **Reese & Dunn (2007)** | To examine the extent of diversity of learning styles, influence of gender on learning style, and whether grade point average (GPA) determines academic success. | N=1500 entering freshmen | PEPS | Statistical differences among students' styles for sound, light, temperature, motivation, and responsibility. Students with higher GPAs preferred learning alone with an authoritative figure in the late morning or early afternoon. Students with lowest GPAs preferred learning in the evening with sound, bright lights. Significant difference noted in gender preferences for learning. |
| **Ross, Drysdale, & Schulz (1999)** | To investigate the effects of cognitive learning style on academic performance in a first-year kinesiology class. | N=99 students over a four-year period | Gregorc Style Delineator | Academic performance based on dominant and least dominant learning style was found to be significant; dominant sequential learners performed significantly better than did dominant random learners. |
| **Sandmire, Vroman, & Sanders (2000)** | To identify factors that influence interdisciplinary teams. | N=78 occupational and physical therapy students | LSI, watching a video and completing a collaborative exercise | No significant difference between learning style subset pairs in performance. Background knowledge predicted performance more than learning styles did. |

**Table 3.5. Summary of Research-Based Literature on Learning Styles in Nursing and Higher Education (continued)**

| Author(s) | Purpose | Sample | Measurement | Findings |
|---|---|---|---|---|
| Snelgrove & Slater (2003) | To establish the validity of an Approaches to Learning Questionnaire | N=300 nursing students | Approaches to Learning Questionnaire | Questionnaire found to be valid — measures deep, surface, and achievement subscales. Deep learning appears to influence academic performance. |
| Thompson & Bing-You (1998) | To discover what the experience of physicians taking inventories, the relationship of the inventories to daily performance, and what behavioral changes were experienced. | N=9 physicians | LSI; MBTI; Hemispheric Mode Indicator (HMI); semi-structured interview | Physicians thought the inventories were "fun to take," were applicable to patient care and education, practice management, and administration, and medical education |
| Titiloye & Scott (2001) | To identify occupational therapy students' learning styles | N=201 junior level students | LSI | High percentage of Convergers (35%) and Assimilators (25%) |
| Vincent & Ross (2001) | To assist business educators in determining learning styles of students. | N=177 business computer students | Center for New Discoveries online and LSI | Learning styles were primarily auditory, many students have equal preference for styles. Authors made suggestions on how to create/implement instructional strategies to enhance student learning based upon style. |

**Table 3.5. Summary of Research-Based Literature on Learning Styles in Nursing and Higher Education (continued)**

| Author(s) | Purpose | Sample | Measurement | Findings |
|---|---|---|---|---|
| Ward (2003) | To determine whether optimistic attributions are more frequently associated with students at Christian universities vs. state-supported colleges (motivation, problem-solving, emotional well-being, and physical health). | N=100 college students | Academic Attributional Style Questionnaire; Coping with Academic Failures Questionnaire | Significant differences were noted between the groups — the students at the Christian college tended toward explanations for negative events that were external, unstable, and specific; state-supported college students had explanations for negative events that were internal, stable, and global. Students at the Christian university were statistically more optimistic than the state-supported students |
| Wessel, Loomis, Rennie, Brook, Hoddinott, & Aherne (1999) | To determine the learning styles and problem-solving ability of physiotherapy students. | N=158 students from 2 to 4 years in baccalaureate program | LSI, Heppner Problem Solving Inventory (PSI) | Majority of students were Assimilator or Converger; PSI not related to learning style; no significant difference in PSI and LSI between years. |

**Table 3.6. Summary of Research-Based Literature on Learning Environments in Nursing and Higher Education**

| Author(s) | Purpose | Sample | Measurement | Findings |
|---|---|---|---|---|
| Ausburn (2004) | To describe the design elements most desired by adult learners. | N=67 adult learners in college education classes | Assessing the Learning Strategies of Adults (ATLAS) and author-developed questionnaire | Adults value course designs that contain options, personalization, self-direction, variety, and a learning community. Also identified difference in learning emphasis by gender, preferred learning strategies, and previous experiences with technology and self-directed learning. |
| Barker & Garvin-Doxas (2004) | To provide a deeper understanding of the learning environment of a selection of computer classrooms. | N=37 computer students | Ethnographic research | Categories that emerged: impersonal environment and guarded behavior and the creation and maintenance of an informal hierarchy, which resulted in competitive behaviors. |
| Bruyn (2004) | To assess the relationship between the use of asynchronous computer-mediated communication and the degree of convergence and level of social presence. | N=55 student postings in a land evaluation course | Content analysis of online postings in WebCT | The level of social presence and degree of convergence was limited and unequal between students and of varying quality. |
| Cope & Staehr (2005) | To investigate the impact of interventions on student learning approaches. | N=59 students in higher education | Approaches to Studying Questionnaire | Gradual increase in the workload on the subjects annually allowed students to apply deep learning approaches. |

**Table 3.6. Summary of Research-Based Literature on Learning Environments in Nursing and Higher Education (continued)**

| Author(s) | Purpose | Sample | Measurement | Findings |
|---|---|---|---|---|
| **France, Fields, & Garth (2004)** | To explore the lived experience of black nursing students in a predominantly white university in a rural southeastern community. | N=4 BSN nursing students | Open-ended questionnaire and interviewing | Results demonstrated an environment not conducive to learning due to lack of relationships, collegiality, and support among classmates, and poor understanding by the participants on how to navigate the educational system. |
| **Lightfoot (2006)** | To investigate the amount of thought students put into e-mail communication vs. traditional face-to-face communication. | N=596 undergraduate business students | Author-developed survey | Students put significantly more thought into e-mail communication with both the instructor and groups of peers than they do with equivalent face-to-face communication; put the same amount of thought into e-mail compared to verbal communication with individual peers. |
| **Masui & De Corte (2005)** | To examine the relationship between reflection and attribution with self-regulated learning. | N=141 business economic students | Training sessions with interviews | Experimental groups demonstrated a higher degree of reflective behavior and their attribution skills were also measurably improved. |

**Table 3.6. Summary of Research-Based Literature on Learning Environments in Nursing and Higher Education (continued)**

| Author(s) | Purpose | Sample | Measurement | Findings |
|---|---|---|---|---|
| Nganasurian (1999) | To identify factors making a positive contribution to learning within mental health care settings. | N=146 student in Phase I; N=51 mental health nursing students in Phase II – United Kingdom nursing students | Researcher-designed questionnaire | Students identified the following factors as contributing to learning: practice; for staff who teach in the clinical settings to have time to spend on 1:1 activity; provide feedback after any activity; good teamwork or integration of the learner into the team; wide variety of client problems to learn from; and a definite link between theory and practice. |
| Nijhuis, Segers, & Gijselaers (2007) | To determine the relationship between perceptions of the learning environment, personality, and learning strategies. | N=522 international business students | Not specified | Four path analyses determined: (1) conscientiousness and openness to experience are related to learning strategies; (2) perceptions of the various elements of learning environment influences learning strategies; (3) personality traits are only slightly related to perceptions of learning environment; (4) there are both direct and indirect relationships between conscientiousness, openness to experience, and learning strategies. |

**Table 3.6. Summary of Research-Based Literature on Learning Environments in Nursing and Higher Education (continued)**

| Author(s) | Purpose | Sample | Measurement | Findings |
|---|---|---|---|---|
| Rovai, Ponton, Derrick, & Davis (2006) | To compare virtual vs. traditional classrooms. | N=202 undergraduate education students | Open-ended questionnaire | Online courses received more praise and more negative comments. Findings suggest that the online course delivery medium caused misalignment for some students between their preferred learning environment and the actual learning environment. |
| Schelfhout, Dochy, & Janssens (2004) | To assess ways that a learning enterprise can best be supported in order to constitute a powerful learning environment. | N=23 business students | Author-developed questionnaire | Results indicated that the teacher-coach approach creates the most powerful learning environment. |
| Scheyvens, Wild, & Overton (2003) | To determine ways that geographers can support the learning needs of international postgraduate scholarship students in Western universities. | N=88 geography students | Focus-group interviews | Academic success is strongly related to the personal well-being of students. |
| Shea, Li, & Pickett (2006) | To determine the relationship between teaching presence and the development of the learning community in online environments. | N=1067 education students | The Teaching Presence Scale | Significant relationship between students' sense of a learning community and effective instructional design and directed facilitation of learning. |

**Table 3.6. Summary of Research-Based Literature on Learning Environments in Nursing and Higher Education (continued)**

| Author(s) | Purpose | Sample | Measurement | Findings |
|---|---|---|---|---|
| **Snelgrove & Slater (2003)** | To establish validity of an approaches to learning questionnaire. | N=300 nursing students | Approaches to Learning Questionnaire | The process questionnaire is a valid and useful tool for nurse teachers to gain knowledge about student nurses' approach to learning. Deep learning appears to influence academic performance. |
| **Speziale & Jacobson (2005)** | To identify how the practices, methodologies, and strategies used in RN nurse education programs changed in the previous five years and were expected to change in the next five years | N=600 (approximately) nursing faculty | Author-developed questionnaire with 187 items defined | Need to develop a high quality, diverse nursing workforce for the future; technology will continue to be a recurring theme; need for faculty to develop more active learning environments. |
| **Vaatstra & Vries (2007)** | To determine whether graduates from activating learning environments assess themselves as having more generic and reflective competences than graduates from conventional learning environments. | N=1200 higher education graduates in Europe and Japan | Data from project CHEERS, which assessed higher education graduates and employment | Activating environment graduates attribute more generic and reflective competences than conventional graduates; quality of content and curriculum design is significantly related to the presence of generic and reflective competences. |

**Table 3.6. Summary of Research-Based Literature on Learning Environments in Nursing and Higher Education (continued)**

| Author(s) | Purpose | Sample | Measurement | Findings |
|-----------|---------|--------|-------------|----------|
| Wanstreet (2006) | To review the literature related to articles on learning environments. | N=125 articles | Various databases | Identified several "topics": learner-learner interactions; learner-instructor interactions; learner-content interactions; learner-interface interaction; computer-mediated communication; and social/psychological connections. |
| Wong & Chung (2002) | To explore the diagnostic reasoning process among nursing students who learned in different institutional contexts — e.g., university vs. hospital-based setting. | N=20 nursing students | Biggs Study Process Questionnaire | No significant differences in the students' ability to formulate diagnoses. Significant difference in reasoning patterns — university students used data-driven strategies while hospital-based students used hypothesis-driven strategies. |

**Table 3.7. Summary of Research-Based Literature on Technology and Learning in Nursing and Higher Education**

| Author(s) | Purpose | Sample | Measurement | Findings |
|---|---|---|---|---|
| **Arthur, Pang, & Wong (2001)** | To measure the degree of technology influence on caring attributes. | N=1957 nurses working in 11 countries | Global Caring Scale, Technology Influence Scale | The higher the influence of technology, the higher the caring score (p<0.001) — especially caring communication and involvement; Lowest technology group recorded the highest caring advocacy scores (p<0.001). |
| **Atack & Rankin (2002)** | To describe the experience of nurses in a web-based course. | N=57 RNs | Online Learner Support Instrument | Significant gains in learning with e-mail, Internet, keyboarding and word processing skills. |
| **Edwards (2005)** | To examine the relationship between the use of technology and outcomes in computer-mediated courses. | N=49 nursing students | Author-developed questionnaires/ interviews and the Motivated Strategies for Learning Questionnaire | Measures of satisfaction with online learning experiences are not related to any other variables in the study. The tools developed and used can be applied across the curriculum to enhance evaluation of learning and program effectiveness. |
| **Elfrink et al. (2000)** | To describe the use of the Nightingale Tracker (NT) in clinical education. | N=44 students from five nursing schools | Nightingale Tracker Interface Questionnaire; researcher-developed user profile | Significant change over time in reaction to the NT; no other significant differences with respect to other variables. |

**Table 3.7. Summary of Research-Based Literature on Technology and Learning in Nursing and Higher Education (continued)**

| Author(s) | Purpose | Sample | Measurement | Findings |
|---|---|---|---|---|
| Jeffries, Woolf, & Linde (2003) | To compare the effectiveness of an interactive, multimedia CD-ROM with traditional methods of teaching the skills of performing a 12-lead ECG. | N=77 BSN students | Researcher-developed questionnaires; pretests and posttests | No significant differences between traditional group and technology group in pretest and posttest scores, satisfaction with learning method or perception of self-efficacy in performing the skill. |
| Kenny (2002) | To explore the experiences of nursing students with online learning. | N=21 students | Qualitative questionnaire and interviews | Four major themes emerged: computer confidence, flexibility, active learning, and practicalities of teaching. Computer confidence was felt to both enhance and detract from student learning. |
| Klaassens (1992) | To determine if inter-active video (IVD) simulations provide adequate practice in problem-solving skills. | Four IVD simulations used by BSN programs | Researcher-developed questionnaire based on discrete cognitive subcomponents of the nursing process | Three of the four IVDs contained adequate percentages of the steps of the nursing process and were rated adequate for the practice of problem solving. |
| Leasure, Davis, & Thievon (2000) | To compare student outcomes in an undergraduate research course taught using both web-based distance learning technology and traditional pedagogy. | Two classes | Multiple choice grades on course exams | No significant difference on exam scores; students who were self-directed were best suited for web-based courses; these students also reported increased confidence with the computer, and writing skills improved. |

**Table 3.7. Summary of Research-Based Literature on Technology and Learning in Nursing and Higher Education (continued)**

| Author(s) | Purpose | Sample | Measurement | Findings |
|---|---|---|---|---|
| MacIntosh (2001) | To understand the influences of interactive videoconferencing technology on learning experiences via interactive distance education. | One class of BSN nursing students | Phenomenological questionnaire, interview, and focus groups | Themes identified: connecting with others, organization, negative influences, and personal factors as influential to learning |
| Weston (2005) | To examine the experiences of instructors attempting to integrate an innovative software application in their classes. | N=13 instructors of anatomy | Structured and informal interviews | Results discuss how technology was used, motivation for using technology, and obstacles for use of technology. |

**Table 3.8. Summary of Research-Based Literature on Thinking Styles of Teachers in Higher Education**

| Author(s) | Purpose | Sample | Measurement | Findings |
|---|---|---|---|---|
| **Evans & Waring (2006)** | To examine the relationship between students' cognitive style, learning preference, and perceived impact on teaching practices. | N=80 undergraduate education students | Cognitive Styles Analysis; Approaches and Study Skills Inventory for Students (ASSIST); Approaches to Learning; and Preferred Mode of Delivery | Significant difference between three cognitive styles and learning preferences, Wholists being most concerned with speed of delivery and least liking of computer assisted learning. Wholists preferred less structure and claimed to use more images. |
| **Zhang (2001)** | To examine the relationship between teaching approaches and thinking styles. | N=67 in-service teachers | Approaches to Teaching Inventory and Thinking Styles Inventory in Teaching | Thinking styles in teaching and approaches to teaching appear to have an overlapping conceptual role. |
| **Zhang (2004)** | To investigate the role of thinking styles in students' preferences for teaching styles and their conceptions of effective teachers. | N=255 students working toward degrees in education | Thinking Styles Inventory—Revised; Preferred Thinking Styles in Teaching Inventory; Effective Teacher Inventory | Particular thinking styles predispose students to a particular teaching style; students were open to more teaching styles than those that matched their thinking styles; thinking styles made a difference in their conception of effective teachers. |
| **Zhang & Sternberg (2002)** | To investigate the relationship between thinking styles and teachers' characteristics. | N=193 in-service teachers | Thinking Styles Questionnaire for Teachers | Seven teacher characteristics were significantly related to thinking styles: gender; professional work experience outside school settings; the degree of enjoying adoption of new teaching materials; tendency for using group projects; perceived autonomy for determining teaching content; and the rating of the quality of their students. |

**Table 3.9. Summary of Research-Based Literature on Teaching Styles of Teachers in Nursing and Higher Education**

| Author(s) | Purpose | Sample | Measurement | Findings |
|---|---|---|---|---|
| Evans (2004) | To explore the relationship between cognitive styles and teaching style. | N=59 trainee teachers in postgraduate certification program | Cognitive Styles Analysis (CSA), Teaching Styles Questionnaire (TSQ), and structured interviews | Significant relationship between TSQ and verbalizer-imager score on the CSA — verbalizers are more likely to teach in a more analytic way; older students adopted a more intuitive approach in the classroom; males more intuitive in teaching styles than females; age and gender were found to be influential in affecting teaching style in relation to the subject taught. |
| Hativa & Birenbaum (2000) | To examine the relationship between students' approaches to learning with teaching approaches and discipline. | N=175 engineering and education students in Israel | Motivated Learning Strategies Questionnaire (MLSQ) | Most favored teaching approach was the lecturer who is organized, clear, and interesting. Students preferred teaching approaches that served their learning approaches. No statistically significant differences between disciplines. |
| Kreber (2005) | To explore concept of reflection and its relationship to teaching. | N=36 science teachers in Canada | Semistructured interviews, Approaches to Teaching Inventory (ATI) | Concrete indicators of reflection were identified; years of experience and beliefs about teaching may play a role in the extent to which faculty are inclined to engage in reflection. |

**Table 3.9. Summary of Research-Based Literature on Teaching Styles of Teachers in Nursing and Higher Education (continued)**

| Author(s) | Purpose | Sample | Measurement | Findings |
|---|---|---|---|---|
| Lindblom-Ylanne, Trigwell, Nevgi, & Ashwin (2006) | To analyze how academic discipline is related to approaches to teaching and to explore the effects of teaching context on approaches to teaching. | N=340 teachers from a variety of disciplines in Finland and the United Kingdom | Approaches to Teaching Inventory | Teachers in "hard sciences" scored significantly higher in the information transfer/teacher-focused approaches (ITTF); teachers in "soft sciences" scored significantly higher in the conceptual change/student-focused approach (CCSF); overall variation in student- and teacher-focused approaches across disciplines and across teaching contexts. |
| Miley & Gonsalves (2003, 2005) | To explore the students' perception of annoying teaching habits. | N=85 family studies and N=789 psychology undergraduate students | 3 x 5 card with one of three questions: most annoying habits of professors vs. one thing that inhibited your learning vs. 2-3 pet peeves about professor's teaching | Faculty disorganization in class presentations and course goals was the top annoying habit. Other habits mentioned: talking too fast, speaking in a monotone, and degrading or talking to students in a condescending way. |
| Schaefer & Zygmont (2003) | To describe the predominant teaching style of a group of nursing faculty and to compare teaching style to the instructional methods used. | N=187 BSN nursing faculty | Principles of Adult Learning Scale and a demographic questionnaire | Significant positive relationship between ability to be flexible and years of clinical practice; significant negative relationship between consistency and Climate Building, Participation in the Learning Process, and Relating to Experience. Participants were more teacher-centered than student-centered even though student-centered language was used. |

**Table 3.9. Summary of Research-Based Literature on Teaching Styles of Teachers in Nursing and Higher Education (continued)**

| Author(s) | Purpose | Sample | Measurement | Findings |
|-----------|---------|--------|-------------|----------|
| Stes, Gijbels, & Petegem (2008) | To explore the relationship between teachers' approaches to teaching and teacher characteristics. | N=50 teaching staff in Belgium | Approaches to Teaching Inventory and demographic questionnaire | No relationship between teachers' approaches to learning, context variables, teaching discipline, and number of students in the classroom. No relationship between teachers' conceptual approach and teacher characteristics of gender, academic status, teaching experience, age, or intention to participate in teacher training. |
| Yacapsin & Stick (2007) | To examine the relationship between an instructor's leadership type and preferred teaching style. | N=100 graduate teacher education instructors | Kaleidoscope Profile for Educators | Significant relationship between leadership type and teaching style. |

**Table 3.10. Summary of Research-Based Literature on Critical Thinking in Nursing and Higher Education**

| Author(s) | Purpose | Sample | Measurement | Findings |
|---|---|---|---|---|
| **Albert, Albert, & Radsma (2002)** | To study the relationship between bilingualism and critical thinking. | N=111 BSN nursing students | French language Cloze Test (C-test); English language C-test; California Critical Thinking Skills Test (CCTST) and California Critical Thinking Disposition Inventory (CCTDI) | No significant relationship between bilingualism and critical thinking ability or critical thinking disposition. Sufficient evidence to support the existence of a curvilinear relationship between bilingualism and critical thinking disposition. |
| **Beeken (1997)** | To determine if there was a relationship between self-concept and critical thinking in staff nurses. To identify if these characteristics influenced practice. | N=35 nurse managers and N=100 staff nurses | CCTST and Tennessee Self-Concept Scale (TSCS) | A positive correlation between critical thinking and self-concept that was not statistically significant. Significantly higher critical thinking scores of BSN-prepared nurses. No statistical significance regarding self-concept. |
| **Bethune & Jackling (1997)** | To explore students' perceptions of change in their critical thinking skills during the course of postgraduate study. | N=44 nursing students — designated either as students with prior university experience or those without | Researcher-developed questionnaire | For most critical thinking areas, students perceived an overall positive shift in their ability. No difference between groups in their perception of change in skill ability overall For four specific skills, there was a notable difference between the two groups of students: researching topics, thinking through factors in unit materials, communicating ideas coherently, and relating nursing knowledge to practice. |

**Table 3.10. Summary of Research-Based Literature on Critical Thinking in Nursing and Higher Education (continued)**

| Author(s) | Purpose | Sample | Measurement | Findings |
|---|---|---|---|---|
| Brooks & Shepherd (1992) | To investigate the relationship between professionalism and critical thinking abilities. | N=200 students — 50 from diploma, ADN, BSN, and RN-BSN programs, respectively | Watson-Glaser Critical Thinking Appraisal (WGCTA); Health Care Professional Attitude Inventory | Significant, low positive correlation between professionalism and critical thinking in all programs; significant low to moderate correlations between critical thinking and age and professionalism with upper division seniors; significant differences in critical thinking between BSN/RN-BSN students vs. diploma/ADN students. |
| Carini, Kuh, & Klein (2006) | To determine the relationship between student engagement and learning. | N=1058 undergraduate students | National Survey of Student Engagement (NSSE); RAND test; Graduate Record Exam | The lowest ability students benefit more from engagement than their classmates; first-year students vs. seniors convert different forms of engagement into academic achievement, and certain institutions more effectively convert student engagement into performance on critical thinking tests. |
| Chau et al. (2001) | To determine the effects of using videotaped vignettes in promoting nursing students' critical thinking abilities in managing different clinical situations. | N=83 Hong Kong nursing students | Pretest and posttest on critical thinking skills as well as nursing knowledge from specific tests to vignette | No significant difference between pretest scores and posttest scores. |

**Table 3.10. Summary of Research-Based Literature on Critical Thinking in Nursing and Higher Education (continued)**

| Author(s) | Purpose | Sample | Measurement | Findings |
|---|---|---|---|---|
| **Chen & Lin (2003)** | To explore the effect of critical reading/writing assignments on promoting critical thinking. | N=170 two-year nursing students — some control and some experimental | Article critique test before and after course — researcher developed | Significant change in all groups between pretest and posttest scores. Significant difference between students in experimental versus control group. Changes in thinking pattern, learning attitude, and perception of growth and achievement in concept analysis |
| **Clarke & Lane (2005)** | To investigate the effectiveness of providing tutorial support for education students in core modules. | N=51 nursing students in the United Kingdom | Grades in research group vs. control group | Critical thinking skills were improved in all groups, but more significant improvements were noted in research group. Additional tutorial support provided students with opportunities for meaningful engagement with the subject matter, their peers, and the lecturer. |
| **Clayton (2006)** | To examine empirical studies on the use of concept maps. | N=7 research studies | Secondary analysis of literature | Concept mapping results in generally positive effects on academic performance, improves students' critical thinking abilities, and serves as an appropriate teaching method. |
| **Colucciello (1999)** | To determine the relationship between critical thinking dispositions and learning styles. | N=100 BSN nursing students — two groups; convenience sample | CCTDI and Kolb's Learning Style Inventory | Indicated a relationship between specific components of critical thinking dispositions and learning modes. |

**Table 3.10.** *Summary of Research-Based Literature on Critical Thinking in Nursing and Higher Education (continued)*

| Author(s) | Purpose | Sample | Measurement | Findings |
|---|---|---|---|---|
| **DiVito (2000)** | To identify critical thinking behaviors in clinical judgments. | Not stated | Not specified | Provides insights into specific objective criteria of critical thinking behaviors of domain-specific knowledge, critical reflection, critical thinking competency, intellectual virtues, and action involvement. |
| **Duchscher (2003)** | To explore the development of thinking. | N=5 newly graduated BSN RNs | Observation during first 6 months of practice — researcher developed | Provides insights into knowledge development over time, offering insights into the role of undergraduate education in teaching, and fostering critical thinking. |
| **Evans & Bendel (2004)** | To examine the effect of Narrative Pedagogy in nursing education on students' ability to move toward cognitive and ethical maturity, thereby increasing autonomy in nursing practice. | N=566 nursing students; six separate classes | Measure of Intellectual Development; CCTDI | Minor improvements in cognitive and ethical maturity and the disposition to think critically in the intervention group; no significant differences. |
| **Forneis & Peden-McAlpine (2007)** | To determine if a reflective contextual learning intervention would improve novice nurses' critical thinking skills during the first 6 months of practice. | N=6 newly hired nurses and their preceptors (dyads) | Stake's phases of data analysis | Several themes emerged that describe the development of CT in a novice nurse: how anxiety and power influence CT; the concept of "putting pieces together"; how questioning can be CT; how CT moves from sequential thinking to contextual thinking; and how intentional CT emerges. |

**Table 3.10. Summary of Research-Based Literature on Critical Thinking in Nursing and Higher Education (continued)**

| Author(s) | Purpose | Sample | Measurement | Findings |
|---|---|---|---|---|
| Howenstein, Bilodeau, Brogna, & Good (1996) | To assess the critical thinking ability of a convenience sample. | N=160 nurses in two urban hospitals | WGCTA | Age and years of experience were negatively correlated with critical thinking; level of education was positively correlated to critical thinking. |
| Ip et al. (2000) | To explore whether undergraduate students display a disposition toward critical thinking. | N=122 nursing students in Hong Kong | CCTDI | Significant positive relationship between critical thinking dispositions and term grade point average. Third-year students scored significantly lower than second-year students. |
| Jones (2004) | To investigate the understanding of critical thinking of academic staff vs. tutors. | N=2 academics and N=7 tutors | Focus group interviews | Tutors used the same way of understanding critical thinking as academics, but they also discussed broader notions of CT. |
| Ketefian (1981) | To study the relationship between critical thinking, educational preparation, and level of moral judgment. | N=79 practicing nurses | WGCTA; Rest's Defining Issues Test | Significant positive relationship between critical thinking and moral judgment; significant difference in moral judgment between professional and technical nurses; critical thinking and education together accounted for 32.9% of the variance in moral judgment. |
| Kuh & Klein (2006) | To examine the extent of student engagement and academic performance with the development of CT. | N=1058 students at 14 universities | Multiple instruments | Student engagement positively linked to critical thinking and grades; lowest ability students benefit more from engagement than classmates |

**Table 3.10. Summary of Research-Based Literature on Critical Thinking in Nursing and Higher Education (continued)**

| Author(s) | Purpose | Sample | Measurement | Findings |
|---|---|---|---|---|
| Kuiper (2005) | To test the efficacy of audiotapes as a method of recording reflections of nursing students and their clinical preceptorship. | N=40 BSN nursing students | Audiotapes versus journaling in clinical course | Tape recording resulted in longer narratives; higher order thinking causal statements were used by tape group; greater self-monitoring and environment structuring compared with journaling. |
| Ladyshewsky (2006) | To explore the concept of peer coaching. | N=43 postgraduate business students | Self-reports | Participants reported "powerful learning effects" with peer coaching. |
| Laird (2005) | To determine the relationship between self-confidence, social agency, and disposition to critical thinking. | N=289 college students in general education courses | Classroom-Based Survey and Interacting (CBSTI) and California Critical Thinking Disposition Inventory (CCTDI) | Increased experiences with diversity — especially enrollment in diversity courses or positive interactions with peers — results in higher scores on academic self-confidence, social agency, and critical thinking disposition. Diversity experiences work together to foster development of certain aspects of self. |
| Magnussen, Ishida, & Itano (2000) | To determine if inquiry-based learning (IBL) enhances critical thinking ability | N=228 first semester nursing students and N=257 final semester nursing students | WGCTA — at beginning of program and at the end | Students initially in "low" group demonstrated a significant increase in mean score; students initially in "high" group demonstrated a significant decrease in score. |

**Table 3.10. Summary of Research-Based Literature on Critical Thinking in Nursing and Higher Education (continued)**

| Author(s) | Purpose | Sample | Measurement | Findings |
|---|---|---|---|---|
| **Martin (2002)** | To validate the underlying principle of a Theory of Critical Thinking of Nurses. | N=149 – ADN and BSN students and graduates and experienced RNs; convenience sample | Elements of Thought Instrument | Significant difference in the critical thinking among the three levels of clinical expertise. No significant difference in critical thinking between ADN and BSN at any level of clinical expertise. Significant difference in quality of decisions made between the three levels of clinical expertise. Significant relationship between age, GPA, number of years in nursing and critical thinking. |
| **Maynard (1996)** | To determine the relationship between critical thinking and professional nursing competence. | N=30 nursing graduates | Researcher developed | No significant change in critical thinking during the educational experience. Significant increase in critical thinking scores for practicing nurses. No relationship between critical thinking and professional competence. |
| **Myrick & Yonge (2004)** | To examine the preceptorship experience and its role in the enhancement of critical thinking in graduate nursing education. | N=45 graduate nursing students | Interviews using grounded theory method | A relational process that occurred between the preceptor and student enhanced the critical thinking ability of the graduate nursing student. |

**Table 3.10. Summary of Research-Based Literature on Critical Thinking in Nursing and Higher Education (continued)**

| Author(s) | Purpose | Sample | Measurement | Findings |
|---|---|---|---|---|
| Nelms & Lane (1999) | To determine the "way of knowing" for women and the relationship this might have with critical thinking. | N=21 initially; N=14 during junior year; N=10 by senior year | Researcher-developed, qualitative study | Separate knowing was incongruent with nursing except for critical thinking purposes. Procedural knowing was the principle used to determine nursing actions that moved them to constructed knowers and caring critical thinkers. |
| Perciful & Nester (1996) | To determine the effect of an experimental clinical teaching method on nursing students' knowledge and critical thinking skills in psychiatric rotation. | N=83 nursing students — compared two classes from different years using different methods | Psychiatric Component of the Mosby Assess Test and two parts of the NLN Psychiatric Exam | Significant increase in critical thinking for the experimental group using computer-assisted instruction and a collaboration model; no significant increase in knowledge. |
| Phillips & Bond (2004) | To explore whether CT is a generic vs. embedded skill. | N=13 Australian management students | Semistructured interviews | Indicated there were four experiences of critical thinking ranging from a prescribed process to an evaluation that looked beyond what is evident. |
| Profetto-McGrath (2003) | To investigate the critical thinking skills (CTS) and critical thinking dispositions (CTD). | N=228 BSN nursing students | CCTST and CCTDI | Critical thinking scores increased between the first and fourth year in a BSN program — although no statistically significant differences; significant relationship between critical thinking skills and critical thinking disposition. |

**Table 3.10. Summary of Research-Based Literature on Critical Thinking in Nursing and Higher Education (continued)**

| Author(s) | Purpose | Sample | Measurement | Findings |
|---|---|---|---|---|
| Profetto-McGrath, Hesketh, Lang, & Estabrooks (2003) | To determine the relationship of critical thinking to research utilization. | N=141 nurses on an acute surgical unit vs. pediatric unit | CCTDI and researcher-developed tool | Significant positive correlation between critical thinking disposition score and overall research utilization. |
| Rapps, Reigel, & Glaser (2001) | To test a model of cognitive development using knowledge base, critical thinking skills, critical thinking dispositions and experience. | N=232 practicing RNs | Researcher-developed questionnaire | Critical thinking skill was a significant contributor to the dualistic level of cognitive development. |
| Saarmann, Freitas, Rapps, & Reigel (1992) | To compare critical thinking ability and values. | N=128 total; 4 groups of N=32 each–ADN-prepared RNs, BSN-prepared RNs, nursing faculty, and nursing students | WGCTA | Critical thinking of faculty not significantly higher than students when age controlled statistically. Faculty valued achievement most highly ($p \leq 0.0001$), students valued goal orientation most highly ($p \leq 0.001$). |

**Table 3.10. Summary of Research-Based Literature on Critical Thinking in Nursing and Higher Education (continued)**

| Author(s) | Purpose | Sample | Measurement | Findings |
|---|---|---|---|---|
| Saint Clair (1994) | To explore the relationship between nursing preparatory program types and the achievement of critical thinking. To determine if educational environment influenced the achievement of educational outcomes. To determine if there was a difference in this environment between three program types. | N=250 (N=130 ADN, N=54 diploma, and N=66 BSN) | Five "standardized instruments" | No difference between program types with respect to critical thinking, adaptive style flexibility, and the academic environment in scholarliness, vocational preparation, development of personal and social skills, intellectual skills, and science and technology skills. Significant differences between program types with respect to dependent/independent thinking and academic environment in developing interpersonal skills. |
| Sedlak (1997) | To describe critical thinking of BSN students during first clinical experience. | N=7 students | Case study, qualitative — interviews, journals, observations | Students do think critically. Opportunities to dialogue in a supportive environment facilitate critical thinking. |
| Shin, Lee, Ha, & Kim (2006) | To explore critical thinking disposition in baccalaureate nursing students over time. | N=32 BSN students in Korea | CCTDI | Significant improvement in critical thinking over time; significant improvement in open-mindedness, self-confidence, and maturity over time. |
| Tapper (2004) | To investigate student perceptions of instruction in CT and aspects of its development. | N=21 agricultural students | Interviews | Students recalled instruction on critical thinking and found it to be useful. |

**Table 3.10. Summary of Research-Based Literature on Critical Thinking in Nursing and Higher Education (continued)**

| Author(s) | Purpose | Sample | Measurement | Findings |
|---|---|---|---|---|
| Thompson & Rebeschi (1999) | To determine the critical thinking skills of BSN students. | Nursing students | CCTST and CCTDI | Measured the critical thinking of nursing students upon entry to and exit from a program. |
| Wallace (1996) | To assess critical thinking ethnographically. | Not stated | Ethnographic study | Emphasis on the importance of recognizing positive and negative feelings associated with experiences; no correct model of critical thinking. |
| Yeh & Chen (2003) | To understand and compare affective dispositions toward critical thinking across Chinese and American cultures. | N=214 Taiwan nursing students and N=196 US nursing students | CCTDI | Mean item responses for each subscale were significantly different between groups. Significant differences in truth-seeking, open-mindedness, systematicity, and maturity. |

# REFERENCES

Abu-Moghli, F. A., Khalaf, I. A., Halabi, J. O., & Wardam, L. A. (2005). Jordanian baccalaureate nursing students' perception of their learning styles. *International Nursing Review, 52,* 39-45.

Adams, B. L. (1999). Nursing education for critical thinking: An integrative review. *Journal of Nursing Education, 38,* 111-119.

Adams, M. H. (1996). Critical thinking as an educational outcome: An evaluation of current tools of measurement. *Nurse Educator, 21,* 23-32.

Akerjordet, K., & Severinsson, E. (2007). Emotional intelligence: A review of the literature with specific focus on empirical and epistemological perspectives. *Journal of Clinical Nursing,* 16, 1405-1416.

Albert, R. T., Albert, R. E., & Radsma, J. (2002). Relationships among bilingualism, critical thinking, and critical thinking disposition. *Journal of Professional Nursing,* 18, 220-229.

Alexander, M. K., & Giguere, B. (1996). Critical thinking in clinical learning: A holistic perspective. *Holistic Nursing Practice,* 10(3), 15-22.

Allinson, C. W., & Hayes, J. (1988). The learning styles questionnaire: An alternative to Kolb's inventory? *Journal of Management Studies,* 25, 269-281.

Allinson, C. W., & Hayes, J. (1990). The validity of the learning styles questionnaire. *Psychological Reports,* 67, 859-866.

American Association for Higher Education, American College Personnel Association, and National Association of Student Personnel Administration. (1998). *Powerful partnerships: A shared responsibility for learning.* [Online]. Available: http://www.myacpa.org/pub/documents/taskforce.pdf.

Amerson, R. (2006). Engergizing the nursing lecture: Application of the theory of multiple intelligence learning. *Nursing Education Perspectives,* 27, 194-196.

Anderson, J. K. (1998). Orientation with style: Matching teaching/learning style. *Journal of Nurses in Staff Development,* 14, 192-197.

Andrews, C. A., Ironside, P. M., Nosek, C., Sims, S. L., Swenson, M. M., Yeomans, C., et al. (2001). Enacting narrative pedagogy: The lived experiences of students and teachers. *Nursing and Health Care Perspectives,* 22, 252-259.

Andrusyszyn, M., Cragg, C. E., & Humbert, J. (2001). Nurse practitioner preferences for distance education methods related to learning style, course content, and achievement. Journal of Nursing Education, 40, 163-170.

Arthur, D., Pang, S., & Wong, T. (2001). The effect of technology on the caring attributes of an international sample of nurses. International Journal of Nursing Students, 38(1), 37-43.

Atack, L., & Rankin, J. (2002). A descriptive study of registered nurses' experiences with web-based learning. Journal of Advanced Nursing, 40, 457-465.

Ausburn, L. J. (2004). Course design elements most valued by adult learners in blended online education environments: An American perspective. Educational Media International, 41, 327-337.

Baker, C. R. (1996). Reflective learning: A teaching strategy for critical thinking. Journal of Nursing Education, 38(1), 19-22.

Bandura, A. (1977). Social learning theory. Englewood Cliffs, NJ: Prentice-Hall.

Bandura, A. (1986). Foundations of thought and action: A social-cognitive theory. Englewood Cliffs, NJ: Prentice-Hall.

Bandura, A. (2001). Social cognitive theory: An agentic perspective. Annual Review of Psychology, 52(1), 1-26.

Bankert, E. G., & Kozel, V. V. (2005). Transforming pedagogy in nursing education: A caring learning environment for adult students. Nursing Education Perspectives, 26, 227-229.

Barbe, W., & Swassing, R. (1979). Teaching through modality strengths: Concepts and practices. Columbus, OH: Zner-Bloser.

Barker, L. J., & Garvin-Doxas, K. (2004). Making visible the behaviors that influence learning environment: A qualitative exploration of computer science classrooms. Computer Science Education, 14, 119-145.

Bastable, S. B. (2003). Nurse as educator: Principles of teaching and learning for nursing practice. Boston: Jones & Bartlett.

Baumberger-Henry, M. (2003). Practicing the art of nursing through student-designed continuing case study and cooperative learning. Nurse Educator, 28, 191-195.

Beck, S. E., Bennett, A., McLeod, R., & Molyneaux, D. (1992). Review of research on critical thinking in nursing education. In L. R. Allen (Ed.), Review of research in nursing education, Vol. V (pp. 1-30). New York: National League for Nursing.

Beckie, T. M., Lowry, L. W., & Barnett, S. (2001). Assessing critical thinking in baccalaureate nursing students: A longitudinal study. Holistic Nursing Practice, 15(3), 18-26.

Beckman, S., Boxley-Harges, S., Bruick-Sorge, C., & Salmon, B. (2007). Five strategies that heighten nurses' awareness of spirituality to impact client care. Holistic Nursing Practice, 21, 135-139.

Beeken, J. (1997). The relationship between critical thinking and self-concept in staff nurses and the influence of these characteristics on nursing practice. Journal of Nursing Staff Development, 13, 272-278.

Beeken, J. E., Dale, M. L., Enos, M. F., & Yarbrough, S. (1997). Teaching critical thinking skills to undergraduate nursing students. Nurse Educator, 22, 37-39.

Bethune, E. & Jackling, N. (1997). Critical thinking skills: The role of prior experience. Journal of Advanced Nursing, 26, 1005-1012.

Beyer, B. K. (1987). Practical strategies for teaching critical thinking. Boston: Allyn & Bacon.

Billings, D. M. (2000). A framework of assessing outcomes and practices in web-based courses in nursing. Journal of Nursing Education, 39, 60-67.

Billings, D. M., & Rowles, C. J. (2001). Development of continuing nursing education offerings for the World Wide Web. Journal of Continuing Education in Nursing, 32, 107-113.

Bondy, K. N., Koenigseder, L. A., Ishee, J. H., & Williams, B. G. (2001). Psychometric properties of the California Critical Thinking Tests. Journal of Nursing Measurement, 9, 309-328.

Braten, I., & Olaussen, B. S. (2007). The motivational development of Norwegian nursing students over the college years. Learning in Health & Social Care, 6(1), 27-43.

Brock, A., & Butts, J. B. (1998). On target: A model to teach baccalaureate nursing students to apply critical thinking. Nursing Forum, 33(3), 5-10.

Brookfield, S. D. (1987). Developing critical thinkers: Challenging adults to explore alternative ways of thinking and acting. San Francisco: Jossey-Bass.

Brooks, A., & Shepherd, J. M. (1992). Professionalism versus general critical thinking abilities of senior nursing students in four types of nursing curricula. *Journal of Professional Nursing, 8,* 87-95.

Brown, G. (1999). Technology in nurse education: A communication teaching strategy. *Association of Black Nursing Faculty Journal,* 10(1), 9-13.

Brown, J. M., Alverson, E. M., & Pepa, C. A. (2001). The influence of a baccalaureate program on traditional, RN-BSN, and accelerated students' critical thinking abilities. *Holistic Nursing Practice,* 15(3), 4-8.

Brown, H. N., & Sorrell, J. M. (1993). Use of clinical journals to enhance critical thinking. *Nurse Educator,* 18, 6-19.

Brown, H. N., & Sorrell, J. M. (1999). Connecting across the miles: Interdisciplinary collaboration in the evaluation of critical thinking. *Nursing Connections,* 12(2), 43-48.

Bruyn, L. L. (2004). Monitoring online communication: Can the development of convergence and social presence indicate an interactive learning environment? *Distance Education,* 25(1), 67-81.

Caine Learning Institute (2005). How People Learn. [Online]. Available: http://www. cainelearning.com.

Caine, R. N., & Caine, G. (1990). Understanding a brain-based approach to learning and teaching. *Educational Leadership,* 48(2), 66-70.

Campeau, A. G. (1998). Distribution of learning styles and preferences for learning environment characteristics among emergency medical care assistants. *Prehospital and Disaster Medicine,* 13(1), 47-54.

Candela, L., Michael, S. R., & Mitchell, S. (2003). Ethical debates: Enhancing critical thinking in nursing students. *Nurse Educator,* 28, 37-39.

Carini, G., Kuh, G., & Klein, S. (2006). Student engagement and student learning: Testing the linkages. *Research in Higher Education,* 47(1), 1-32.

Carkhuff, M. H. (1996). Reflective learning: Work groups as learning groups. *Journal of Continuing Education in Nursing,* 27, 209-214.

Carnwell, R. (2000). Pedagogical implications of approaches to study in distance learning: Developing models through qualitative and quantitative analysis. *Journal of Advanced Nursing,* 31, 1018-1028.

Carpio, B., Illesca, M., Ellis, P., Crooks, D., Droghetti, J., Tompkins, C., et al. (1999). Student and faculty learning styles in a Canadian and a Chilean self-directed, problem-based nursing program. Canadian Journal of Nursing Research, 31(3), 31-50.

Carter, B. (2000). Complexity, critical thinking and intellectual virtues. Journal of Child Health Care, 4, 136.

Cartwright, J. C., & Menkens, R. (2002). Student perspectives on transitioning to new technologies for distance learning. Computer Informatics in Nursing, 20, 143-149.

Celia, L. M., & Gordon, P. R. (2001). Using problem-based learning to promote critical thinking in an orientation program for novice nurses. Journal of Nurses in Staff Development, 17(1), 12-17.

Chaffee, E., & Tierney, W. (1988). Collegiate culture and leadership strategies. New York: American Council on Education/Macmillan.

Chaffee, J. (1985). Thinking critically. Boston: Houghton Mifflin.

Chan, S. W., & Wai-Tong, C. (2000). Implementing contract learning in a clinical context: Report on a study. Journal of Advanced Nursing, 31, 298-305.

Chau, J. P., Chang, A. M., Lee, I. F., Ip, W. Y., Lee, D. T., & Wootton, Y. (2001). Effects of using videotaped vignettes on enhancing students' critical thinking ability in a baccalaureate nursing program. Journal of Advanced Nursing, 36, 112-119.

Chen, F. C., & Lin, M. C. (2003). Effects of a nursing literature reading course on promoting critical thinking in two-year nursing program students. Journal of Nursing Research, 11, 137-146.

Chen, S., & Lee, W. (2000). The impact of learning styles of nursing students and clinical instructors on academic achievement and teaching satisfaction. Nursing Research (China), 8, 313-324.

Chenowith, L. (1998). Facilitating the process of critical thinking for nursing. Nurse Education Today, 18, 281-292.

Chickering, A. (1969). Education and identity. San Francisco: Jossey-Bass.

Chiu, L. H. (2005). Motivation for nurses undertaking a post-registration qualification in Malaysia. International Nursing Review, 52, 46-51.

Chubinski, S. (1996). Creative critical-thinking strategies. Nurse Educator, 21, 23-27.

Clark, D. J. (1998). Course redesign. Incorporating an Internet web site into an existing nursing class. *Computers in Nursing,* 16, 219-222.

Clarke, K., & Lane, A. M. (2005). Seminar and tutorial sessions: A case study evaluating relationships with academic performance and student satisfaction. *Journal of Further & Higher Education,* 29(1), 15-23.

Clayton, L. H. (2006). Concept mapping: An effective, active teaching-learning method. *Nursing Education Perspectives,* 27, 197-203.

Cody, W. K. (2002). Critical thinking and nursing science: Judgment, or vision? *Nursing Science Quarterly,* 15, 184-189.

Cohen, S., & Milone-Nuzzo, P. (2001). Advancing health policy in nursing education through service learning. *Advances in Nursing Science,* 23(3), 28-40.

Coker, C. A. (2000). Consistency of learning styles of undergraduate athletic training students in the traditional classroom versus the clinical setting. *Journal of Athletic Training,* 35, 441-444.

Colucciello, M. L. (1997). Critical thinking and dispositions of baccalaureate nursing students — A conceptual model for evaluation. *Journal of Professional Nursing,* 13, 236-245.

Colucciello, M. L. (1999). Relationships between critical thinking dispositions and learning styles. *Journal of Professional Nursing,* 15, 294-301.

Cooper, N. J. (2000). The use of narrative in the development of critical thinking. *Nurse Education Today,* 20, 513-518.

Cope, C., & Staehr, L. (2005). Improving students' learning approaches through intervention in an information systems learning environment. *Studies in Higher Education,* 30, 181-197.

Copp, S. L. (2002). Using cooperative learning strategies to teach implications of the nurse practice act. *Nurse Educator,* 27, 236-241.

Cross, K. P. (1981). *Adults as learners.* San Francisco: Jossey-Bass.

Daley, B. J., Shaw, C. R., Balistrieri, T., Glasenapp, K., & Piacentine, L. (1999). Concept maps: A strategy to teach and evaluate critical thinking. *Journal of Nursing Education,* 38, 42-47.

Daly, W. M. (2001). The development of an alternative method in the assessment of critical thinking as an outcome of nursing education. *Journal of Advanced Nursing, 36,* 120-130.

Degazon, C. E., & Lunney, M. (1995). Clinical journal: A tool to foster critical thinking for advanced levels of competence. *Clinical Nurse Specialist, 9,* 270-274.

Dexter, P., Applegate, M., Backer, J., Clayton, K., Keffer, J., Norton, B., et al. (1997). A proposed framework for teaching and evaluating critical thinking in nursing. *Journal of Professional Nursing, 13,* 160-167.

Diaz, D. P., & Cartnal, R. B. (1999). Students' learning styles in two classes: Online distance learning and equivalent on-campus. *College Teaching, 47,* 130-135.

DiBartola, L. M., Miller, M. K., & Turley, C. L. (2001). Do learning styles and learning environment affect learning outcome? *Journal of Allied Health, 30,* 112-115.

Diekelmann, N. (2000). Being prepared for class: Challenging taken-for-granted assumptions. *Journal of in Nursing Education, 39,* 291-293.

Diekelmann, N. (2001). Narrative pedagogy: Heideggerian hermeneutical analyses of the lived experiences of students, teachers, and clinicians. *Advances in Nursing Science, 23,* 53-71.

Diekelmann, N. (2002a). Teacher talk: New pedagogies for nursing. "Pitching a lecture" and "reading the faces of students": Learning lecturing and the embodied practices of teaching. *Journal of Nursing Education, 41(3),* 97-99.

Diekelmann, N. (2002b). Teacher talk: New pedagogies for nursing. Engendering community: Learning and sharing expertise in the skills and practices of teaching. *Journal of Nursing Education, 41(6),* 241-242.

Diekelmann, N. (2002c). Teacher talk: New pedagogies for nursing. "Too much content…" Epistemologies' grasp and nursing education. *Journal of Nursing Education, 41(11),* 469-470.

Diekelmann, N. (2003). Teacher talk: New pedagogies for nursing. Engendering community: Learning to live together. *Journal of Nursing Education, 42(6),* 243-244.

Diekelmann, N., & Diekelmann, J. (2000). Learning ethics in nursing and genetics: Narrative pedagogy and the grounding of values. *Journal of Pediatric Nursing, 15,* 226-231.

Diekelmann, N., & Mikol, C. (2003). Teacher talk: New pedagogies for nursing. Knowing and connecting: Competing demands and creating student-friendly and teacher-friendly curricula. _Journal of Nursing Education,_ 42(9), 385-389.

Diekelmann, N., & Scheckel, M. (2003). Teacher talk: New pedagogies for nursing. Teaching students to apply nursing theories and models: Trying something new. _Journal of Nursing Education,_ 42(5), 195-197.

Diekelmann, N., Ironside, P. M., & Gunn, J. (2005). Recalling the curriculum revolution: Innovation with research. _Nursing Education Perspectives,_ 26(2), 70-77.

Diekelmann, N., Swenson, M. M., & Sims, S. L. (2003). Teacher talk: New pedagogies for nursing. Reforming the lecture: Avoid what students already know. _Journal of Nursing Education,_ 42(3), 103-105.

Diseth, A. (2002). The relationship between intelligence, approaches to learning and academic achievement. _Scandinavian Journal of Educational Research,_ 46, 219-230.

DiVito, T. P. (2000). Identifying critical thinking behaviors in clinical judgments. _Journal of Nurses in Staff Development,_ 16, 174-180.

Dobrzykowski, T. M. (1994). Teaching strategies to promote critical thinking in nursing staff. _Journal of Continuing Education in Nursing,_ 25, 272-276.

Drevdahl, D., Dorcy, K., & Grevstad, L. (2001). Integrating principles of community-based practice in a community health nursing practicum. _Nurse Educator,_ 26, 234-239.

Duchscher, J. E. (2003). Critical thinking: Perceptions of newly graduated female baccalaureate nurses. _Journal of Nursing Education,_ 42(1), 14-27.

Dunn, M., Dunn, R., & Price, G. (1991). _Productivity environmental preference survey_ (PEPS). Lawrence, KS: Price Systems.

Dunn, R., & Dunn, K. (1978). _Teaching students through their individual learning styles: A practical approach._ Reston, VA: National Association of Secondary School Principals.

Eble, K. E. (Ed.). (1980). _Improving teaching styles._ San Francisco: Jossey-Bass.

Edwards, P. A. (2005). Impact of technology on the content and nature of teaching and learning. _Nursing Education Perspectives,_ 26(6), 344-347.

Edwards, S. L. (1998). Critical thinking and analysis: A model of written assignments. _British Journal of Nursing,_ 7, 159-166.

Elfrink, V. L., Davis, L. S., Fitzwater, E., Castleman, J., Burley, J., Gorney-Moreno, M.J., et al. (2000). A comparison of teaching strategies for integrating information technology into clinical nursing education. *Nurse Educator,* 25, 136-144.

Elliott, D. (1996). Promoting critical thinking in the classroom. *Nurse Educator,* 21(2), 49-52.

Entwistle, J. J., & Tait, H. (1994). *The revised Approaches to Studying Inventory.* Edinburgh, Scotland: University of Edinburgh, Centre for Research into Learning and Instruction.

Evans, B. C., & Bendel, R. (2004). Cognitive and ethical maturity in baccalaureate nursing students: Did a class using narrative pedagogy make a difference? *Nursing Education Perspectives,* 25, 188-195.

Evans, C. (2004). Exploring the relationship between cognitive style and teaching style. *Educational Psychology,* 24, 509-530.

Evans, C., & Waring, M. (2006). Towards inclusive teacher education: Sensitizing individuals to how they learn. *Educational Psychology,* 26, 395-407.

Facione, N. C., & Facione, P. A. (1994). Critical thinking disposition as a measure of competent clinical judgment: The development of the California Critical Thinking Disposition Inventory. *Journal of Nursing Education,* 33, 345-350.

Facione, N. C., & Facione, P. A. (1996a). Assessment design issues for evaluating critical thinking in nursing. *Holistic Nursing Practice,* 10(3), 41-53.

Facione, N. C., & Facione, P. A. (1996b). Externalizing the critical thinking in knowledge development and clinical judgment. *Nursing Outlook,* 44, 129-136.

Fang-Chiao, C., & Ming-Chen, L. (2003). Effects of a nursing literature reading course on promoting critical thinking in two-year nursing program students. *Journal of Nursing Research,* 11, 137-148.

Ferrari, E. (2006). Academic education's contribution to the nurse-patient relationship. *Nursing Standard,* 21(10), 35-40.

Forneis, S. G., & Peden-McAlpine, C. (2007). Evaluation of a reflective learning intervention to improve critical thinking in novice nurses. *Journal of Advanced Nursing,* 57, 410-421.

France, N., Fields, A., & Garth, K. (2004). "You're just shoved to the corner:" The lived experience of Black nursing students being isolated and discounted, a pilot study. *Visions,* 12(1), 28-36.

Freeman, V. S., Fell, L. L., & Muellenberg, P. (1998). Learning styles and outcomes in clinical laboratory science. *Clinical Laboratory Science,* 11, 287-290.

Freeman, V. S., & Tijerina, S. (2000). Delivery methods, learning styles, and outcomes of physician assistant students. *Physician Assistant,* 24, 43-44, 47-48, 50.

Friedman, P., & Alley, R. (1984). Learning/teaching styles: Applying the principles. *Theory into Practice,* 23(1), 77-81.

Fritz, S., Speth, C., Barbuto, J. E., & Boren, A. (2004). Exploring relationships between college students' learning styles and motivation. *Psychological Reports,* 95, 969-974.

Frye, B., Alfred, N., & Campbell, M. (1999). Use of the Watson-Glaser Critical Thinking Appraisal with BSN students. *Nursing & Health Care Perspectives,* 20, 253-255.

Gagne, R. M. (1965). *The conditions of learning.* New York: Holt, Rinehart & Wilson.

Gardner, H. (1983). *Frames of mind: The theory of multiple intelligences.* New York: Basic Books.

Garrett, M., Schoener, L., & Hood, L. (1996). Debate: A teaching strategy to improve verbal communication and critical-thinking skills. *Nurse Educator,* 21, 37-40.

Gendrop, S. C., & Eisenhauer, L. A. (1996). A transactional perspective on critical thinking. *Scholarly Inquiry of Nursing Practice,* 10, 329-345.

Gillespie, M. (2002). Student-teacher connection in clinical nursing education. *Journal of Advanced Nursing,* 37, 566-576.

Gillespie, M. (2005). Student-teacher connection: A place of possibility. *Journal of Advanced Nursing,* 52, 211-219.

Gordon, J. M. (2000). Congruency in defining critical thinking by nurse educators and non-nurse scholars. *Journal of Nursing Education,* 39, 340-351.

Gottleib, J. A. (2002). Designing and implementing an RN refresher course for the acute care hospital: Development of the nurses' critical thinking skills. *Journal of Nurses in Staff Development,* 18, 86-91.

Graham, I., & Richardson, E. (2008). Experiential gaming to facilitate cultural awareness: Its implication for developing emotional caring in nursing. _Learning in Health & Social Care,_ 7(1), 37-45.

Grasha, A. F. (2000). Integrating teaching styles and learning styles with instructional technology. _College Teaching,_ 48(1), 2-11.

Gray, M. T. (2003). Beyond content: Generating critical thinking in the classroom. _Nurse Educator,_ 28, 136-140.

Gregorc, A. F. (1982). _An adult's guide to style._ Maynard, MA: Gabriel Systems.

Guild, P. B., & Ganger, S. (1998). _Marching to different drummers_ (2nd ed.). Alexandria, VA: Association for Supervision and Curriculum Development.

Gulpinar, M. A. (2005). The principles of brain-based learning and contructivist models in education. _Educational Sciences: Theory and Practice,_ 5, 299-306.

Halstead, J. A. (Ed.). (2007). _Nurse educator competencies: Creating an evidence-based practice for nurse educators._ New York: National League for Nursing.

Halstead, J. A., & Coudret, N. A. (2000). Implementing web-based instruction in a school of nursing: Implications for faculty and students. _Journal of Professional Nursing,_ 16, 273-281.

Hansten, R. I., & Washburn, M. J. (2000). Facilitating critical thinking. _Journal of Nurses in Staff Development,_ 16, 23-30.

Harrelson, G. L., Leaver-Dunn, D., & Wright, K. E. (1998). An assessment of learning styles among undergraduate athletic training students. _Journal of Athletic Training,_ 33(1), 50-53.

Hart, L. A. (1983). _Human brain, human learning._ New York: Longman.

Hativa, N., & Birenbaum, M. (2000). Who prefers what? Disciplinary differences in students' preferred approaches to teaching and learning styles. _Research in Higher Education,_ 41, 209-236.

Heath, L. S. (2000). _An investigation of critical thinking, critical thinking dispositions, and preferred learning styles of nursing students in a baccalaureate program._ Unpublished doctoral dissertation, Walden University, Minneapolis, MN.

Heibert, J. L. (1996). Learning circles: A strategy for clinical practicum. *Nurse Educator,* 21, 37-42.

Heinrich, K. T. (1992). The intimate dialogue: Journal writing by students. *Nurse Educator,* 17, 17-21.

Heller, B. A., Ortos, M. T., & Crowley, J. D. (2000). The future of nursing education: Ten trends to watch. *Nursing and Health Care Perspectives,* 21, 9-13.

Hendry, G., Heinrich, P., Lyon, P. M., Barratt, A. L., Simpson, J. M., Hyde, S. J., et al. (2005). Helping students understand their learning styles: Effects on study self-efficacy, preference for group work, and group climate. *Educational Psychology,* 25, 395-407.

Hickman, J. S. (1993). A critical assessment of critical thinking in nursing education. *Holistic Nursing Practice,* 7(3), 36-47.

Hicks, F. D. (2001). Critical thinking: Toward a nursing science perspective. *Nursing Science Quarterly,* 14, 14-21.

Higuchi, K., & Donald, J. (2002). Thinking processes used by nurses in clinical decision making. *Journal of Nursing Education,* 41, 145-153.

Hilgard, E. R. (1956). *Theories of learning* (2nd ed.). New York: Appleton-Century-Crofts.

Hoisington, D. L. (2000). *Use of technology by nursing students: Learning styles, age, and experience.* Unpublished doctoral dissertation, Michigan State University, Lansing.

Honey, P., & Mumford, A. (1986). *The manual of learning styles.* Maidenhead, England: Peter Honey.

Honigsfeld, A., & Schiering, M. (2004). Diverse approaches to the diversity of learning styles in teacher education. *Educational Psychology,* 24, 487-507.

Howard, D., Hayes, M., Solomonides, I., & Swannell, M. (2001). Changes in student nurses' approaches to studying. *Nursing Times Research,* 6, 921-935.

Howenstein, M. A., Bilodeau, K., Brogna, M. J., & Good, G. (1996). Factors associated with critical thinking among nurses. *Journal of Continuing Education for Nurses,* 27, 100-103.

Ip, W. Y., Lee, D. T., Lee, I. F., Chau, J. P., Wootton, Y. S., & Chang, A. M. (2000). Disposition towards critical thinking: A study of Chinese undergraduate nursing students. *Journal of Advanced Nursing,* 32, 84-90.

Ironside, P. M. (2001). Creating a research base for nursing education: An interpretive review of conventional, critical, feminist, postmodern, and phenomenologic pedagogies. *Advances in Nursing Science, 23(3)*, 72-87.

Ironside, P. M. (2003). Trying something new: Implementing and evaluating narrative pedagogy using a multimethod approach. *Nursing Education Perspectives, 24*, 122-128.

Ironside, P. M. (2006). Using narrative pedagogy: Learning and practicing interpretive thinking. *Journal of Advanced Nursing, 55*, 478-486.

Jaeger, A. J. (2003). Job competencies and the curriculum: An inquiry into emotional intelligence in graduate professional education. *Research in Higher Education, 44*, 615-639.

Jeffries, P. R., Woolf, S., & Linde, B. (2003). Technology-based vs. traditional instruction: A comparison of two methods for teaching the skill of performing a 12-lead ECG. *Nursing Education Perspectives, 24*, 70-74.

Jensen, E. (2000). Brain-based learning: A reality check. *Educational Leadership, 57(7)*, 76-80.

Jensen, E. P. (2008). A fresh look at brain-based education. *Phi Delta Kappan, 89*, 408-417.

Jensen, G. (1987). Learning styles. In J. Provost & S. Anchors (Eds.), *Applications of the Myers-Briggs type indicator in higher education* (pp. 45-55). Palo Alto, CA: Consulting Psychologist Press.

Jie, L., & Xiaoqing, Q. (2006). Language learning styles and learning strategies of tertiary-level English learners in China. *Regional Language Centre Journal, 37(1)*, 69-90.

Johannsson, S. L., & Wertenberger, D. H. (1996). Using simulation to test critical thinking skills of nursing students. *Nurse Education Today, 16*, 323-327.

Johnson, D. W., & Johnson, R. T. (1975). *Learning together and alone.* Englewood Cliffs, NJ: Prentice-Hall.

Jones, A. (2004). Teaching critical thinking: An investigation of a task in introductory macroeconomics. *Higher Education Research & Development, 23*, 167-181.

Jones, S. A. (1991). Critical thinking: Impact on nursing education. *Journal of Advanced Nursing, 16*, 529-533.

Jones, T. H., & Paolucci, R. (1999). Research framework and dimensions for evaluating the effectiveness of educational technology systems on learning outcomes. Journal of Research on Computing in Education, 32(1), 17-28.

Joshua-Amadi, M. (2003a). Recruitment and retention: A study of motivation – part 1. Nursing Management (London), 9(8), 17-21.

Joshua-Amadi, M. (2003b). Recruitment and retention: A study of motivation – part 2. Nursing Management (London), 9(9), 14-19.

Kataoka-Yahiro, M., & Saylor, C. (1994). A critical thinking model for nursing judgment. Journal of Nursing Education, 33, 351-356.

Kawashima, A. (2005). The implementation of narrative pedagogy into nursing education in Japan. Nursing Education Perspectives, 26(3), 168-171.

Kenny, A. (2002). Online learning: Enhancing nurse education? Journal of Advanced Nursing, 38, 127-135.

Ketefian, S. (1981). Critical thinking, education preparation, and development of moral judgment among selected groups of practicing nurses. Nursing Research, 30, 98-103.

Kim, J. (2003). Graduate students' experiences in web site development: A project assignment for nursing informatics class. Computers, Informatics, Nursing, 21, 143-149.

Kintgen-Andrews, J. (1993). Critical thinking and nursing education. Journal of Nursing Education, 30, 99-100.

Kirkpatrick, M. K., & Brown, S. (2004). Narrative pedagogy: Teaching geriatric content with stories and the "make a difference" project (MADP). Nursing Education Perspectives, 25, 183-187.

Kitchener, K., & King, P. (1990). The reflective judgment model: Transforming assumptions about knowing. In J. Bass (Ed.), Fostering critical reflection in adulthood (pp. 159-176). San Francisco: Jossey-Bass.

Klaassens, E. L. (1992). Evaluation of interactive videodisc simulations designed for nursing to determine their ability to provide problem-solving practice based on the use of the nursing process. Unpublished doctoral dissertation, Northern Illinois University, DeKalb.

Klindworth, D. (1998). Using multiple intelligences: Collaboratively planning a unit of study. Labtalk, October, 25-26.

Knowles, M. S. (1978). *The adult learner: A neglected species* (2nd ed.). Houston, TX: Gulf.

Kolb, D. A. (1984). *Experiential learning: Experience as the source of learning and development.* London: Prentice Hall.

Kreber, C. (2005). Reflection on teaching and the scholarship of teaching: Focus on science majors. *Higher Education,* 50, 323-359.

Kuh, G., & Klein, S. (2006). Student engagement and student learning: Testing the linkages. *Research in Higher Education,* 47(1), 1-32.

Kuhn, M. A. (1995). Gaming: A technique that adds spice to learning? *Journal of Continuing Education in Nursing,* 26, 35-39.

Kuiper, R. (2000). A new direction for cognitive development in nursing to prepare the practitioners of the future. *Nursing Leadership Forum,* 4, 116-124.

Kuiper, R. (2005). Self-regulated learning during a clinical preceptorship: The reflections of senior baccalaureate nursing students. *Nursing Education Perspectives,* 26(6), 351-356.

Kuramoto, A. M. (1999). The challenges and rewards of institutional collaboration in distance education. *Journal of Nurses in Staff Development,* 15, 236-240.

Ladyshewsky, R. (2006). Peer coaching: A constructivist methodology for enhancing critical thinking in postgraduate business education. *Higher Education Research & Development,* 25, 67-84.

Laird, T. F. N. (2005). College students' experiences with diversity and their effects on academic self-confidence, social agency, and disposition toward critical thinking. *Research in Higher Education,* 46, 365-387.

Lassiter, K. S., Matthews, T. D., Bell, N. L., & Maher, C. M. (2002). Comparison of the General Ability Measure for Adults and the Kaufman Adolescent and Adult Intelligence Test with college students. *Psychology in Schools,* 39, 497-506.

Lauterbach, S. S., & Becker, P. H. (1996). Caring for self: Becoming a self-reflective nurse. *Holistic Nursing Practice,* 39, 149-154.

Leasure, A. R., Davis, L., & Thievon, S. L. (2000). Comparison of student outcomes and preferences in a traditional vs. world wide web-based baccalaureate nursing research course. *Journal of Nursing Education,* 39, 149-154.

Lee, J. E. M., & Ryan-Wenger, N. (1997). The "Think Aloud" seminar for teaching clinical reasoning: A case study of a child with pharyngitis. Journal of Pediatric Health Care, 11, 101-110.

Lightfoot, J. M. (2006). A comparative analysis of e-mail and face-to-face communication in an educational environment. Internet & Higher Education, 9, 217-227.

Linares, A. Z. (1999). Learning styles of students and faculty in selected health care professions. Journal of Nursing Education, 38, 407-414.

Lindblom-Ylanne, S. (2004). Raising students' awareness of their approaches to study. Innovations in Education & Teaching International, 41, 405-421.

Lindblom-Ylanne, S., Trigwell, K., Nevgi, A., & Ashwin, P. (2006). How approaches to teaching are affected by discipline and teaching context. Studies in Higher Education, 31, 285-298.

Locsin, R. C. (2001). The dilemma of decision-making: Processing thinking critical to nursing. Holistic Nursing Practice, 15(3), 1-3.

Loving, G. L., & Wilson, J. S. (2000). Infusing critical thinking into the nursing curriculum through faculty development. Nurse Educator, 25, 70-75.

Lusk, M. (2003). Collaborative testing to promote learning. Journal of Nursing Education, 42, 121-124.

MacDonald, J., & Mason, R. (1999). Refining assessment for resource based learning. Assessment and Evaluation in Higher Education, 24, 345-355.

MacIntosh, J. (2001). Learner concerns and teaching strategies for video-conferencing. Journal of Continuing Education in Nursing, 32, 260-265.

Magnussen, L., Ishida, D., & Itano, J. (2000). The impact of the use of inquiry-based learning as a teaching methodology on the development of critical thinking. Journal of Nursing Education, 39, 360-364.

Marcy, V. (2001). Adult learning styles: How the VARK learning style inventory can be used to improve student learning. Perspective on Physician Assistant Education, 12, 117-120.

Martin, C. (2002). The theory of critical thinking of nursing. Nursing Education Perspectives, 23, 243-247.

Martin, G. W. (1996). An approach to the facilitation and assessment of critical thinking in nurse education. *Nurse Education Today,* 16, 3-9.

Martin, I. G., Stark, P., & Jolly, B. (2000). Benefiting from clinical experience: The influence of learning style and clinical experience on performance in an undergraduate objective structured clinical examination. *Medical Education,* 34, 530-534.

Maslow, A. (1954). *Motivation and personality.* New York: Harper & Row.

Maslow, A. (1987). *Motivation and personality* (3rd ed.). New York: Harper & Row.

Mastrian, K. G., & McGonigle, D. (1999). Using technology-based assignments to promote critical thinking. *Nurse Educator,* 24, 45-47.

Masui, C., & De Corte, E. (2005). Learning to reflect and to attribute constructively as basic components of self-regulated learning. *British Journal of Educational Psychology,* 75, 351-372.

Mau, W.C. (2001). Gender differences on the Scholastic Aptitude Test, the American College Test and college grades. *Educational Psychology,* 21, 133-137.

May, B. A. (2000). *Relationships among basic empathy, self-awareness, and learning styles of baccalaureate pre-nursing students within King's personal system.* Unpublished doctoral dissertation, University of Tennessee, Knoxville.

Mayer, R. E. (2003). Learning environments: The case for evidence-based practice and issue-driven research. *Educational Psychology Review,* 15, 359-366.

Maynard, C. A. (1996). Relationship of critical thinking ability to professional nursing competence. *Journal of Nursing Education,* 35, 12-18.

McColgin, C. C. (2000). *Match between learning styles and teaching methods: An exploratory study of the effects on nursing students' academic performance, perceived learning, and course evaluations.* Unpublished doctoral dissertation, Syracuse University, Syracuse, NY.

McDade, D. C. (1999). *Relationships between learning styles and critical thinking ability among health professional students.* Unpublished doctoral dissertation, University of Georgia, Athens.

McKenna, G. (1995a). Learning theories made easy: Behaviorism. *Nursing Standard,* 9(29), 29-31.

McKenna, G. (1995b). Learning theories made easy: Cognitivism. _Nursing Standard,_ 9(30), 25-28.

McKenna, G. (1995c). Learning theories made easy: Humanism. _Nursing Standard,_ 9(31), 29-31.

McLaughlin, D. G. (2001). _Research on learning styles of students who are taking Web-based courses._ Unpublished doctoral dissertation, Idaho State University, Pocatello.

Merritt, S. L. (1989). Learning styles: Theory and use as a basis for instruction. In W. L. Holzemer (Ed.), _Review of research in nursing education, Vol. II_ (pp. 1-31). New York: National League for Nursing.

Meyer, J. H., & Eley, M. G. (2006). The Approaches to Teaching Inventory: A critique of its development and applicability. _British Journal of Educational Psychology,_ 76, 633-649.

Miley, W. M., & Gonsalves, S. (2003). What you don't know can hurt you: Students' perceptions of professors' annoying teaching habits. _College Student Journal,_ 37, 447-456.

Miley, W. M., & Gonsalves, S. (2005). A simple way to collect data on how students view teaching styles. _College Teaching,_ 53(1), 20.

Miller, J. A. (1998). Enhancement of achievement and attitudes through individualized learning-style presentations of two allied health courses. _Journal of Allied Health,_ 27, 150-156.

Miller, M. A. (1992). Outcomes evaluation: Measuring critical thinking. _Journal of Advanced Nursing,_ 17, 1401-1407.

Miller, M. A., & Malcolm, N. S. (1990). Critical thinking in the nursing curriculum. _Nursing and Health Care,_ 11, 67-73.

Mogale, N. M., & Botes, A. C. (2001). Problem-based case study to enhance critical thinking in student nurses. _Curationis,_ 24(3), 27-35.

Morton-Rias, D., Dunn, R., Terregrossa, R., Geisert, G., Mangione, R., Ortiz, S., et al. (2007). Allied health students' learning styles identified with two different assessments. _Journal of College Student Retention: Research, Theory & Practice,_ 9, 233-250.

Mupinga, D. M., Nora, R. T., & Yaw, D. C. (2006). The learning styles, expectations, and needs of online students. _College Teaching,_ 54, 185-189.

Myers, I. B. (1980). *Gifts differing.* Palo Alto, CA: Consulting Psychologists Press.

Myrick, F., & Yonge, O. (2004). Enhancing critical thinking in the preceptorship experience in nursing education. *Journal of Advanced Nursing,* 45, 371-380.

National League for Nursing. (2000). *Guidelines for item writing.* New York: Author.

National League for Nursing, Task Group on Nurse Educator Competencies. (2005a). *Core competencies of nurse educators with task statements.* New York: Author. [Online]. Available: http://www.nln.org/facultydevelopment/pdf/corecompetencies.pdf.

National League for Nursing. (2005b). *The scope of practice for nurse educators.* New York: Author

Neill, K. M., Lachat, M. F., & Taylor-Panek, S. (1997). Enhancing critical thinking with case studies and nursing process. *Nurse Educator,* 22, 30-32.

Nelms, T. P., & Lane, E. B. (1999). Women's ways of knowing in nursing and critical thinking. *Journal of Professional Nursing,* 15, 179-186.

Nganasurian, W. E. (1999). Evaluating learning opportunities offered to mental health nursing students. *Journal of Psychiatric and Mental Health Nursing,* 5, 393-402.

Niedringhaus, L. K. (2001). Using student writing assignments to assess critical thinking skills: A holistic approach. *Holistic Nursing Practice,* 15(3), 9-17.

Nijhuis, J., Segers, M., & Gijselaers, W. (2007). The interplay of perceptions of the learning environment, personality, and learning strategies: A study amongst international business studies students. *Studies in Higher Education,* 32(1), 59- 77.

Oermann, M. H. (1990). Research on teaching methods. In G. M. Clayton & P. A. Baj (Eds.), *Review of research in nursing education, Vol. III* (pp. 1-31). New York: National League for Nursing.

Oermann, M. H. (1997). Evaluating critical thinking in clinical practice. *Nurse Educator,* 22, 25-28.

Oermann, M., Truesdell, S., & Ziolkowski, L. (2000). Strategy to assess, develop, and evaluate critical thinking. *Journal of Continuing Education for Nurses,* 31, 155- 160.

Olson, V. G., & Scanlan, C. L. (2002). Physical therapy students' learning styles and their teaching method and instructional activity preferences. *Journal of Physical Therapy Education,* 16(2), 24-31.

Ornstein, R. E. (1972). *The psychology of consciousness.* New York: Viking Press.

O'Sullivan, P. S., Blevins-Stephens, W. L., Smith, F. M., & Vaughan-Wrobel, B. (1997). Addressing the National League for Nursing critical thinking outcome. *Nurse Educator, 22,* 23-29.

Patton, J. G., Woods, S. J., Agarenzo, T., Brubacker, C., Metcalf, T., & Sherrer, L. (1997). Enhancing the clinical practicum experience through journal writing. *Journal of Nursing Education, 36,* 238-240.

Perciful, E. G., & Nester, P. A. (1996). The effect of an innovative clinical method on nursing students' knowledge and critical thinking skills. *Journal of Nursing Education, 35,* 23-38.

Perry, W. (1970). *Forms of intellectual and ethical development in the college years: A scheme.* New York: Holt, Rinehart, & Winston.

Phillips, V., & Bond, C. (2004). Undergraduates' experiences in critical thinking. *Higher Education Research & Development, 23,* 277-294.

Pintrich, P. R. (2004). A conceptual framework for assessing motivation and self-regulated learning in college students. *Educational Psychology Review, 16,* 385-407.

Pless, B. S., & Clayton, G. M. (1993). Clarifying the concept of critical thinking in nursing. *Journal of Nursing Education, 32,* 425-428.

Pozo-Munoz, C., Rebolloso-Pacheco, E., & Fernandez-Ramirez, B. (2000). The "ideal teacher." Implications for student evaluation of teacher effectiveness. *Assessment & Evaluation in Higher Education, 25,* 253-264.

Premkumar, K., Hunter, W., Davison, J., & Jennett, P. (1998). Development and validation of an evaluation tool for multimedia resources in health education. *International Journal of Medical Information, 50,* 243-250.

Profetto-McGrath, J. (2003). The relationship of critical thinking skills and critical thinking dispositions of baccalaureate nursing students. *Journal of Advanced Nursing, 43,* 569-577.

Profetto-McGrath, J., Hesketh, K. L., Lang, S., & Estabrooks, C. A. (2003). A study of critical thinking and research utilization among nurses. *Western Journal of Nursing Research, 25,* 322-337.

Prosser, M., & Trigwell, K. (2006). Confirmatory factor analysis of the Approaches to Teaching Inventory. _British Journal of Educational Psychology,_ 76, 405-419.

Rane-Szostak, D., & Robertson, J. F. (1996). Issues in measuring critical thinking: Meeting the challenge. _Journal of Nursing Education,_ 35, 5-11.

Rao, S., & DiCarlo, S. (2000). Peer instruction improves performance on quizzes. _Advances in Physiology Education,_ 24(1), 51-55.

Rapps, J., Reigel, B., & Glaser, D. (2001). Testing a predictive model of what makes a critical thinker. _Western Journal of Nursing Research,_ 23, 610-626.

Rauen, C. A. (2001). Using simulation to teach critical thinking skills. You can't just throw the book at them. _Critical Care Nursing Clinics of North America,_ 13, 93-103.

Ravert, P. (2002). An integrative review of computer-based simulation in the education process. _Computers, Informatics, Nursing,_ 20, 203-208.

Redding, D. A. (2001). The development of critical thinking among students in baccalaureate nursing education. _Holistic Nursing Practice,_ 15(4), 57-64.

Reese, V. L. & Dunn, R. (2007). Learning-style preferences of a diverse freshman population in a large, private, metropolitan university by gender and GPA. _Journal of College Student Retention: Research, Theory & Practice,_ 9(1), 95-112.

Rempher, K. J., Lasome, C. E. M., & Lasome, T. J. (2003). Leveraging palm technology in the advanced practice nursing environment. _AACN Clinical Issues: Advanced Practice in Acute & Critical Care,_ 14, 363-370.

Ribbons, R. M. (1998). The use of computers as cognitive tools to facilitate higher order thinking skills in nurse education. _Computers in Nursing,_ 16, 223-228.

Richardson, J. T. E. (2005). Students' approaches to learning and teachers' approaches to teaching in higher education. _Educational Psychology,_ 25, 673-680.

Riechmann, S. W., & Grasha, A. F. (1974). A rational approach to developing and assessing the construct validity of a student learning styles scale instrument. _Journal of Psychology,_ 87, 213-223.

Roberts, C. M., Sucher, K., Perrin, D. G., & Rodriguez, S. (1995). Concept mapping: An effective instructional strategy for diet therapy. _Journal of the American Dietetic Association,_ 95, 908-911.

Roberts, J. W. (2002). Beyond learning by doing: The brain compatible approach. _Journal of Experiential Education,_ 25, 281-285.

Rogers, C. H. (1969). _Freedom to learn._ Columbus, OH: Merrill.

Romano, J., Wallace, T. L., Helmick, I. J., Carey, L. M., & Adkins, L. (2005). Study procrastination, achievement, and academic motivation in web-based and blended distance learning. _Internet & Higher Education,_ 8, 299-305.

Rooda, L. A. (1994). Effects of mind mapping on student achievement in a nursing research course. _Nurse Educator,_ 19, 25-27.

Ross, J. L., Drysdale, M. T. B., & Schulz, R. A. (1999). Learning style in the classroom: Towards quality instruction in kinesiology. _Avante,_ 5(3), 31-42.

Rovai, A. P., Ponton, M. K., Derrick, M. G., & Davis, J. M. (2006). Student evaluation of teaching in the virtual and traditional classrooms: A comparative analysis. _Internet & Higher Education,_ 9(1), 23-35.

Saarmann, L., Freitas, L., Rapps, J., & Reigel, B. (1992). The relationship of education to critical thinking ability and values among nurses: Socialization into professional nursing. _Journal of Professional Nursing,_ 8, 26-34.

Sadler-Smith, E. (1997). "Learning style": Frameworks and instruments. _Educational Psychology,_ 17(1/2), 51-64.

Saint Clair, A. J. (1994). _The effect of undergraduate nursing education program type on the achievement of critical thinking, field dependent-independent thinking, adaptive style flexibility, and self-esteem._ Unpublished doctoral dissertation, University of Connecticut, Storrs.

Sandmire, D. A., Vroman, K. G., & Sanders, R. (2000). The influence of learning styles on collaborative performances of allied health students in a clinical experience. _Journal of Allied Health,_ 29, 143-149.

Saucier, B. L. (1995). Critical thinking skills of baccalaureate nursing students. _Journal of Professional Nursing,_ 11, 351-357.

Scanlon, A. (2006). Humanistic principles in relation to psychiatric nurse education: A review of the literature. _Journal of Psychiatric and Mental Health Nursing,_ 13, 758-764.

Schaefer, K. M., & Zygmont, D. (2003). Analyzing the teaching style of nursing faculty: Does it promote a student-centered or teacher-centered learning environment? _Nursing Education Perspectives,_ 24, 238-245.

Scheffer, B. K., & Rubenfeld, M. G. (2000). A consensus statement on critical thinking in nursing. *Journal of Nursing Education,* 39, 352-359.

Schelfhout, W., Dochy, F., & Janssens, S. (2004). The use of self, peer, and teacher assessment as feedback system in a learning environment aimed at fostering skills of cooperation in an entrepreneurial context. *Assessment & Evaluation in Higher Education,* 29, 177-201.

Scheyvens, R., Wild, K., & Overton, J. (2003). International students pursing postgraduate study in geography: Impediments to their learning experience. *Journal of Geography in Higher Education,* 27, 309-323.

Seale, J. K., Chapman, J., & Davey, C. (2000). The influence of assessments on students' motivation to learn in a therapy degree course. *Medical Education,* 34, 614-621.

Sedlak, C. A. (1997). Critical thinking of beginning baccalaureate nursing students during the first clinical nursing course. *Journal of Nursing Education,* 36, 11-18.

Sedlak, C. A. (1999). Differences in critical thinking of nontraditional and traditional nursing students. *Nurse Educator,* 24, 38-44.

Seymour, B., Kinn, S., & Sutherland, N. (2003). Valuing both critical and creative thinking in clinical practice: Narrowing the research-practice gap? *Journal of Advanced Nursing,* 42, 288-296.

Shapiro, E. (2006). Brain-based learning meets PowerPoint. *The Teaching Professor,* 20(5), 5.

Shea, P., Li, C. S., & Pickett, A. (2006). A study of teaching presence and student sense of learning community in fully online and web-enhanced college courses. *Internet & Higher Education,* 9, 175-190.

Shin, K. R., Lee, J. H., Ha, J. Y., & Kim, K. H. (2006). Critical thinking dispositions in baccalaureate nursing students. *Journal of Advanced Nursing,* 56, 182-189.

Simpson, E., & Courtney, M. (2002). Critical thinking in nursing education: Literature review. *International Journal of Nursing Practice,* 8, 89-98.

Simpson, R. L. (1997). The information age: Influencing practice and academic environments. *Nursing Management,* 28(11), 26-27.

Skiba, D.J. (2005). The Millennials: Have they arrived at your school of nursing? _Nursing Education Perspectives,_ 26(6), 370-371.

Skiba, D. J. (2006). Got large lecture hall classes? Use clickers. _Nursing Education Perspectives,_ 27(5), 278-280.

Skiba, D. J. (2007a). Nursing Education 2.0: Second Life. _Nursing Education Perspectives,_ 28(3), 156-157.

Skiba, D. J. (2007b). Nursing Education 2.0: Poke me. Where's your face in space? _Nursing Education Perspectives,_ 28(4), 214-216.

Skiba, D. J. (2007c). Faculty 2.0: Flipping the novice to expert continuum. _Nursing Education Perspectives,_ 28(6), 342-344.

Skiba, D. J., & Barton, A. J. (2006). Adapting your teaching to accommodate the Net generation of learners. _Online Journal of Issues in Nursing,_ 11(2), 15-16.

Skinner, B. F. (1974). _About behaviorism._ New York: Vintage Books.

Smith-Blair, N., & Neighbors, M. (2000). Use of the Critical Thinking Disposition Inventory in critical care orientation. _Journal of Continuing Education in Nursing,_ 31, 251-256.

Snelgrove, S., & Slater, J. (2003). Approaches to learning: Psychometric testing of a study process questionnaire. _Journal of Advanced Nursing,_ 43, 496-505.

Sofaer, B. (1995). Enhancing humanistic skills: An experiential approach to learning about ethical issues in health. _Journal of Medical Ethics,_ 21(1), 31-35.

Sorrell, J. M., Brown, H. N., Silva, M. C., & Kohlenberg, E. M. (1997). Use of writing portfolios for interdisciplinary assessment of critical thinking outcomes of nursing students. _Nursing Forum,_ 32(4), 12-24.

Spelic, S. S., Parson, M., Hercinger, M., Andrews, A., Parks, J., & Norris, J. (2001). Evaluation of critical thinking outcomes in a BSN program. _Holistic Nursing Practice,_ 15, 27-34.

Sperry, R. W. (1977). Bridging science and values: A unifying view of mind and brain. _American Psychologist,_ 32, 237-245.

Speziale, H. J., & Jacobson, L. (2005). Trends in registered nurse education programs 1998-2008. *Nursing Education Perspectives,* 26, 230-235.

Sternas, K., O'Hare, P., Lehman, K., & Milligan, R. (1999). Nursing and medical student teaming for service learning in partnership with the community: An emerging holistic model for interdisciplinary education and practice. *Holistic Nursing Practice,* 13(2), 66-77.

Sternberg, R. (1985). *Beyond IQ: A triarchic theory of intelligence.* New York: Cambridge University Press.

Sternberg, R. J. (1988). Mental self-government: A theory of intellectual styles and their development. *Human Development,* 31, 197-224.

Sternberg, R. J. (1997). *Thinking styles.* New York: Cambridge University Press.

Sternberg, R. J. (2008). The answer depends on the question: A reply to Eric Jensen. *Phi Delta Kappan,* 89, 418-420.

Stes, A., Gijbels, D., & Petegem, P. (2008). Student-focused approaches to teaching in relation to context and teacher characteristics. *Higher Education,* 55, 255-267.

Stone, C. A., Davidson, L. J., Evans, J. L., & Hansen, M. A. (2001). Validity evidence for using a general critical thinking test to measure nursing students' critical thinking. *Holistic Nursing Practice,* 15(4), 65-74.

Takase, M., Maude, P., & Manias, E. (2006). Impact of the perceived public image of nursing on nurses' work behavior. *Journal of Advanced Nursing,* 53, 333-343.

Tanner, C. A. (1999). Evidence-based practice: Research and critical thinking. *Journal of Nursing Education,* 38, 99.

Tapper, J. (2004). Student perceptions of how critical thinking is embedded in a degree program. *Higher Education Research & Development,* 23, 199-222.

Thomas, J., Clarke, B., Pollard, K., & Miers, M. (2007). Facilitating interprofessional enquiry-based learning: Dilemmas and strategies. *Journal of Interprofessional Care,* 21, 463-465.

Thompson, C., & Rebeschi, L. M. (1999). Critical thinking skills of baccalaureate nursing students at program entry and exit. *Nursing and Health Care Perspectives,* 20, 248-252.

Thompson, J. A., & Bing-You, R. G. (1998). Physicians' reactions to learning style and personality type inventories. *Medical Teacher,* 20(1), 10-14.

Tierney, W. (1990). *Assessing academic climates and cultures.* San Francisco: Jossey-Bass.

Titiloye, V. M., & Scott, A. H. (2001). Occupational therapy students' learning styles and application to professional academic training. *Occupational Therapy in Health Care,* 15(1/2), 145-155.

Trigwell, K., & Prosser, M. (2004). Development and use of the Approaches to Teaching Inventory. *Educational Psychology Review,* 16, 409-424.

Trigwell, K., Prosser, M., & Ginns, P. (2005). Phenomenographic pedagogy and a revised Approaches to Teaching Inventory. *Higher Education Research & Development,* 24, 349-360.

Ulsenheimer, J. H., Bailey, D. W., McCullough, E. M., Thornton, S .E., & Warden, E. W. (1997). Thinking about thinking. *Journal of Continuing Education in Nursing,* 28, 150-156.

Vaatstra. R., & Vries, R. (2007). The effect of the learning environment on competences and training for the workplace according to graduates. *Higher Education,* 53, 335-357.

Valle, A., Cabanach, R. G., Nunex, J. C., Gonzalez-Pienda, J., Rodriguez, S., & Pineiro, I. (2003). Cognitive, motivational, and volitional dimensions of learning: An empirical test of a hypothetical model. *Research in Higher Education,* 44, 557-580.

Vandeveer, M. (2005). From teaching to learning: Theoretical foundations. In D. M. Billings & J. A. Halstead (Eds.), *Teaching in nursing: A guide for faculty* (3rd ed.), (pp. 189-223). St. Louis, MO: Saunders.

Vanetzian, E., & Corrigan, B. (1996). "Prep" for class and class activity key to critical thinking. *Nurse Educator,* 21, 45-48.

Vanhanen, L., & Janhonen, S. (2000). Change in students' orientations to nursing during nursing education. *Nurse Education Today,* 20, 654-661.

Vaughan-Wrobel, B. C., O'Sullivan, P., & Smith, L. (1997). Evaluating critical thinking skills of baccalaureate nursing students. *Journal of Nursing Education,* 36, 485-488.

Videbeck, S. L. (1997a). Critical thinking: A model. *Journal of Nursing Education,* 36, 23-28.

Videbeck, S. L. (1997b). Critical thinking: Prevailing practice in baccalaureate schools of nursing. *Journal of Nursing Education,* 36, 5-10.

Vincent, A., & Ross, A. (2001). Learning style awareness: A basis for developing teaching and learning strategies. *Journal of Research on Computing in Education,* 33(5), 1-10.

Wallace, D. (1996). Experiential learning and critical thinking in nursing. *Nursing Standard,* 10(3), 43-47.

Wanstreet, C. E. (2006). Interactions in online learning environments. *Quarterly Review of Distance Education,* 7, 399-411.

Ward, C. W. (2003). Explanatory styles among undergraduate students in a Christian and a state-supported institution of higher learning, and learning orientations. *Christian Higher Education,* 2, 353-365.

Ward, R. (1997). Implications of computer networking and the Internet for nurse education. *Nurse Educator Today,* 17, 178-183.

Weiss, R. P. (2000). Brain-based learning. *Training & Development,* 54(7), 20-24.

Wessel, J., Loomis, J., Rennie, S., Brook, P., Hoddinott, J., & Aherne, M. (1999). Learning styles and perceived problem-solving ability of students in a baccalaureate physiotherapy programme. *Physiotherapy Theory and Practice,* 15(1), 17-24.

Weston, T. (2005). Why faculty did — and did not — integrate instructional software in their undergraduate classrooms. *Innovative Higher Education,* 30, 99-115.

Willingham, D. (2008). When and how neuroscience applies to education. *Phi Delta Kappan,* 89, 421-423.

Willis, J. (2008). Building a bridge from neuroscience to the classroom. *Phi Delta Kappan,* 89, 424-427.

Wlodkowski, R. C. (1978). *Motivation and teaching: A practical guide.* Washington, DC: National Education Association.

Wonder, J., & Donovan, M. (1984). *Whole-brain thinking.* New York: Ballantine.

Wong, F. K. Y., Kember, D., Chung, L. Y. F., & Yan, L. (1995). Assessing the level of student reflection from reflective journals. *Journal of Advanced Nursing,* 22, 48-52.

Wong, T. K. S., & Chung, J. W. Y. (2002). Diagnostic reasoning processes using patient simulation in different learning environments. *Journal of Clinical Nursing, 11*(1), 65-72.

Yacapsin, M., & Stick, S. L. (2007). Study discovers link between instructor's leadership type and teaching styles in the higher education classroom. Online submission for ERIC (ED495250).

Yeh, M. L. (2002). Assessing the reliability and validity of the Chinese version of the Critical Thinking Disposition Inventory. *International Journal of Nursing Students, 39*, 123-132.

Yeh, M. L., & Chen, H. H. (2003). Comparison of affective disposition toward critical thinking across Chinese and American baccalaureate nursing students. *Journal of Nursing Research, 11*, 39-46.

Young, P. K. (2004). Trying something new: Reform as embracing the possible, the familiar, and the at-hand. *Nursing Education Perspectives, 25*, 124-130.

Zalon, M. L. (2000). A prime-time primer for distance education. *Nurse Educator, 25*(1), 28-33.

Zhang, L. (2001). Approaches and thinking styles in teaching. *Journal of Psychology, 135*, 547-561.

Zhang, L. (2004). Thinking styles: University students' preferred teaching styles and their perceptions of effective teachers. *Journal of Psychology, 138*, 233-252.

Zhang, L., & Sternberg, R. J. (2002). Thinking styles and teachers' characteristics. *International Journal of Psychology, 37*(1), 3-12.

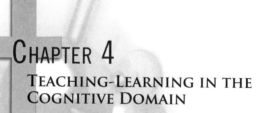

# CHAPTER 4

## TEACHING-LEARNING IN THE COGNITIVE DOMAIN

*Cesarina Thompson, PhD, RN*

"The teachers of this country, one may say,
have its future in their hands."

**William James**

This chapter focuses on teaching and learning in the cognitive domain. It is acknowledged, however, that the cognitive domain is related to the affective and psychomotor domains and that teaching-learning experiences focusing on one domain will often also impact the other domains of learning. Moreover, as noted in the previous chapter, learning is a complex process that is affected by a multitude of factors, such as teacher behaviors, student characteristics, and sociocultural variables. Although this chapter focuses on teaching strategies or teacher behaviors, student characteristics, desired learning outcomes, and the environment or context in which learning takes place also must be considered when selecting and evaluating the effectiveness of any teaching strategy.

## REVIEW OF THE LITERATURE

The following databases were used to search the literature: CINAHL, Academic Search Premier, and ERIC. Initially, the search was limited to literature published between 1995 and 2007. However, given the paucity of literature found during this time period, the search was subsequently expanded to include all relevant literature, regardless of publication date.

As previously noted, there are obvious interrelationships among the three domains of learning. When reviewing teaching-learning methods, it is difficult to identify any strategy that impacts solely on one domain of learning. In addition, there are numerous strategies that are and can be used to promote cognitive learning. However, an exhaustive review of research covering the myriad of cognitive strategies is beyond the scope of this chapter. Being mindful of these challenges, a decision was made to focus the review of literature on three of the most commonly used teaching strategies that promote or enhance cognitive learning: lecture, discussion, and collaborative learning methods.

The following key words and phrases were entered to retrieve relevant research: cognitive learning strategies, critical thinking strategies, lecture method and effects on learning, group work method and effects on learning outcomes, group work and learning, group work and learning in higher education, collaborative learning and higher education, problem-based learning, discussion method and learning, teaching strategies and learning, effective teaching, and effective teaching in higher education. It is interesting to note that the electronic search using these terms yielded very few nursing education research studies, yet research studies in other disciplines were retrieved. A second manual search was subsequently conducted to determine if relevant articles had been missed through the electronic search. A decision was made to review more recent issues (1998-2007) of the *Journal of Nursing Education, Nursing Education Perspectives,* and *Nurse Educator* as these journals specifically publish research in nursing education. As a result, several additional nursing education studies were found using this search method.

As evidence-based articles in nursing education were reviewed, it became evident that some of the studies did not fit into any of the previously established categories (lecture, discussion, collaborative methods), yet the purpose of the studies was to examine the effects of a specific teaching-learning activity on cognitive learning. Thus, these studies are reviewed in a separate section, "Other Teaching Strategies." Similarly, the small number of evidence-based nursing research articles on critical thinking are reviewed in a separate section called "Strategies to Promote Critical Thinking," as they did not clearly fall within the previously established categories of lecture, discussion, or collaborative methods.

## GENERAL OBSERVATIONS

There is no question that research on effective cognitive learning methods has been scarce. As Entwistle and Ramsden (1983) noted, "little direct attention has been given by researchers to the process of student learning and the effects of teaching on it.... Although research into teaching methods is well represented...inquiries relating the teaching to students' learning are much less common" (p. 2). As will be evident in this review, the same conclusion currently applies to research in nursing education. Although the nursing literature is replete with articles that advocate for the use of various teaching methods, there are very few evidence-based articles describing the effectiveness of specific teaching methods. Of the evidence-based articles reviewed, each examined different teaching approaches, making it difficult to formulate general conclusions and implications for nursing education. Interestingly, observations made by Oermann (1990) following a comprehensive review of research on teaching methods in nursing still hold true today, "as seen in other *Nursing Research,* there is a lack of replication of studies on teaching methods in nursing education...few nurse educators have extended their work. One time studies dominate..." (p. 24). Thus, the literature reviewed in this section also reflects educational research conducted in other disciplines. Of the 37 evidenced-based articles reviewed, 21 were conducted by nurse researchers. These are compiled in Table 4.1 which begins on page 162 at the end of this chapter.

What evidence exists to support the effectiveness of teaching strategies focused on promoting learning in the cognitive domain? Early studies of effective teaching in higher education relied on student ratings of teaching effectiveness. Over the past three decades, several educational researchers have conducted comprehensive reviews of the literature on student ratings of teaching effectiveness (Dunkin, 1986; Feldman, 1976; Murray, 1985; Sherman, Armistead, Fowler, Barksdale, & Reif, 1987; Thompson & Sheckley, 1997). These reviews have generally shown that knowledge of the subject matter often is ranked among the top five categories of effective teaching by students across disciplines. In addition, clarity of presentation and organization of material have been consistently associated with characteristics of effective teaching.

In addition to these commonly identified characteristics of effective teaching, Chickering and Gamson (1987) developed a framework known as the Seven Principles for Effective Teaching Practices in Undergraduate Education. These principles are as follows: 1) encourage student-faculty contact, 2) encourage cooperation among students, 3) encourage active learning, 4) give prompt feedback, 5) emphasize time on task, 6) communicate high expectations, and 7) respect diverse talents and ways of learning. According to these researchers, these principles "rest on 50 years of research on the way teachers teach and students learn, how students work and play with one another, and how students and faculty talk to each other" (p. 4). Chickering and Gamson maintain that when all seven principles are present in the learning environment "their effects multiply" (p. 4). Although the literature to support these principles is voluminous, empirical evidence to validate their effectiveness in higher education is not as compelling (Sorcinelli, 1991; Thompson, 1993). While there is ample evidence to support the use of some of the principles in higher education (e.g., encourage cooperation among students), more research is needed to clearly understand the effects of other principles (e.g., emphasize time on task) and to understand how the interaction of selected principles (e.g., prompt feedback combined with high expectations) affects learning.

Thompson (1993) used Chickering and Gamson's seven principles as a framework in her doctoral dissertation to identify the teaching preferences of traditional and nontraditional undergraduate nursing students. Results of this study showed nursing students, regardless of age, preferred teaching practices that included these seven principles (Thompson & Sheckley, 1997). However, as the study did not examine student learning outcomes, it is unknown whether the use of these principles in the classroom had a positive effect on learning.

Although student ratings are commonly used in higher education as a measure of teaching effectiveness, we must question whether the use of students' preferred practices in the classroom necessarily leads to enhanced learning. Garrison and Archer (2000) argue that "measures of effective teaching should be designed so that they are appropriate to the nature of the intended learning outcomes, rather than relying on student ratings, which tend to be closely linked to presentation techniques" (p. 117). In addition, research indicates that what constitutes effective teaching is discipline-specific. Entwistle and Ramsden (1983) studied 2208 students in 66 departments and concluded that "no general recipe for better teaching and assessment can be given" (p. 209) as learning is dependent on individual student differences and on the context in which it takes place. For example, in the sciences "good teaching seems to depend more on operation learning, on relating evidence and conclusions, and on the appropriate use of a certain amount of initial rote learning to master the terminology" (p. 209). In contrast, informal teaching methods, such as discussion, seem to be more effective for students in the arts since they foster the search for personal meaning, which frequently is a goal of arts courses and curricula (Entwistle & Ramsden, 1983).

It also has become clear that teaching practices need to match assessment procedures (Garrison & Archer, 2000). Research indicates that students judged teaching effectiveness based on the type of assessment used. If assessment procedures emphasized recall of facts, then good teaching had to be clearly structured and offered at the right pace. Teaching was rated more highly if the teacher "assumed full responsibility for organizing and presenting content in a way that could be easily reproduced on an exam" (p. 121). Garrison and Archer further indicate that a "connection" is needed between learning outcomes and effective teaching. The ultimate goal of research on teaching is to identify teaching practices that will "have a high probability of realizing desired outcomes" (p. 120). "Approaches to learning reflect a complex relationship between personal and situational factors that lead to differing approaches to learning and the quality of learning outcome" (p. 55).

Based on the review of the literature, research in nursing education is still in its infancy. It is difficult to formulate any conclusions or generalizations about which cognitive teaching strategies are more effective in nursing education because very few articles that describe teaching approaches are evidence-based. Of those that are, most are one-time, isolated studies that do not build on previous research. Moreover, there has been a lack of attention to the relationship among the context of learning, teaching strategies, and desired learning outcomes. The nursing literature is replete with articles advocating the use of the discussion method to promote learning. Although several of these articles suggest that students are more satisfied when this teaching method is used, no evidence is provided to indicate if and when this method might be more effective than another in terms of learning outcomes and when it might be less effective. Ferguson and Day (2005) note that there is wide support among nurse educators for the need to integrate evidence-based practice into the nursing curriculum. Yet, there has been little focus on examining if the teaching and curricular practices employed by nursing faculty themselves are, in fact, evidence-based. The increasing diversity of nursing students and the rapidly expanding knowledge base of the discipline challenge nurse educators to examine teaching practices and determine the most effective ways to help students achieve desired learning outcomes.

# EFFECTS OF TEACHING PRACTICES ON STUDENT PERFORMANCE AND COGNITIVE LEARNING OUTCOMES

## *Lecture*

The lecture method is perhaps the most frequently used teaching strategy in higher education. When using this method, the teacher is primarily responsible for organizing the content and presenting it to students (Rowles & Brigham, 2005). Although some educators have argued that the use of lecture promotes passivity among students and should not be used as a primary teaching strategy, the literature indicates that the lecture can be effective in certain learning situations (McKeachie, Pintrich, Lin, Smith, & Sharma, 1986). Experts caution that the lecture method may not be the preferred method for fostering cognitive (and affective) learning (Menges, Weimer & Associates, 1996). However, it should be noted that this conclusion may only be true when using the most traditional, strictest definition of lecture, where the teacher simply delivers the content without promoting any teacher-student or student-student interactions. Oermann (2004) argues for an integrated approach to teaching nursing that incorporates active learning strategies within lectures to enhance learning outcomes. Although it has been suggested that the use of active learning strategies, such as problem-based learning and discussion, may enhance critical thinking skills, these types of strategies are not always appropriate in a given learning situation. Depending on the curriculum content, the level of student, and the time allotted, the lecture method may be a more appropriate strategy. As Oermann notes, the lecture may be a more effective method to review difficult concepts and illustrate their application in practice, and she provides examples of how faculty can integrate active learning strategies into their lectures so students can gain the benefits of both methods.

Research on the use of the lecture method has focused on teacher characteristics or behaviors in the classroom. Researchers note that student performance in relation to the use of lectures is dependent on two variables: presentation characteristics of the lecturer and student characteristics (Menges et al., 1996). One of the more important lecturer characteristics associated with greater student learning is teacher organization and clarity in presenting the content. Research has shown that highlighting the structure of the content and emphasizing the relationships among concepts throughout the lecture enhances student achievement (Menges et al.). Lecture can be effective if cognitive involvement is fostered by using reflection during the presentation, illustrating points with relevant examples, and providing a framework for organizing the information (Garrison & Archer, 2000).

Oulette (1986) describes how to apply and evaluate the use of the Ausubel Model to facilitate nursing students' retention of information presented through lecture. The model, originally described by David Ausubel in 1963, provides a framework for selecting essential information to be presented and organizing that information in a logical and sequential manner (e.g., simple to complex) to facilitate student learning and integration of new content with information previously learned (Ausubel, 2000). **Advanced organizers** are teaching tools that help learners "bridge the gap" between existing and new knowledge (Ausubel, 2000, p. 11). Ausubel's model consists of two types of advanced organizers that are used to frame the content to be taught. **Comparative organizers** are used to explain new concepts that may share similarities with familiar concepts, and **expository organizers** are used when new information is introduced to provide the learner with an outline of topics and how these topics relate to each other. Advanced organizers provide the learner with ideas and concepts about the new material to be learned, but at a higher level of abstraction. Thus, they serve as anchors for new ideas that are introduced (Ausubel, 2000).

Gillies (1984) reported on a quasi-experimental study in which expository advanced organizers were used before presenting content in a medical-surgical nursing course. The sample consisted of 43 baccalaureate students, 21 of whom were in the experimental group that received the advanced organizers and 22 of whom were in the control group that received the placebo treatment. Prior to presenting the content on peripheral circulatory disorders, students in the experimental group were provided with a 300-word written advanced organizer that described more general information and principles related to the class content, such as consequences of cellular ischemia, possible causes of ischemia, and treatment modalities. The control group was given a 300-word written passage of historical information related to a topic such as Harvey's discovery of how blood travels throughout the body. Student performance was measured through the use of quizzes at the end of each class, unit exams, and final course exams. Findings showed that the use of advanced organizers increased initial learning for some students, but was not effective in promoting retention of content.

In the field of education, Kiewra et al. (1997) compared the effects of lecture presentation in combination with various types of advanced organizers on the learning outcomes of 109 students enrolled in an educational psychology course. Results showed that organizers facilitated information recall and an ability to relate topics to one another.

According to Ausubel (2000), the effective use of advanced organizers contributes to meaningful rather than rote learning. Meaningful learning results in a "modification of both the newly acquired information and of the specifically relevant aspect of cognitive structure to which the new information is linked" (p. 3). The use of advanced organizers requires educators to carefully assess the learners' readiness for learning (e.g., cognitive maturity and existing knowledge base) as a basis for organizing and presenting materials. Ausubel acknowledges that some educators have rejected the use of the expository, or lecturing, method because they presume this strategy does not promote meaningful learning. He argues, however, that since educators have not paid enough attention to the process of knowledge acquisition and retention and how to best construct and present materials to foster meaningful learning, discarding lecture as a teaching strategy may be premature. According to Ausubel, the following are ineffective expository teaching practices:

1.  premature use of pure verbal techniques with cognitively immature pupils

2.  arbitrary presentation of unrelated facts without any organizing or explanatory principles

3.  failure to integrate new learning tasks with previously presented materials

4.  use of evaluation procedures that merely measure ability to recognize discrete facts or to reproduce ideas in the same words or in the identical context as originally encountered (p. 7).

Although much of the more recent research on the use and effectiveness of the lecture method has been conducted in other disciplines, most investigations have been in disciplines that provide a foundation for nursing education (e.g., physics and communication) or for other health professions (e.g., occupational therapy). Thus, these findings may be quite relevant to nursing education.

Some researchers have focused on student characteristics or behaviors when listening to a lecture. For example, studies show that learning outcomes are improved when note taking is used with a lecture. Titsworth (2001) found that when students enrolled in a basic communication course (N=233) used note taking, their performance on detail and concept tests increased. Findings from other studies show that the act of note taking itself forces students to encode the information, rather than just recording it, and thus improves learning (Menges et al., 1996). These findings suggest that it is more beneficial for students to take and review their own notes rather than rely on the instructors' or other students' notes (Menges et al.). Better note taking, and, ultimately, better cognitive outcomes may be achieved by students when note taking is guided by the instructors' questions and reflections throughout the lecture.

In addition, studies have shown that the use of a matrix format (a diagram showing the complex relationships among concepts), rather than the traditional linear outline format, when taking notes enhances learning. A study conducted in nursing supports this assertion. Rooda (1994) examined the effects of mind mapping on the achievement of students in a nursing research course. A quasi-experimental design was used to compare achievement of students exposed to mind mapping (N=24) with that of students not introduced to this method (N=36). Each unit of content was presented using the traditional lecture method and was followed by mind mapping activities. These activities involved students mapping the content presented on the blackboard with help from classmates. Results showed that the group using mind mapping did significantly better on course exams than the group not using this method. A number of articles in the nursing literature have been published in the last few years that advocate the use of mind mapping or concept mapping as a method to enhance critical thinking. This area of literature is reviewed in the "Strategies to Promote Critical Thinking" section of this chapter.

Researchers in other disciplines have compared the effectiveness of the lecture to other teaching/learning methods. For example, Dal Bello-Haas, Bazyk, Ekelman, and Milidonis (1999) compared the effectiveness of the feedback lecture method with the traditional lecture method among occupational and physical therapy students enrolled in a neurology medicine class. The students in the traditional lecture class (N=16) were given a reading assignment to complete before class and then attended an 80-minute class in which the instructor presented the content on traumatic brain injuries (TBI). The students in the feedback lecture group (N=15) were given study guides four days prior to the class on TBI with specific learning objectives. The students then attended the class, which was divided into two 30-minute segments: each segment included two, 10-minute segments for small-group discussion. All students completed a pre-test and post-test following the class. Students were again tested four months after the class to measure long-term retention of content. Results showed that there were no significant differences in pre-test and post-test scores between the two groups. The authors identified several study limitations, such as small sample size, that may have influenced the results. The authors also note that the type of content covered in this class is at the lower level of the cognitive domain and thus could "be learned just as effectively with less active teaching methods" (p. 39). This observation is consistent with that of McKeachie et al. (1986) and other researchers (Garrison & Archer, 2000) who emphasize that any teaching method may be effective if it is appropriate for the desired learning outcomes.

Similarly, Zitzmann (1996) compared the learning outcomes of students in an introductory course in clinical parasitology (N=29) by teaching the first half of the course using the traditional lecture method and using self-instructional modules for the second half of the course. Students were given an objective exam at the end of each half of the course. Results showed that there were no significant differences in exam scores when comparing the two methods. As identified by the author, the particular course examined in this study "involves a large amount of memorization, which lends itself to self-instuction" (p. 198).

Moreover, Liotta-Kleinfeld and McPhee (2001) compared the use of the traditional lecture method and the problem-based learning method in a neuroscience course for occupational therapy students. Learning outcomes were measured through an 85-item multiple choice final exam consisting of questions written at various levels of Bloom's cognitive domain taxonomy. Results showed that there were no significant differences in test scores between the traditional lecture group (N=18) and the problem-based learning group (N=25).

In contrast, Hwang & Kim (2006) reported that baccalaureate nursing students in Korea who were taught adult health nursing content using the problem-based learning (PBL) method (N =35) scored significantly higher on a knowledge test than students who were taught using the traditional didactic method (N=36). The authors further examined the data by students' GPA and found that students in the problem-based method who had lower GPAs demonstrated the greatest gains in scores. The authors note that this study is one of only a few that show a positive effect of problem-based learning on student learning outcomes and suggest that this may be a particularly beneficial method for students with lower GPAs. However, the strategies used with students in the PBL group may have had an effect on the results. Based on the authors' description of the methodology, students in the PBL group were presented case scenarios and were asked to work in small groups to identify clinical issues and then develop concept maps of the nursing and medical concepts. Each session was then followed by a 10-20 minute feedback session. It is unclear what was discussed in these sessions. In addition, each of the seven PBL modules was supplemented by two to three 2-hour class sessions conducted by one of the investigators. Although what was presented in these 2-hour sessions is not described by the authors, it would appear that the students in the PBL group benefited from the use of a mixed method of learning — group activities and discussion typical of PBL method and the more traditional didactic method. Thus, the higher scores received by the PBL group on the post-test cannot be attributed solely to the use of the PBL method. The combination of the PBL method and the didactic sessions may also explain the greater gains achieved by students with lower GPAs.

More recently, Carrero, Gomar, Penzo, and Rull (2007) used a randomized, controlled method to compare the effectiveness of using problem-based learning and the traditional lecture method with a group of first-year anesthesia residents who completed a class on "pre-anesthesia assessment" over two consecutive years. Participants were randomly assigned to the problem-based class (total for two years, N=25) or lecture class (total for two years, N=29). Four tests (two pre-tests and two post-tests) were developed based on four similar cases that simulated preoperative patients. Both groups were given a pre-test immediately prior to the teaching session and a post-test immediately following the class sessions. The tests measured six knowledge areas of relevance to pre-anesthesia assessment, including recognizing clinical data and clinical reasoning. Results showed that participants in both groups improved their scores on the post-tests. However, there were no significant differences in the overall achievement between the two groups when scores of pre- and post-tests were compared. The authors concluded that both methods are effective when measuring short-term knowledge acquisition and retention.

Beers (2005) compared the effectiveness of two teaching methods — lecture and problem-based learning — on test scores of nursing students. Two groups of students enrolled in Adult Health I during two consecutive semesters (fall 2001, N=18; spring 2002, N=36) participated in the study. Students who enrolled in the fall course were taught diabetes content using the lecture method only. Students enrolled in the spring course were taught the content using problem-based learning. Both groups were given a pre-test and a post-test following the class sessions. The 10-item objective tests used before and after the teaching sessions were developed by Health Education Systems, Inc. (HESI). Results showed that there was no statistically significant difference in the pre-test scores of the two groups and no statistically significant difference between the two groups on the post-test.

Menges et al. (1996) note that "the available research on learning from lecture suggests that it is no better or worse than other methods on a very gross level" (p. 263). Based on evidence, these researchers further suggest that the use of the lecture method can be enhanced by encouraging students to take and review notes and by helping students build connections among concepts.

The effectiveness of the lecture as a teaching method may also be related to the lecturing skills of faculty. Expertise in a subject area does not necessarily result in teaching expertise. Although faculty may be prepared as content experts, not all have had teacher preparation. Diekelmann (2002) contends that teachers must engage in reflective thinking about their lecturing skills to facilitate learning. Teachers need to assess what students know, what they do not know, and how they experience learning to develop effective lectures (Diekelmann, 2002; Diekelmann, Swenson, & Sims, 2003). "Lecturing...is more about following students' thinking and learning than about presenting and applying knowledge in problem-solving situations" (Diekelmann, 2002, p. 98). Young and Diekelmann (2002) conducted a qualitative study to describe how new teachers in nursing learned to lecture. Findings revealed that many of the new teachers interviewed concentrated on the process of teaching rather than on student learning. Lecturing skills can be enhanced by being reflective about one's teaching and assessing students' understanding by "reading" students' faces, questioning students, engaging them in dialogue, and constructing learning experiences to facilitate student learning (Diekelmann, 2002).

## Discussion

There are a variety of teaching-learning strategies that can be included under the category of discussion. The literature indicates that this teaching method has received much support in higher education because "it appears to place teachers and students on equal footing" (Brookfield, 1990, p. 88). This teaching method has been recommended especially for adult learners to help students integrate new knowledge with their previous experiences. In fact, research shows that relating class topics to students' lives and experiences is perceived as an effective teaching method by adult learners (Thompson, 1993).

McKeachie et al. (1986) describe many methods with the common goal of encouraging greater student participation in the classroom. These various methods have been also commonly referred to as "student-centered" approaches. Research in this area indicates that discussion methods may be more effective for long-term retention of concepts and for promoting learning in the cognitive (and affective) domain (Menges et al., 1996). Refer to Chapter 6 for further findings on the interconnectedness of the affective and cognitive domains.

According to Menges et al., how teachers and students relate to each other is an important element of discussion. The types of questions posed by the teacher and the type of feedback given to students have an impact on learning; however, there is debate among researchers as to how significant this impact may be. House, Chassie, and Spohn (1992) maintain that, "the more difficult and complex the question, the higher the thinking level demanded" (p. 197). The authors describe various types of questioning techniques to facilitate learning including, delivery, wait time, and feedback. Although this article was published in a nursing journal, no application was made to nursing education.

While the use of this method is widely supported by educators, Brookfield (1990) cautions that its use and purpose must be well planned to promote meaningful discussions and avoid potential detriments to learning within a group (e.g., a sense of competitiveness among students or a tendency for extroverted students to monopolize the discussion). Brookfield describes various elements to consider in planning and facilitating an effective discussion, such as dealing with overtalkative students, reducing analytical confusion, and protecting minority viewpoints.

Although the use of "active" teaching strategies, such as the discussion method, has been widely encouraged by nurse educators to enhance learning and critical thinking abilities, there is very little empirical evidence demonstrating the effect of discussion on learning. Gray (2003) reports on the use of a teaching strategy to develop students' thinking and discussion skills in a senior seminar on Trends and Issues in Nursing. Although the author notes that the strategy facilitated accomplishments of course objectives that addressed leadership, communication, and critical thinking, it is unknown from the information presented how this strategy specifically facilitated cognitive learning.

Rossignol (1997) examined the relationship between discourse strategies used by teachers and students and student critical thinking abilities. According to this researcher, discourse strategies are teacher-centered and student-centered techniques. Both techniques are used in dialogue to foster critical thinking (e.g., probing questions, elaboration, and high level questions). A total of 57 senior baccalaureate nursing students enrolled in a clinical course participated in all phases of the study. Surprisingly, findings showed that teacher use of probing questions and elaborations was significantly associated with low level of student critical thinking abilities as measured by the Watson-Glaser Critical Thinking Appraisal (WGCTA). In addition, greater student participation in the discussion was associated with lower levels of student critical thinking. Rossignol notes that the findings contradict the common assumption that greater student participation in discussion leads to higher levels of critical thinking abilities. The author concludes that faculty should focus on the quality, rather than the quantity, of student participation to promote the development of critical thinking.

### Collaborative Learning

Slavin (1980) describes cooperative learning as classroom techniques that require students to work in small groups and receive rewards or recognition based on their group's performance. "Collaborative learning restructures the classroom away from the traditional lecture to small group work requiring intensive interactions between students and the faculty member while working through complex projects" (Cabrera, Nora, Bernal, Terenzini, & Pascarella, 1998, p. 2).

Research suggests that the use of collaborative strategies has a positive effect on students' cognitive development and long-term knowledge retention as well as their personal development. In addition, the use of collaborative learning may be especially beneficial for women and minorities, because research indicates that these groups prefer learning styles that emphasize connected learning and collaborative learning (Adams, 1992).

The use and benefits of cooperative learning strategies have been extensively researched and advocated in primary and secondary levels. However, research on the effect of collaborative learning strategies across various disciplines in higher education has been limited and yielded inconsistent results. One explanation for these disparate results is that, for the most part, studies have focused on examining the effects of a specific collaborative teaching strategy in an individual course. Typically, these studies have been isolated investigations in a specific discipline. As evidenced by the examples provided below, most studies have been conducted with small samples, limiting the generalizability of findings and limiting the ability to synthesize findings across studies. More recent research is highlighted here to illustrate these points.

A study of 2,050 second-year college students enrolled in 23 institutions in spring 1994 (sample drawn from the National Study of Student Learning, which is a longitudinal investigation of factors influencing learning and development in college) revealed that collaborative learning was the single best predictor for the cognitive (and affective) outcomes that had been defined: personal development, understanding of science and technology, appreciation for art, analytic skills, and openness to diversity (Cabrera et al., 1998).

The impact of participating in various types of collaborative learning experiences (e.g., working in groups in and out of class, participating in internships) was examined by conducting interviews with 65 engineering students from 7 institutions participating in the Engineering Coalition of Schools for Excellence in Education and Leadership (ECSEL) (Colbeck, Campbell, & Bjorklund, 2000). Study participants reported that working in groups enhanced their ability to communicate, solve problems, and manage conflict. Students were especially positive about internship experiences that gave them the opportunity to work with industry partners. However, they also described the challenges of working in groups when individual group members' goals vary (e.g., some are interested only in the grade, while others are more interested in learning as much as they can from the experience) and when there is lack of guidance from instructors. Although the authors conclude that students benefit from participating in group projects, academic achievement of students was not examined in this study. The authors do recommend that future research examine the relationship of participating in group work to student gains in professional skills.

In the field of mathematics, Lane and Aleksic (2002) redesigned a section of a traditional, lecture-based statistics course to include laboratory sessions in which students worked in groups to solve problems. A pre- and post-test design was used to measure content knowledge in all sections of the course. Scores for students in the experimental section (N=140) were compared to scores of students who were enrolled in sections using the traditional, lecture-based format (N=340). There were no differences in students' pre-test scores, but students in the experimental section did significantly better on the content knowledge post-test.

Similarly, Duncan and Dick (2000) examined the effectiveness of offering supplemental collaborative learning groups in four mathematics courses. A total of 291 students enrolled in four different math courses volunteered to participate in these workshops led by graduate students and former program participants. Participating students worked with one another to solve challenging math problems related to the content of the course in which they were enrolled. Data were collected over five academic semesters. Data analysis included a comparison of predicted course grade (calculated based on math SAT scores) to the actual grade received as a result of participating in the workshops. Results showed that course grades for students who participated in the program were more than one-half point better than the predicted grade (p<.001).

In the field of physics, Cox and Junkin (2002) examined learning outcomes of students in an introductory physics lab. The experimental group consisted of 59 students, and the control group consisted of 70 students; each group was divided into two sections. A pre-test and post-test consisting of 10 multiple choice items was used to measure learning gains. Results showed that students in the experimental group, who worked with group members and others outside their group to answer lab questions, scored significantly higher on the post-test than the control group students, who completed the labs individually.

In contrast, studies have shown that although many students prefer collaborative teaching methods, the use of these methods does not necessarily affect cognitive achievement. Booth and James (2001) modified a traditional physics class by including cooperative learning techniques. The content of the lectures was not modified from the previous year to allow for group comparisons. During the course of the lecture, questions were posed to the class. Students were asked to think about each question individually and then discuss it with a partner to formulate an answer. The aim of this strategy was to enhance deep learning rather than surface understanding of concepts. A 30-item test of conceptual knowledge of mechanics was used to measure performance. Performance of students in the revised course (N=52) was compared to that of students who had completed the same course the previous two years (N=60; combined total for both years). Results showed that while students gave positive ratings to the new teaching method, their performance scores were not significantly different than scores attained by students in the previous year.

Wathen and Resnick (1997) examined the effectiveness of using explanations and "talking aloud" on learning biology content by comparing (a) individual student achievement using these two collaborative learning strategies (N=16 using each strategy) with (b) students using the same learning strategies but working in dyads (N=16 dyads using each strategy). The incorporation of collaborative learning through the use of dyads had no effect on cognitive achievement as evaluated by a factual learning measure given to the subjects at the beginning and at the end of a learning module on the circulatory system. This study's findings addresses the question posed earlier in this section, namely, whether the use of students' preferred teaching style means they will learn more. Wathen and Resnick suggest that this may not be the case; but they do support the assertion that intended learning outcomes should guide the selection of teaching practices.

As noted in a review of the literature conducted by McKeachie et al. (1986), collaborative/cooperative strategies may not show up as more effective when student achievement is measured by an objective exam. Cooperative/collaborative teaching methods are designed to foster group membership skills, promote more positive interpersonal relationships among students, and make the learning situation less threatening (Johnson & Johnson, 1987; McKeachie et al.). Thus, teachers may be doing good things and having positive results, but researchers may be using the wrong instruments to measure relevant outcomes.

The inconsistent findings reported here also may be due to the various definitions and descriptions that researchers have ascribed to "cooperative/collaborative learning strategies." For example, the term "collaborative learning" has been used to describe students working in pairs or in groups on in-class or out-of-class assignments, students tutoring other students, and students leading in-class discussions or seminars (Thompson, 1993). The variability in the structures and processes of these learning situations may have much to do with the studies' results.

Given the nature of the health care delivery system, there is a need for nurses to work collaboratively with other health care professionals to promote positive patient outcomes. Although support for the use of collaborative learning strategies can be found in the nursing literature (Reuland, 2000), there is a lack of empirical evidence that demonstrates the effects of these strategies on learning. One empirical study found in the nursing literature focused on the frequency with which staff development educators used collaborative teaching strategies in teaching nurses (Viau, 1994). Results showed that staff development educators used a combination of teacher-centered and learner-centered strategies. In addition, staff development educators with master's and doctoral degrees were more likely than baccalaureate-prepared educators to use learner-centered strategies (Viau). This finding is not surprising, as content for adult education and adult learning strategies (of which collaborative learning is a key component) is more likely to be incorporated in graduate nursing programs.

Another, more recent study explored the effectiveness of using collaborative testing to facilitate learning in a Fundamentals of Nursing course (Lusk & Conklin, 2003). Students (N=25) completed all unit exams by answering test questions individually for the first 40 minutes of the testing period and then were allowed to discuss their answers with a randomly assigned partner for the last 20 minutes of the testing period. Based on this discussion, students could change their answers or retain their original answer. All students completed the final exam using the traditional, individualized method to assess comprehension of course content. Performance of students using the collaborative testing method was compared to that of students who had completed the course the previous year using the traditional testing method (N=24). Results showed that while students using the collaborative method performed better on the unit exams, final exam scores did not differ between the two groups. Although the use of the collaborative testing method did not result in higher scores on final exams, there were some unexpected benefits derived from this method. Students reported that they spent more time studying, and they learned to respect and value the opinions of other students (Lusk & Conklin).

Goodfellow (1995) used cooperative learning strategies in a nursing research course. Students were required to meet for one hour each week with their group to develop a research poster. In addition, students were grouped informally during class to work on specific learning tasks related to the class topic. Results showed that students achieved higher midterm and final exam grades than previous students who were taught using traditional methods.

Elberson, Vance, Stephenson, and Corbett (2001) examined the effectiveness of using cooperative learning strategies in an undergraduate pathophysiology course. Nursing students were assigned to groups consisting of three to five participants. Each group was required to research a course-related topic, develop a creative teaching strategy for the topic, and display their project for evaluation. The majority of students reported that the cooperative learning strategy facilitated retention of content, increased motivation to learn, and promoted teamwork. A small number of students identified concerns with group dynamics. Although Elberson et al. contend that "cooperative learning is an effective strategy for learning difficult content" (p. 261), no objective measures for evaluating learning outcomes are reported.

Dickerson, Peters, Walkowiak, and Brewer (1999) reported on the use of active learning strategies to teach case management to RN-BSN students. As part of the course requirements, students worked in pairs to develop a clinical pathway. Although the authors stated that the active learning approach used to teach case management "can be effective in an educational setting" (p. 57), the data presented suggested that the method was not necessarily successful in fostering achievement of learning outcomes. The authors reported that the papers "did not reflect a thorough understanding about identifying outcomes and variance tracking" (p. 55), an important concept to understand in relation to critical pathways.

## STRATEGIES TO PROMOTE CRITICAL THINKING

Critical thinking has been a topic of discussion in the educational literature for many years. Although educators outside the discipline of nursing have proposed various definitions of critical thinking, there are underlying similarities among these definitions (Halpern, 1996). A widely known and referenced definition is that produced by the Delphi study sponsored by the American Philosophical Association (APA) (Facione, 1990). Facione surveyed 53 experts from various disciplines to arrive at a consensus statement of critical thinking:

> We understand critical thinking to be purposeful, self-regulatory judgment which [sic] results in interpretation, analysis, evaluation, and inference as well as explanation of the evidential, conceptual, methodological, criteriological, or contextual considerations upon which judgment is based (p. 2).

Scriven and Paul (2007) define critical thinking to be an "intellectually disciplined process of actively and skillfully conceptualizing, applying, analyzing, synthesizing and/or evaluating information gathered from, or generated by, observation, experience, reflection, reasoning, or communication as a guide to belief and action." Similarly, Halpern defined critical thinking as "purposeful, reasoned, and goal directed — the kind of thinking involved in solving problems, formulating inferences, calculating likelihoods, and making decisions when the thinker is using skills that are thoughtful and effective for the particular context and type of thinking task" (p. 5). According to Brookfield (1990), the development of critical thinking should be a goal of college teaching. He explains that educators should help learners develop "a critically alert cast of mind — one that is skeptical of claims to final truths or ultimate solutions to problems, is open to alternatives, and acknowledges the contextuality of knowledge" (pp. 21-22).

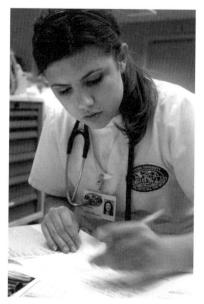

Although critical thinking is not new to nursing education, the concept became a focus of scholarly discussion and debate among nurse educators after it was incorporated in the National League for Nursing's accreditation criteria in the 1990s (NLN, 1996). The American Association of Colleges of Nursing also includes critical thinking as a core competency of professional nursing practice at the baccalaureate level and defines it as "independent and interdependent decision making...that includes questioning, analysis, synthesis, interpretation, inference, inductive and deductive reasoning, intuition, application and creativity" (AACN, 1998, p. 9). In addition, critical thinking is identified as a core competency of advanced practice nursing (AACN, 1996). A study by Valiga and Bruderle (1994) in fact showed that faculty in associate degree and baccalaureate programs rated critical thinking as a concept critical to the nursing curriculum.

Although a thorough review of the literature in this area is beyond the scope of this chapter, an overview of more recent nursing literature is provided in this section. (See Chapter 3 for further information about critical thinking research findings.) A number of articles have been published in the nursing literature focusing on teaching and measuring critical thinking abilities of nursing students. However, the majority of these articles are not evidence-based, but simply describe the use of specific strategies thought to promote the development of critical thinking, such as group activities, discussion, journaling, concept/ mind mapping, and inquiry-based learning (Abegglen & O'Neill Conger, 1997; Bell et al., 2002; Daley, Shaw, Balistrieri, Glasenapp, & Piacentine, 1999; Lierman, 1997).

More recently, Ellerman, Kataoka-Yahiro, and Wong (2006) described the use of logic models in one nursing program to enhance students' critical thinking skills. The authors describe the use of several instructional methods — concept mapping, concept papers, conceptual linking and substruction (a tool used to evaluate concepts in a research study) — to facilitate integration of concepts across the curriculum. Each instructional tool is introduced at a specific point in the curriculum, with concept mapping and concept papers used earlier in the program and conceptual linking and substruction used in the senior year. The faculty introduced these new ways of looking at clinical data to "stimulate continuous input with a dynamic flow of ideas that prompts relationships and influences to be considered in multiple directions" (p. 221), rather than promote only a linear approach to data analysis that is reinforced by strictly using the nursing process. The first cohort of students who were exposed to all four methods (N=33) were asked to rate their level of critical thinking at the beginning and at the end of the nursing program. Data showed that students believed their level of critical thinking had significantly increased and a majority felt capable of making clinical decisions. However, findings of the study are based only on students' self-reports. There was no objective method used to evaluate gains in critical thinking skills. While the concept of logic models seem to have obvious applications to the discipline of nursing, more research in this area is needed.

Some nurse educators have argued that a definition of critical thinking needs to be discipline-specific and have attempted to develop such a definition that reflects thinking skills needed in nursing practice. Scheffer and Rubenfeld (2000) used a similar approach as that used in the APA consensus study to survey nursing experts in 10 countries and develop a definition of critical thinking in nursing. The Delphi study included five rounds of surveys with the number of respondents in each round ranging from 42 to 72 experts.

The following consensus statement was developed and agreed upon by 88% (45) of the 51 experts who responded to the final round of surveys:

*Critical thinking in nursing is an essential component of professional accountability and quality of nursing care. Critical thinkers in nursing exhibit these habits of the mind: confidence, contextual perspective, creativity, flexibility, inquisitiveness, intellectual integrity, intuition, open-mindedness, perseverance, and reflection. Critical thinkers in nursing practice the cognitive skills of analyzing, applying standards, discriminating, information seeking, logical reasoning, predicting and transforming knowledge, and using logical standards (p. 357).*

Although this definition was derived from nursing experts, the thinking abilities identified in this definition are not unlike those found in the APA consensus statement. However, a general observation that can be made from the available literature is that no consensus has been achieved to date on how to define and measure critical thinking in nursing (Angel, Duffey, & Belyea, 2000; Riddell, 2007; Walsh & Seldomridge, 2006). From a research perspective, this lack of consensus has significantly impacted the development and growth of a scientific base of knowledge in this area.

Given the expectations of professional nursing organizations that publish educational guidelines and standards and nursing accrediting bodies, there has been a focus in nursing education on measuring critical thinking as a program outcome. A number of nurse educators have conducted studies to evaluate the critical thinking gains of nursing students. However, these types of studies have yielded inconsistent findings (Adams, 1999; Shin, Lee, Ha, & Kim, 2006; Thompson & Rebeschi, 1999). One explanation for these findings is that, in most cases, the method used to measure critical thinking has not been appropriate given the definition of critical thinking used in a particular program. For example, the California Critical Thinking Skills Test (CCTST) and the California Critical Thinking Dispositions Inventory (CCTDI) have been used by faculty in a number of nursing programs to measure critical thinking outcomes. However, these instruments are based on a specific definition of critical thinking (Facione, 1990).

The use of these instruments to measure critical thinking outcomes is not appropriate unless the definitions on which these instruments are based are in fact employed and integrated in the nursing curriculum. The measurement of critical thinking outcomes provides little useful data unless the process (teaching strategies) by which they were achieved can also be documented and examined. Recent studies designed to examine the effectiveness of teaching strategies on student learning and critical thinking abilities are reviewed in this section.

Magnussen, Ishida, and Itano (2000) examined the effects of inquiry-based learning (a modification of problem-based learning) during clinical conferences on the critical thinking abilities of students in a baccalaureate nursing program. The Watson-Glaser

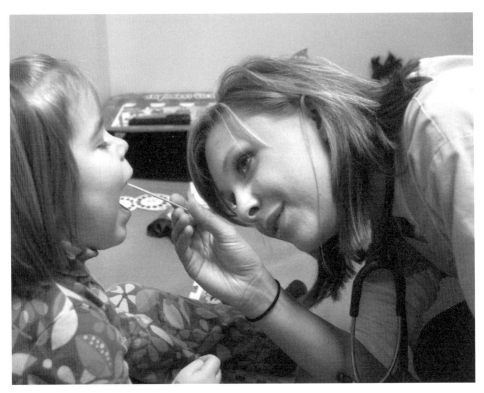

Critical Thinking Appraisal (WGCTA) was administered to students upon entry into the nursing program and again at exit from the program to measure critical thinking gains. A total of 150 students completed both the pre- and the post-test. Results showed that only students whose scores on the pre-test were considered low showed significant gains on the post-test. Students who had scored in the medium and high ranges on the pre-test actually showed a drop in scores on the post-test. The authors offer several explanations for these inconsistent findings that also have been noted by other researchers (e.g., Thompson & Rebeschi, 1999). Two of these concerns that warrant mention and consideration by researchers are the timing of testing and the validity of measurement instruments. Although the pre-test/post-test design is methodologically sound, student motivation to do well on the post-test may be limited if there are no consequences for poor performance. Thus, scores obtained on the post-test may not be a valid reflection of students' abilities.

Perhaps a more important issue for nurse educators to consider is that the method of evaluation must be appropriate for the teaching methodologies employed. The inquiry-based learning strategy described by Magnussen et al. (2000) may in fact be effective in enhancing critical thinking. However, the WGCTA may not be a valid instrument to assess its effectiveness.

Stewart and Dempsey (2005) conducted a longitudinal study of baccalaureate nursing students to determine if critical thinking dispositions were related to students' GPA and performance on the NCLEX-RN licensure exam. The California Critical Thinking Disposition Inventory (CCTDI) was used to measure critical thinking dispositions as students progressed through the program. The sample initially consisted of all sophomore level students (N=55), but due to significant attrition, the senior level sample consisted of 34 students. Results showed that although scores improved from the sophomore to the junior levels, overall scores did not increase significantly from the sophomore to the senior levels. Interestingly, there were no significant differences between the CCTDI scores of students who passed the NCLEX-RN and those who did not. In fact, the CCTDI scores of students who did not pass were 11 points higher than the scores of students who did pass. The findings of this study further support the idea that standardized instruments to measure critical thinking abilities may not be valid to measure thinking skills relevant to nursing practice. The authors agree with others who have suggested that discipline-specific instruments may more accurately measure nursing students' thinking abilities (Stewart & Dempsey).

Angel et al., (2000) conducted a longitudinal study to compare the effectiveness of two learning strategies on the knowledge acquisition and critical thinking abilities of baccalaureate nursing students in their first clinical semester. A total of 142 students participated in the study. Data were collected from students enrolled in a beginning level nursing course, Basic Theories, Concepts, and Skills for Clinical Nursing. Students' critical thinking abilities were measured at the beginning of the semester using the WGCTA. In addition, initial critical thinking abilities were assessed using a case study designed to determine students' knowledge and thinking processes. One group (N=72) completed weekly health patterns assessments on their patients using a form designed by the faculty (structured format). The other group (N=70) completed the same assignment, but was required to conduct and record the assessment using a format designed by the students (unstructured format). Results indicated that knowledge and critical thinking abilities (measured through case study) increased significantly for all students, regardless of strategy used.

Although there were no overall differences in knowledge and critical thinking between the two groups, there were some differences found when the variables of age and previous educational background of students were examined. Older students benefited more from the use of the unstructured format, while younger students benefited more from the use of the structured format. This finding is consistent with adult learning literature and adult development theory (e.g., Perry's [1970] stages of intellectual development) that suggests tolerance for ambiguity increases as one advances in age. The authors conclude that, "it is not the learning strategy alone that influences educational outcomes; perhaps it is the interaction between learning strategy and characteristics of the learner that influences gain in knowledge outcomes" (Angel et al., 2000, p. 227).

Another area of investigation related to critical thinking development has been the use of concept mapping, particularly in the clinical setting (Schuster, 2000). Although not all of these articles are based on empirical evidence, findings from more recent research as well as previous research conducted by Rooda (1994) suggest that this may be a useful strategy to incorporate in the classroom as well as clinical teaching. Daley et al. (1999) introduced concept mapping to senior baccalaureate nursing students enrolled in their final clinical course. Students developed three concept maps during the semester that were scored based on hierarchical organization, differentiation of concepts, and cross linkages among concepts. These criteria and scoring methodology have been established by researchers in the area of concept mapping (Novak & Gowin, 1984, as cited in Daley et al., 1999). Findings showed that over the course of the semester students' concept maps became increasingly more complex, illustrating a greater number of interrelationships among client data, pathophysiological and pharmacological factors, and nursing interventions. Results showed a statistically significant difference in conceptual and critical thinking between the first map and the final concept map created by students. The authors do caution that this was a preliminary study. Only the work of 18 students was analyzed across the semester. However, these students were randomly selected from 6 clinical groups. The authors recommend replication of the study and further research to assess the construct validity of concept maps as a measurement of critical thinking (Daley et al.).

McGovern and Valiga (1997) examined the cognitive development of freshmen nursing students and evaluated the effects of using developmental instructional strategies on cognitive growth. The Learning Context Questionnaire (LCQ), an instrument based on Perry's (1970) scheme of cognitive development, was used to assess stages of development of nursing students enrolled in first-year nursing courses. A total of 66 students completed the survey in the fall semester and 71 completed the survey in the spring semester. Of the 66 students who participated in the study during the fall, 14 received the experimental treatment, while 52 participated in the traditional class format. In the spring semester, 17 students received the experimental treatment, while 54 served as the control group. The goal of developmental instruction by educational theorists is to foster learning by using a mix of strategies that supports students' current level of development, yet challenges them to go beyond their current capabilities (McGovern & Valiga). According to this framework, the degree of personalism (e.g., trust and respect) demonstrated by the teacher and the degree of structure provided (e.g., directions for assignments, grading criteria, etc.) reflect support strategies, while the degree of diversity and types of learning experiences represent strategies that challenge students. As the learner grows and develops, the degree of support provided is decreased, while the degree of challenge offered is increased.

Students in the experimental groups were exposed to instructional strategies based on this developmental framework. For example, students were challenged through engaging discussions of issues that incorporated a variety of perspectives (diversity) and they learned through direct experiences as well as from each other (types of experiences). Support strategies were incorporated into the learning environment by providing students with a high degree of structure for their assignments (e.g., clear directions and evaluation criteria), but, at the same time, structure was minimized by varying the seating arrangements in the classroom. Personalism was emphasized by the use of "One-Minute Papers" that allowed faculty to assess students' understanding/misconceptions about topics discussed and the use of extensive feedback on all written assignments.

Results showed that all students, despite teaching strategy used, demonstrated an increase in their cognitive development. However, there were no differences in mean level of cognitive development between the treatment and control groups. All students were found to be at Perry's level of multiplicity (accepting that there is uncertainty in the world and that there are multiple points of views/opinions and one point of view may be just as legitimate as another). Although increases were noted, subjects remained within the same level at the end of the course. The authors note that despite the lack of statistically significant differences, students' verbal and written comments suggested a movement toward higher levels of cognitive development. Lack of an observable statistical difference could be attributed to the small sample size and nonrandom assignment to groups. The authors note several other design limitations and offer suggestions for future research.

Walsh and Seldomridge (2006) provide a summary of the literature in defining, promoting, and measuring critical thinking abilities. They agree with others that findings from studies focusing on critical thinking are "for the most part, mixed and of unclear direction" (p. 214). The authors argue that time constraints in the classroom setting, the increased use of classroom technology, and the complexities of today's health care environment may make it difficult for educators to effectively use strategies that promote critical thinking. Nurse educators are urged to rethink the concept of critical thinking in nursing, identify which elements are important to foster in the classroom setting and which are more relevant to clinical practice, and then select and implement appropriate teaching and evaluation strategies to promote and measure thinking skills.

There is clearly a need to expand the evidence base in this area. Although various definitions of critical thinking have been proposed in nursing, the available literature indicates that strong similarities exist between nursing-specific definitions (Scheffer & Rubenfeld, 2000) and those developed in other disciplines (Facione, 1990). The challenge to nurse educators is to design methodologically sound studies to measure the growth of critical thinking abilities of students as they progress through the nursing program. To accomplish this, faculty must first reach a consensus as to how critical thinking will be defined in their program, select strategies designed to foster the particular skills identified in the definition, strategically decide how these thinking skills will be taught consistently across the curriculum, and determine the most appropriate methods to measure students' thinking abilities. Although this may seem like a daunting task, existing literature (Angel et al., 2000; Daley et al., 1999; McGovern & Valiga, 1997) can be used as starting points to design future studies.

## OTHER TEACHING STRATEGIES

Several articles were found in the nursing literature addressing the use of teaching-learning strategies that did not fit in any of the three categories of lecture, collaborative learning, and discussion. These are labeled "other teaching strategies." As was the case with literature reviewed in the other categories, a number of articles were found to support the use of specific strategies. However, only evidence-based articles are reviewed in this section.

Zorn, Ponick, and Peck (1995) examined the effects of participating in an international study program on the cognitive development of senior baccalaureate nursing students. A total of 28 students participated in the study. Eight of these students spent 12 weeks studying in England, while 20 comprised the control group. The experimental group completed two courses abroad: a theory and clinical course focusing on management of nursing care and one focusing on the role of the nurse as a researcher and member of the profession. Students in the control group took the same courses at the home university using the same course outlines.

Cognitive development was measured at the beginning and at the end of the study using the Measurement of Epistemological Reflection (MER), an instrument based on Perry's (1970) scheme of intellectual development. There were no significant differences in age or GPA between the experimental and the control groups. In addition, there was no significant difference between the two groups in MER scores at the beginning of the semester. Results showed that students who participated in the study abroad program were more likely to advance in Perry's positions than students who did not participate. However, the authors do note that results of this study must be interpreted with caution due to the small sample size and other study design limitations (Zorn et al., 1995).

Myer, Brenner, and Wood (1995) compared the learning outcomes of RN students enrolled in a traditionally taught classroom course (N=10) on management and leadership to the outcomes of RNs exposed to videotaped classes (N=16) of the same course. Results showed that students did equally well in terms of grades, but students who were exposed to the videotaped classes rated the course less favorably than students who participated in the traditional classroom taught course.

A number of articles can be found in the literature on using games as a teaching method. However, most of these articles are not evidence-based and do not describe the effects of using this strategy on learning. De Tornyay and Thompson (1987) asserted that, "there is limited empirical evidence to substantiate the superiority of simulations and games over traditional methods for cognitive learning" (p. 29). Although this assertion is still valid with respect to the use of games, there is a growing body of research focusing on the use of simulations, and this research is reported in Chapter 5.

The limited research that is reported documents inconsistent findings. Cowen and Tesh (2002) examined the effects of using a game to teach pediatric cardiovascular dysfunction to nursing students. Both the treatment group (N=42) and the comparison group (N=43) were introduced to the content using traditional strategies of lecture, overhead transparencies, and class discussion. The treatment group also played a teacher-developed game the last 30 minutes of class. A pre-test/post-test design was used to compare learning outcomes. Results showed that the treatment group scored 1.56 points higher on the post-test than the comparison group (p=.0002), a small numerical difference that was statistically significant, and post-test scores were higher in both groups. The authors note that these findings suggest that both teaching methods were effective in facilitating learning, but they did conclude that, although creating a game may be more time consuming than developing a lecture on a topic, the use of interactive strategies may be more effective in increasing student comprehension and retention of complex concepts. They also note that this strategy increases student involvement in the learning activity, an outcome they suggest is desirable.

Roberts (1993) compared the effects of educational gaming to that of the traditional lecture on the achievement of occupational therapy students. Using a pre-test/post-test design, students who participated in the lecture groups (two groups, N=90 total) scored significantly higher on the post-test administered immediately after the class than the students who participated in the game groups (two groups, N=86 total). Follow-up post-testing was also conducted two weeks and eight weeks after the initial post-test to determine knowledge retention. Results were mixed, demonstrating that "overall there is no particular benefit to either method in terms of learning scores. It could be argued that both the gaming and the lecture methods are acceptable ways of teaching the material" (p. 373).

The use of humor in the classroom has been described as an effective strategy to decrease student anxiety, energize students, and facilitate learning (Ulloth, 2002). Several studies to examine the effects of humor were reported in the literature during the 1980s and early 1990s. However, most of these studies were conducted in other disciplines. Recently, Ulloth conducted a qualitative study to describe the benefits of using humor in the nursing classroom. Three faculty in three associate degree nursing programs who intentionally used humor in their classrooms were selected for the study. Their classes were videotaped and their students were subsequently interviewed. Students reported that the use of humor helped to relieve stress, focused their attention, made learning fun, facilitated learning, and enhanced the student-teacher relationship (Ulloth).

Cullen and Johnston (1999) report on the use of quality circles in the classroom to improve student learning and satisfaction. The project was conducted with 40 baccalaureate nursing students enrolled in a medical-surgical course. Representatives from the class were randomly selected from a group of volunteers to meet biweekly with faculty and discuss course-related issues and concerns raised by their classmates. The purpose of using this technique was to increase teacher-student communication and satisfaction with the course and enable faculty to implement course modifications as warranted during the course of the semester. At the end of the semester, students were asked their perceptions about the strategy. Students were highly satisfied with the course content, tests, grading, and student-faculty interactions. To determine if learning improved, course grades for students enrolled in the course were compared to grades achieved by students who completed the same course the previous semester using the traditional format. Although there were no significant differences in class means, the authors report that "this was one of the few semesters [the semester of the study] in which everyone passed the course" (p. 370).

Koenig and Zorn (2002) describe the use of storytelling as a teaching strategy in nursing. The authors contend that storytelling is an effective teaching method in nursing education because the process of storytelling encourages active learning, facilitates thinking, promotes caring communities, and creates a connection between students and teachers. Although not empirically tested, they provide an example of how storytelling could be used to present content. The authors further suggest that as nursing students become increasingly diverse, storytelling may be especially beneficial to facilitate learning among students who differ in terms of age, academic preparation, cultural heritage, and physical abilities (Koenig & Zorn). Several articles can be found in the nursing literature describing the benefits of storytelling as a teaching strategy, but there is a lack of empirical evidence to support the effectiveness of this strategy.

## CONCLUSIONS

So what is the state of the science of nursing education with respect to facilitating learning in the cognitive domain? Is there adequate evidence that certain teaching methods will in fact contribute to better cognitive learning outcomes? Table 4.1 (presented at the end of the chapter) provides a summary of research discussed in this chapter, highlighting the methodology and major findings of each study.

Much of the literature reported in this chapter reflects small samples and one-time, isolated studies that examined the effect of a specific teaching strategy or technique (e.g., traditional lecture vs. lecture with group work) on learner outcomes (measured primarily by course or exam grades). Studies reviewed vary widely in design and methodology, limiting the ability to derive meaningful conclusions from the findings and develop implications to enhance teaching and learning. In terms of nursing education, there is little empirical evidence demonstrating the effectiveness of teaching methods in facilitating the achievement of cognitive learning outcomes. Moreover, in many of the studies reviewed, learning outcomes were measured with teacher-made exams that may or may not be valid and reliable measures of the desired outcomes.

A review of the literature indicates that although certain teaching practices have been strongly advocated in nursing education (e.g., abandoning the lecture method for more "active" learning strategies), these recommendations have not been evidence-based. In fact, the literature reviewed on the use of the lecture method suggests that, when done skillfully, lecturing can be quite effective in promoting learning. Existing evidence contradicts the belief of some educators that the lecture method does not promote student learning. As Menges et al. (1996) noted, scholarship in teaching should shift away from focusing on teaching techniques to examining how students learn. Any method could be effective if supported with knowledge of cognitive processes and use of strategies to facilitate knowledge construction (e.g., advanced organizers, questioning students during lecture, etc.). The work of Diekelmann (2002) reviewed in this chapter supports this view. Findings from Diekelmann's research indicates that to enhance student learning, nurse educators should frequently reflect on the effectiveness of their lectures and continuously assess student understanding. Admittedly, the existing evidence is not without limitations. The paucity of research in nursing education on the lecture method challenges nurse educators to further investigate how that method can best be used to achieve learning outcomes.

In terms of critical thinking development, a variety of reports were found in the nursing literature describing teaching methods that foster critical thinking, including concept mapping, case studies, and developmental instructional strategies. However, only a small portion of these articles were evidence-based. Existing evidence suggests that, contrary to some nurse educators' beliefs, engaging students in more "active" teaching strategies (e.g., discussion) does not automatically result in better thinking skills. For example, Rossignol's (1997) research showed that greater student participation was associated with lower levels of student critical thinking. More research is needed in this area to formulate guidelines for effectively teaching and measuring critical thinking in nursing education.

Although the use of collaborative learning strategies has been advocated by nurse educators, existing research in nursing and other disciplines does not provide clear evidence that collaborative strategies improve learning. A major limitation of the research in this area stems from the multitude of definitions used to describe collaborative learning. In addition, not all studies specifically examined the impact of collaborative strategies on learning outcomes. Existing evidence suggests that although students may rate the use of collaborative learning strategies positively, their academic performance may not be affected positively.

The use of the discussion method and its effect on the cognitive learning outcomes of students has received very little attention in the nursing literature. The commonly articulated assumption, that the use of discussion enhances learning and promotes the development of critical thinking, is not supported by existing research. In fact, one study in nursing revealed that increased student participation was associated with lower levels of critical thinking. This finding challenges nurse educators to carefully consider the characteristics of the learners, the learning task, and the learning context before employing the discussion method.

There is limited and inconsistent evidence on the effectiveness of "other teaching strategies" in promoting cognitive learning. For example, the use of gaming was found to be beneficial in one study, yet in another it was found to be no better than the lecture method. Again, these inconsistent findings may be related to the use of measurement instruments that are not appropriate for the intended learning outcome. While the use of humor as a teaching strategy has received considerable attention in the nursing literature, its effects on cognitive learning outcomes have not been adequately measured.

## IMPLICATIONS FOR RESEARCH IN NURSING EDUCATION

Overall, the research on cognitive learning in nursing education is in its infancy and needs significant development. Based on the literature reviewed in this chapter, nurse educators are faced with a number of issues and concerns that need to be addressed to build the science of nursing education, enhance the educational preparation of future nurses, and ultimately improve the care provided to clients.

An important issue raised in the literature is that in order to improve learning outcomes, educators need to focus more on how students process and assimilate information and use this as a guide for selecting appropriate teaching strategies. As aptly stated by Menges et al. (1996), "It is true that better teaching does frequently produce more and better learning, but a focus on learning is just as likely to make for better teaching. It's not that one is more important than the other. The two are inseparably linked, which we understand in theory, but often ignore in practice" (p. 3).

Research in nursing education needs to examine the effectiveness of specific teaching practices, but it also needs to help faculty determine which methods are associated with the best learning outcomes based on learner characteristics and learning goals. For example, using discussion as a teaching method may make for a more interactive classroom, but if students do not have a well-developed knowledge base about a topic and/or they are at lower levels of intellectual development, it is unlikely that meaningful learning will result. As a first step, studies using qualitative and quantitative methods are needed to explore how nursing students process information and "make meaning" in various learning situations. Young and Diekelmann's (2002) qualitative study of how new teachers learn lecturing skills may be a helpful model to use in designing studies focusing on how nursing students learn.

Results from these studies can then be used as a basis for comparing the effectiveness of various teaching strategies on learning outcomes.

In addition, research in the area of intellectual development needs to be expanded to determine which teaching methods result in greater intellectual gains. Future studies should expand on the work already conducted in nursing (e.g., McGovern & Valiga, 1997) to expand the science base. In keeping with a student-centered model of research in education, future studies should also explore which methods, and in which sequence/combination, are most effective in maximizing cognitive learning and the intellectual growth of nursing students as they progress through nursing programs.

To adequately assess the effectiveness of collaborative strategies in nursing education, studies using clear and consistent definitions of "collaborative teaching strategies" and "collaborative learning" in nursing education need to be conducted. To maximize the generalizability of findings, a series of well-designed studies using adequate sample sizes should be conducted examining if and when collaborative learning can be effective in promoting cognitive learning outcomes in nursing.

**Table 4.1. Summary of Research on Teaching Methods Designed to Enhance Cognitive Learning**

| Authors | Description | Sample Size | Measures | Findings |
|---|---|---|---|---|
| Angel et al. (2000) | Compared two methods for completing health patterns assessment on critical thinking | N=142 nursing students in first semester of a clinical course | Watson-Glaser Critical Thinking Appraisal (WGCTA) | No significant difference in achievement between two methods. |
| Beers (2005) | Compared two teaching methods: problem-based learning and lecture to present diabetes content | Two groups of nursing students (fall semester group N=18 and spring semester group N=36) enrolled in Adult Health course | Pretest and posttest; 10-item multiple choice tests related to diabetes content developed by HESI | No significant difference in achievement between two groups. |
| Booth & James (2001) | Compared use of traditional lecture to use of modified lecture in a physics course (students asked to do collaborative work on questions posed by instructor at various times during class) | Two groups of physics students; N=52 in modified course; N=60 in traditional course (combined total of students who had completed same course in the previous two years) | Pretest and posttest | No significant difference in achievement between two groups. However, students in modified course gave positive ratings to teaching method. |
| Cabrera et al. (1998) | Examined relationship of collaborative learning to perceived gains in learning and openness to diversity | N=2050 drawn from 23 institutions (from larger national study on student learning) | Self-reported questionnaires | Participation in collaborative learning activities found to be best predictor of cognitive and affective learning outcomes. |

**Table 4.1. Summary of Research on Teaching Methods Designed to Enhance Cognitive Learning (continued)**

| Authors | Description | Sample Size | Measures | Findings |
|---------|-------------|-------------|----------|----------|
| Carrero et al. (2007) | Compared effectiveness of lecture method and case/problem-based method | Two groups of first-year anesthesia residents: N=29 lecture method; N=25 case/problem-based method | Pretest and posttest | No significant differences in overall achievement between the two groups. |
| Colbeck et al. (2000) | Explored engineering students' perception of working in groups | N=65 students drawn from 7 institutions | Focus group and individual interviews | Students reported that group work had a positive effect on their communication skills, problem-solving skills, and ability to work with others; achievement not examined. |
| Cowen & Tesh (2002) | Explored use of gaming on students' knowledge of pediatric cardiac dysfunctions | Two groups: N=42 treatment and N=43 control; nursing students | Pretest and posttest | Treatment group scored significantly higher on exam. |
| Cox & Junkin (2002) | Compared traditional physics lab (students work individually) to group work | Two groups, total N=129 (experimental N=59 and control N=70); each group divided into 2 sections | Pretest and posttest | Experimental group (collaborative group work) scored significantly higher on posttest than control group (worked individually). |
| Cullen & Johnston (1999) | Explored use of quality circles | N=40 BSN students | Course grades | Use of quality circles associated with better grades. |

**Table 4.1. Summary of Research on Teaching Methods Designed to Enhance Cognitive Learning (continued)**

| Authors | Description | Sample Size | Measures | Findings |
|---|---|---|---|---|
| **Dal Bello-Haas et al. (1999)** | Compared effectiveness of traditional lecture to feedback lecture in physical therapy class | N=16 (traditional lecture); N=15 (feedback lecture) | Pretest and posttest on class content (students tested immediately after class and 4 months later) | No significant differences in test scores between two groups. |
| **Daley et al. (1999)** | Examined use of concept maps to foster critical thinking | N=18 senior BSN nursing students | First and last concept maps created by students | Significant differences in conceptual and critical thinking between first and final concept maps developed during the semester. |
| **Dickerson et al. (1999)** | Examined effect of various "active" strategies to teach case management | N=33 RN-BSN students | Exam | Authors report that strategies were effective, but exam results as described in report do not support conclusion. |
| **Duncan & Dick ) (2000)** | Examined effectiveness of supplemental collaborative learning groups in 4 math courses | N=291 students enrolled in 4 different math courses | Actual course grade vs. predicted course grade based on math SAT score | Actual grades significantly higher than predicted grade as a result of participating in collaborative learning groups. |
| **Elberson et al. (2001)** | Looked at use of collaborative learning to teach pathophysiology to nursing students | Not reported | None described | No actual measure of cognitive learning reported, but authors report that approach increased knowledge and understanding. |

**Table 4.1. Summary of Research on Teaching Methods Designed to Enhance Cognitive Learning (continued)**

| Authors | Description | Sample Size | Measures | Findings |
|---|---|---|---|---|
| Ellerman et al. (2006) | Examined effect of logic models on critical thinking skills | N=33 BSN nursing students | Students' self-reports | Critical thinking significantly increased with use of logic models. |
| Gillies (1984) | Examined effect of advanced organizers on learning | N=43 BSN students: N=21 experimental and N=22 control | Quizzes, exams | Advanced organizers effective with initial learning of content, but not effective for long-term retention. |
| Goodfellow (1995) | Studied use of cooperative learning (group work) to teach nursing research | Students in nursing research course; sample size not reported | Midterm and final exams | Group work associated with higher midterm and final exam grades. |
| Hwang & Kim (2006) | Compared problem-based learning (PBL) to lecture method | N=71 BSN students in Korea: N=35 (PBL) and N=36 (didactic) | Pretest and posttest | PBL group scored significantly higher on posttest; but PBL group also received supplemental sessions conducted by one of the authors. |
| Kiewra et al. (1997) | Studied effect of advanced organizers on learning | N=109 educational psychology students | Posttest only | Use of organizers facilitated recall of facts and relationships among topics. |
| Koenig & Zorn (2002) | Used storytelling with diverse students | Not an empirical study | Not an empirical study | Authors advocate the use of this strategy with students of diverse backgrounds. |

**Table 4.1. Summary of Research on Teaching Methods Designed to Enhance Cognitive Learning (continued)**

| Authors | Description | Sample Size | Measures | Findings |
|---|---|---|---|---|
| Lane & Aleksic (2002) | Compared traditional lecture course in statistics to modified course that included group sessions | N=480; two groups: (experimental group N=140; control group N=340) | Pretest and posttest | Experimental group scored significantly higher on posttest. |
| Liotta-Kleinfeld & McPhee (2001) | Compared traditional lecture to PBL in neuroscience course | Two groups of OT students: N=18 (traditional lecture); N=25 (PBL) | Final exam | No significant differences in test scores between two groups. |
| Lusk & Conklin (2003) | Studied effect of collaborative testing | N=25 nursing students | Unit and final exams | Collaborative testing significantly improved unit exam, but not final exam, grades. |
| Magnusses et al. (2000) | Examined effects of inquiry-based learning on critical thinking abilities | N=150 BSN nursing students | Entry and exit measure of critical thinking using WGCTA | Only students who had low scores on entry measure showed significant gains on posttest. Those in mid to high ranges showed a drop in CT scores. |
| McGovern & Valiga (1997) | Studied effect of development strategies on cognitive development level | N=159 nursing students: N=151 control and N=45 treatment (over 2 semesters) | Learning Context Questionnaire | No statistical difference in mean level of cognitive development between treatment and control. |

**Table 4.1. Summary of Research on Teaching Methods Designed to Enhance Cognitive Learning (continued)**

| Authors | Description | Sample Size | Measures | Findings |
|---|---|---|---|---|
| **Myer et al. (1995)** | Compared learning outcomes between traditional class and videotaped class in nursing | N=10 (traditional class); N=16 (videotaped class) | Course and final exam grades | No significant differences in outcomes. |
| **Roberts (1993)** | Used games in occupational therapy course | N=86 OT students | Pretest and posttest | No significant difference in achievement between games and lecture methods. |
| **Rooda (1994)** | Examined effects of using mind mapping on achievement in nursing research course | N=36 (traditional method); N=24 (mind mapping used) | Multiple choice exams | Group using mind mapping scored significantly higher than group using traditional method. |
| **Rossignol (1997)** | Studied effect of discourse strategies on critical thinking | N=57 senior nursing students | WGCTA | Increased levels of student participation associated with lower levels of critical thinking. |
| **Shin et al. (2006)** | Examined critical thinking disposition of BSN students | N=32 BSN students in Korea | CCTDI | Significant improvement in CT dispositions over time; significant improvement in open-mindedness, self-confidence, and maturity. |

**Table 4.1. Summary of Research on Teaching Methods Designed to Enhance Cognitive Learning (continued)**

| Authors | Description | Sample Size | Measures | Findings |
|---|---|---|---|---|
| Stewart & Dempsey (2005) | Looked at critical thinking dispositions on entry and exit and relationship of CT scores to NCLEX performance | N=34 BSN students who completed longitudinal study | CCTDI and NCLEX-RN exam | No overall significant improvement in scores from sophomore to senior year; no significant difference between the CCTDI scores of students who passed NCLEX-RN and those who did not. |
| Thompson & Rebeschi (1999) | Studied critical thinking skills and dispositions on entry and exit | 38 BSN students who completed longitudinal study | CCTST and CCTDI | Significant increases on CCTST and CCTDI from entry to exit. |
| Titsworth (2001) | Examined effect of note taking, teacher immediacy, and organizational cues on cognitive learning of communication students during a lecture | N=233 divided into 4 groups, each exposed to a different treatment condition (teaching strategy) | Detail and concept tests immediately after class and one week later | Students who took notes scored significantly higher than students who did not take notes; providing organizational cues only impacted scores on detail test. |
| Ulloth (1992) | Looked at benefits of humor | N=3 faculty; number of students not reported | Interview | Students reported humor decreased stress, focused attention; no specific measures of learning reported. |

**Table 4.1. Summary of Research on Teaching Methods Designed to Enhance Cognitive Learning (continued)**

| Authors | Description | Sample Size | Measures | Findings |
|---|---|---|---|---|
| Viau (1994) | Surveyed nursing staff development educators to assess frequency of use of collaborative teaching-learning methods | N=124 staff development educators | Questionnaire | Staff development educators tend to use a combination of teacher-centered and learner-centered strategies; educators with master's and doctoral degrees were significantly more likely to use learner-centered strategies. |
| Wathen & Resnick (1997) | Studied effects of collaborative learning | N=16 student dyads (total of 32) in biology course | Pretest and posttest | No significant effect on cognitive achievement. |
| Young & Diekelmann (2002) | Explored how new teachers learn to lecture | N=17 novice nurse educators | Interview | Seven themes were derived using this method. |
| Zitzmann (1996) | Compared lecture to self-instructional module | N=29 students in clinical parasitology | Exam | No significant differences in scores. |
| Zorn et al. (1995) | Looked at effects of study abroad program on cognitive development | Two groups: N=28 nursing students (N=8 participated in study abroad; N=20 in control group) | Measure of epistemological reflection | Students who participated in study abroad more likely to advance in cognitive level. |

## REFERENCES

Abegglen, J., & O'Neill Conger, C. (1997). Critical thinking in nursing: Classroom tactics that work. *Journal of Nursing Education*, 36, 452-458.

Adams, B. L. (1999). Nursing education for critical thinking: An integrative review. *Journal of Nursing Education*, 38, 111-119.

Adams, M. (1992). Cultural inclusion in the American college classroom. *New Directions for Teaching and Learning*, 49, 5-17.

American Association of Colleges of Nursing. (1996). *The essentials of master's education for advanced practice nursing*. Washington, DC: Author.

American Association of Colleges of Nursing. (1998). *The essentials of baccalaureate education for professional nursing practice*. Washington, DC: Author.

Angel, B., Duffey, M., & Belyea, M. (2000). An evidence-based project for evaluating strategies to improve knowledge acquisition and critical-thinking performance in nursing students. *Journal of Nursing Education*, 39, 219-228.

Ausubel, D. P. (2000). *The acquisition and retention of knowledge*. Boston: Kluwer Academic.

Beers, G. W. (2005). The effect of teaching method on objective test scores: Problem-based learning versus lecture. *Journal of Nursing Education*, 44, 305-309.

Bell, M., Heye, M., Campion, L., Hendricks, P., Owens, B., & Schoonover, J. (2002). Evaluation of a process-focused learning strategy to promote critical thinking. *Journal of Nursing Education*, 41(4), 175-177.

Booth, K., & James, B. (2001). Interactive learning in higher education level 1 mechanics module. *International Journal of Science Education*, 23, 955-967.

Brookfield, S. (1990). *The skillful teacher*. San Francisco: Jossey-Bass.

Cabrera, A., Nora, A., Bernal, E., Terenzini, P., & Pascarella, E. (1998). *Collaborative learning: Preferences, gains in cognitive and affective outcomes, and openness to diversity among college students.* Paper presented at the Annual Meeting of the Association for the Study of Higher Education, November 5-8, 1998, Miami, FL. (ERIC Document Reproduction Service No. ED427589)

Carrero, E., Gomar, C., Penzo, W., & Rull, M. (2007). Comparison between lecture-based and case/problem-based learning discussion for teaching pre-anaesthetic assessment. *European Journal of Anaesthesiology*, 24, 1008-1015.

Chickering, A. W., & Gamson, Z. F. (1987). Seven principles for good practice in undergraduate education. *American Association for Higher Education Bulletin*, 39(7), 3-7.

Colbeck, C., Campbell, S., & Bjorklund, S. (2000). Grouping in the dark: What college students learn from group projects. *Journal of Higher Education,* 71(1), 60-83.

Cowen, K., & Tesh, A. (2002). Effects of gaming on nursing students' knowledge of pediatric cardiovascular dysfunction. *Journal of Nursing Education,* 41, 507-509.

Cox, A. J., & Junkin, W. F. (2002). Enhanced student learning in the introductory physics laboratory. *Physics Education,* 37(1), 37-44.

Cullen, J., & Johnston, L. (1999). Using quality circles in the classroom to improve student learning and satisfaction. *Journal of Nursing Education,* 38, 368-370.

Dal Bello-Haas, V., Bazyk, S., Ekelman, B., & Milidonis, M. (1999). A study comparing the effectiveness of the feedback lecture method with the traditional lecture method. *Journal of Physical Therapy Education,* 13(2), 36-40.

Daley, B., Shaw, C., Balistrieri, T., Glasenapp, K., & Piacentine, L. (1999). Concept maps: A strategy to teach and evaluate critical thinking. *Journal of Nursing Education,* 38, 42-47.

De Tornyay, R., & Thompson, M. (1987). *Strategies for teaching nursing.* New York: Wiley.

Dickerson, S. S., Peters, D., Walkowiak, J. A., & Brewer, C. (1999). Active learning strategies to teach case management. *Nurse Educator,* 24(5), 52-57.

Diekelmann, N. (2002). "Pitching a lecture" and "reading the faces of students": Learning, lecturing and the embodied practices of teaching. *Journal of Nursing Education,* 41, 97-99.

Diekelmann, N., Swenson, M., & Sims, S. (2003). Reforming the lecture: Avoiding what students already know. *Journal of Nursing Education,* 42, 103-105.

Duncan, H., & Dick, T. (2000). Collaborative workshops and student academic performance in introductory college mathematics courses: A study of a Treisman model math excel program. *School Science and Mathematics,* 100, 365-373.

Dunkin, M. J. (1986). Research on teaching in higher education. In M. C. Wittrock (Ed.), *Handbook of research on teaching* (3rd ed.). New York: Macmillan.

Elberson, K. L., Vance, A. R., Stephenson, N. L., & Corbett, R. W. (2001). Cooperative learning: A strategy for teaching pathophysiology to undergraduate nursing students. *Nurse Educator,* 26, 259-261.

Ellerman, C. R., Kataoka-Yahiro, M. R., & Wong, L. C. (2006). Logic models used to enhance critical thinking. *Journal of Nursing Education,* 45, 220-227.

Entwistle, N. J., & Ramsden, P. (1983). *Understanding student learning.* London: Croom Helm.

Facione, P. (1990). *Critical thinking: A statement of expert consensus for purposes of educational assessment and instruction. Research findings and recommendations* (The Delphi Report). Newark, DE: American Philosophical Association. (ERIC Document Reproduction Service No. ED315423)

Feldman, K. A. (1976). The superior college teacher from the students' view. *Research in Higher Education,* 5, 243-288.

Ferguson, L., & Day, R. A. (2005). Evidence-based nursing education: Myth or reality? *Journal of Nursing Education,* 44, 107-115.

Garrison, D. R., & Archer, W. (2000). *A transactional perspective on teaching and learning: A framework for adult and higher education.* Oxford, UK: Elsevier Science.

Gillies, D. A. (1984). Effect of advanced organizers on learning medical surgical nursing content by baccalaureate nursing students. *Research in Nursing and Health,* 7, 173-180.

Goodfellow, L. M. (1995). Cooperative learning strategies: An effective method of teaching nursing research. *Nurse Educator,* 20, 26-29.

Gray, M. T. (2003). Beyond content: Generating critical thinking in the classroom. *Nurse Educator,* 28, 136-140.

Halpern, D. F. (1996). *Thought & knowledge: An introduction to critical thinking* (3rd ed.). Mahwah, NJ: Lawrence Erlbaum.

House, B., Chassie, M., & Spohn, B. (1992). Questioning: An essential ingredient in effective teaching. *Journal of Continuing Education in Nursing,* 21, 196-201.

Hwang, S. Y., & Kim, M. J. (2006). A comparison of problem-based learning and lecture-based learning in an adult health nursing course. _Nursing Education Today,_ 26, 315-321.

Johnson, D. W., & Johnson, R. (1987). Research shows the benefits of adult cooperation. _Educational Leadership,_ 45, 29-32.

Kiewra, K., Mayer, R., Dubois, N., Christiansen, M., Kim, S., & Risch, N. (1997). Effects of advance organizers and repeated presentations on students' learning. _Journal of Experimental Education,_ 65(2), 147-159.

Koenig, J. M., & Zorn, C. R. (2002). Using storytelling as an approach to teaching and learning with diverse students. _Journal of Nursing Education,_ 41, 393-399.

Lane, J., & Aleksic, M. (2002). _Transforming elementary statistics to enhance student learning._ Paper presented at the Annual Meeting of the American Educational Research Association, April 1-5, 2002, New Orleans, LA. (ERIC Document Reproduction Service No. ED463332)

Lierman, J. (1997). _Effects of instructional methods upon the development of critical thinking skills in baccalaureate nursing students._ Doctoral dissertation, University of Missouri, Columbia. (ProQuest Digital Dissertations database publication no. AAT 9726191)

Liotta-Kleinfeld, L., & McPhee, S. (2001). Comparison of final exam test scores of neuroscience students who experienced traditional methodologies versus problem-based learning methodologies. _Occupational Therapy in Health Care,_ 14(3/4), 35-53.

Lusk, M., & Conklin, L. (2003). Collaborative testing to promote learning. _Journal of Nursing Education,_ 42, 121-124.

Magnussen, L., Ishida, D., & Itano, J. (2000). The impact of the use of inquiry-based learning as a teaching methodology on the development of critical thinking. _Journal of Nursing Education,_ 39, 360-364.

McGovern, M., & Valiga, T. (1997). Promoting the cognitive development of freshman nursing students. _Journal of Nursing Education,_ 36(1), 29-35.

McKeachie, W. J., Pintrich, P. R., Lin, Y., Smith, D., & Sharma, R. (1986). _Teaching and learning in the college classroom: A review of the literature_ (2nd ed.). Ann Arbor: University of Michigan.

Menges, R., Weimer, M., & Associates (1996). _Teaching on solid ground._ San Francisco: Jossey-Bass.

Murray, H. G. (1985). Classroom teaching behaviors related to college teaching effectiveness. In J. G. Donald & A. M. Sullivan (Eds.), Using research to improve teaching. _New Directions for Teaching and Learning,_ 23, 21-34.

Myer, S., Brenner, Z., & Wood, K. (1995). A comparison of learner outcomes to traditional and videotaped classes. _Nurse Educator,_ 20(2), 29-33.

National League for Nursing (1996). _Criteria and guidelines for the evaluation of baccalaureate and higher degree programs._ New York: Author.

Oermann, M.H. (2004). Using active learning in lecture: Best of "both worlds." _International Journal of Nursing Education Scholarship,_ 1(1), 1-9.

Oermann, M.H. (1990). Research on teaching methods. In G. M. Clayton & P. A. Baj (Eds). _Review of Research in Nursing Education_ (Vol. III). New York: National League for Nursing.

Oulette, F. (1986). Facilitating classroom learning: The Ausubel model. _Nurse Educator,_ 11(6), 16-19.

Perry, W. G., Jr. (1970). _Forms of intellectual and ethical development in the college years: A scheme._ New York: Holt, Reinhart & Winston.

Reuland, M. (2000). _Collaborative learning as professional socialization._ Paper presented at the Annual Meeting of the American Educational Research Association, April 24-28, 2000, New Orleans, LA. (ERIC Document Reproduction Service No. ED440274)

Riddell, T. (2007). Critical assumptions: Thinking critically about critical thinking. _Journal of Nursing Education,_ 46, 121-126.

Roberts, A. E. (1993). An evaluation of the effectiveness of educational gaming as a teaching method for therapists. _British Journal of Occupational Therapy,_ 56, 371-375.

Rooda, L. (1994). Effects of mind mapping on student achievement in a nursing research course. _Nurse Educator,_ 19(6), 25-27.

Rossignol, M. (1997). Relationship between selected discourse strategies and student critical thinking. _Journal of Nursing Education,_ 36, 467-475.

Rowles, C. J., & Brigham, C. (2005). Strategies to promote critical thinking and active learning. In D. M. Billings & J. A. Halstead (Eds.), Teaching in nursing: A guide for faculty (pp. 283-315). St. Louis, MO: Elsevier Saunders.

Schuster, P. M. (2000). Concept mapping: Reducing clinical care plan paperwork and increasing learning. Nurse Educator, 25, 76-81.

Scheffer, B. K., & Rubenfeld, M. G. (2000). A consensus statement on critical thinking in nursing. Journal of Nursing Education, 39, 352-359.

Scriven, M., & Paul, R. (2007). Defining critical thinking. [Online]. Available: http://www.criticalthinking.org/aboutCT/definingCT.cfm.

Sherman, T. M., Armistead, L. P., Fowler, F., Barksdale, M. A., & Reif, G. (1987). The quest for excellence in university teaching. Journal of Higher Education, 48, 66-84.

Shin, K. R., Lee, J. H., Ha, J. Y., & Kim, K. H. (2006). Critical thinking dispositions in baccalaureate nursing students. Journal of Advanced Nursing, 56, 182-189.

Slavin, R. E. (1980). Cooperative learning. Review of Educational Research, 50, 315-342.

Stewart, S., & Dempsey, L. F. (2005). A longitudinal study of baccalaureate nursing students' critical thinking dispositions. Journal of Nursing Education, 44, 81-84.

Sorcinelli, M. D. (1991). Research findings on the seven principles. In A. W. Chickering & Z. P. Gamson (Eds.), Applying the seven principles for good practice in undergraduate education. New Directions for Teaching and Learning, 47, 13-25.

Thompson, C. (1993). Best and worst classroom learning experiences as perceived by adult undergraduates in baccalaureate nursing programs. Doctoral dissertation, University of Connecticut, Storrs. (ProQuest Digital Dissertations database publication no. AAT 9332901)

Thompson, C., & Rebeschi, L. (1999). Critical thinking skills of baccalaureate nursing students at program entry and exit. Nursing & Health Care Perspectives, 20, 248-252.

Thompson, C., & Sheckley, B. (1997). Difference in teaching preferences between traditional and adult BSN students. Journal of Nursing Education, 36, 163-170.

Titsworth, B. S. (2001). The effects of teacher immediacy, use of organizational lecture cues, and students' notetaking on cognitive learning. Communication Education, 50, 283-297.

Ulloth, J. K. (2002). The benefits of humor in nursing education. *Journal of Nursing Education, 41,* 476-481.

Valiga, T., & Bruderle, E. (1994). Concepts included in and critical to nursing curricula: An analysis. *Journal of Nursing Education, 33,* 118-124.

Viau, P. (1994). Collaborative teaching-learning: A potential framework for staff development educators. *Journal of Nursing Staff Development, 10(4),* 195-201.

Walsh, C. M., & Seldomridge, L. A. (2006). Critical thinking: Back to square two. *Journal of Nursing Education, 45,* 212-219.

Wathen, S. H., & Resnick L. B. (1997). *Collaborative versus individual learning and the role of explanations.* Paper presented at the Annual Meeting of the American Educational Research Association, Chicago, IL.

Young, P., & Diekelmann, N. (2002). Learning to lecture: Exploring the skills, strategies, and practices of new teachers in nursing education. *Journal of Nursing Education, 41,* 405-412.

Zitzmann, M. B. (1996). Comparing the learning outcomes of lecture and self-instruction methods in a senior clinical laboratory science course. *Clinical Laboratory Science, 9(4),* 198-201.

Zorn, C., Ponick, D., & Peck, S. (1995). An analysis of the impact of participation in an international study program on the cognitive development of senior baccalaureate nursing students. *Journal of Nursing Education, 34,* 67-70.

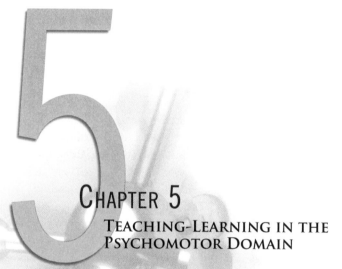

# Chapter 5

## Teaching-Learning in the Psychomotor Domain

*Pamela R. Jeffries, DNS, RN, FAAN, ANEF*
*Gail Kost, MSN, RN, CNE*
*Vema Sweitzer, MN, RN, CNE*

"Education is not a preparation for life,
education is life itself."

John Dewey

In the 1960s, Benjamin Bloom and a team of educational psychologists analyzed academic learning behaviors. The analysis results led to what is known today in the field of education as "Bloom's taxonomy." This taxonomy, or hierarchy of learning behaviors, was categorized into three interrelated and overlapping learning domains: the cognitive (knowledge), affective (attitudes), and psychomotor (skills) (Yoder, 1993). This chapter describes the psychomotor domain and addresses skill attainment by nursing students. The domain, research-based literature, conclusions, and recommendations for further research in the psychomotor domain are discussed.

## THE PSYCHOMOTOR DOMAIN

The psychomotor domain includes the development of basic motor skills, coordination, and physical movement. In Bloom's early research (1953), this domain was not explicated as clearly as the cognitive domain, because the scholars lacked experience in teaching these skills. In subsequent work, however, Harrow (1972) outlined six categories to describe the taxonomy in this area of learning. These six categories are reflex movements (the lowest level of the hierarchy), basic fundamental movements, perceptual abilities, physical abilities, skilled movements, and nondiscursive movements (the highest level in the hierarchy). Harrow asserted that it is through repetitive practice that one learns physical skills and progresses along the hierarchy. In 1990, Reilly and Oermann suggested a psychomotor taxonomy that was more useful for nursing. It was published in *Psychomotor Levels in Developing and Writing Objectives* (Dave, 1970) and was based on neuromuscular movement and coordination. The Reilly and Oermann taxonomy described five levels of progression: imitation, manipulation, precision, articulation, and naturalization, and also described criteria for each of those levels. Table 5.1 outlines the criteria associated with all the levels of the psychomotor taxonomy. Menix (2003) helped clarify that as one progresses from one level to the next, skills are performed with greater precision, speed, coordination, and increased independence.

Psychomotor learning is demonstrated by the performance of two types of physical skills, each of which can be judged in terms of the student's coordination, dexterity, manipulation, grace, strength, and speed. **Fine-motor skills** are demonstrated by the use of precision instruments or tools (e.g., suturing, inserting a Foley catheter), and **gross motor skills** are demonstrated by the use of the body in dance or athletic performance. In educational arenas, verbs associated with the psychomotor domain include bend, grasp, operate, handle, differentiate, express, or perform skillfully.

### Table 5.1. Levels in Psychomotor Taxonomy, with Criteria (Reilly & Oermann, 1999)

| Psychomotor Categories | Criteria |
|---|---|
| Imitation | Necessary actions are taken with some errors; weaknesses appear in the smoothness of the gross motor actions and the time to complete the skill. |
| Manipulation | Written directives are followed with some degree of accuracy; however, there will be some variance in the coordination of movements and time taken to perform the action. |
| Precision | Actions are completed in a logical, sequential order with few errors occurring at noncritical times. Movements are well-coordinated, but the time taken to perform the action is variable. |
| Articulation | Coordinated actions are performed in a logical, sequential manner with limited errors; time to perform the action is improving and is reasonable. |
| Naturalization | Professional competence is demonstrated when performing the action or skill that is automatic, with good coordination and reasonable timing. |

The literature at http://utut.essortment.com/psychomotordeve_pqs.htm (2008) suggests there are three stages through which an individual progresses when learning psychomotor skills: cognitive, associative, and autonomic. The beginning stage is the cognitive stage, where the learner is consciously trying to "control" psychomotor movement. Initially, the movements are awkward, slow, and deliberate, because the learner must think about each step before doing the movement or task. Performance often is poor, and the person frequently makes errors during this choppy, slow performance. The frustration level is high, but diligent practice allows the learner to move on to the next stage.

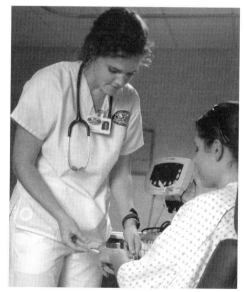

In the second stage of psychomotor development, the *associative stage*, the learner spends less time thinking about every detail and begins to associate the movement being learned with another movement already known. For now, the movements are not internalized nor are they automatic. A learner in this stage thinks about most movements, but performance of the skill begins to look smoother or more "natural," and the student feels less awkward.

The final stage of psychomotor development is the *autonomic stage,* when learning is complete, although the learner often continues to refine the skill through practice. No longer does the learner need feedback about the performance, because the movements are spontaneous, natural, and no longer require thinking about the steps involved since they are almost "second nature."

# REVIEW OF THE LITERATURE

Using key words such as clinical skills, basic nursing skills, selected skills, simulations, and psychomotor skills, as well as specific clinical skill procedures such as medication administration, urinary catheterization, injections, and tracheal suctioning, nursing (CINAHL), education (ERIC, CARL), and medical (MEDLINE) databases from 1998 to 2008 were searched for reports of research on teaching psychomotor skills. Additional sources were found in references cited in the resources identified through the search. Since the search yielded only 30 research studies on teaching psychomotor skills (all of which are summarized in Table 5.2 which begins on page 198 at the end of this chapter), other articles contributing to the understanding of teaching psychomotor skills in nursing also were reviewed and included here to clarify and enrich the research-based reports. Finally, findings of the research-based articles were categorized into common themes using content analysis procedures.

# GENERAL COMMENTS AND CRITIQUE

The 30 research reports identified through the electronic search of the literature included 14 that focused on instructional strategies to teach psychomotor skills, one that addressed lecture, one focusing on the work-based learning approach (described later in this chapter), six on using simulations (including use of simulators and objective structured clinical examinations [OSCEs] to teach skills), one using a problem-based learning (PBL) approach, two on student-centered/self-directed learning, three addressing the use of multimedia (including CD-ROMs, CAI, and DVDs), one using a web-based platform, and another using peer learning partnerships. Nine of the 30 articles discussed teaching psychomotor skills in countries other than the United States, specifically the United Kingdom, Australia, Canada, Sweden, and New Zealand.

Research on teaching psychomotor skills is in an early stage. Generally, the studies reported to date have been descriptive and evaluative; few have been guided by a theoretical framework. Sample sizes tend to be small in most studies, with faculty evaluating or discussing instructional delivery in one course or module. In addition, the literature cited in the studies reported and supporting the work tends to be more than 10 years old, suggesting an insufficient current knowledge base to support the studies. Finally, the measurement instruments used in the studies (e.g., checklists, questionnaires, competency checks) tend to be instructor-developed and used only in one study, and information about their validity and reliability typically was not provided.

A content analysis of this research literature revealed three major areas: a) *faculty roles* when teaching psychomotor skills; b) *instructional strategies* when teaching psychomotor skills (e.g., lecture, online instruction, work-based learning approach, simulations [OSCEs and use of simulations]), and c) *evaluation* of psychomotor skill performance (e.g., checklists, "skillimeters," and questionnaires/interviews). Each of these major areas is discussed separately.

# THE FACULTY ROLE

Tanner (1993) recommended that teaching could be improved by initiating more conversations about teaching and building a community with colleagues. Maeve (1994) supported this recommendation by asserting that sharing successes and failures of teachers helps explicate what good practice is, and promotes scholarship in teaching. To avoid burnout and enhance feelings of self-worth, she noted, teachers need to be aware of the good aspects of practice. The Minnesota Baccalaureate Psychomotor Skills Faculty Group (1998) was one group that accepted Tanner's challenge to "tell teacher tales."

In order to share "teacher tales," the baccalaureate nursing faculty at the University of Minnesota who taught psychomotor skills in a laboratory setting convened for three hours on Saturday mornings for several weeks to discuss their shared world. A question that quickly became foundational from this sharing of ideas was "How can we best teach psychomotor skills?" The intent was not for all to teach in the same manner but to be united in, clarify, and explain the value of psychomotor skills to students in preparing them for entry into practice.

Through this dialogue, it was discovered that some faculty taught only psychomotor skills, while others combined this responsibility with additional didactic and/or clinical assignments. Among the group members, a number of abilities needed to teach psychomotor skills were identified (see Table 5.3).

> **Table 5.3. Teacher Abilities Needed to Enhance the Teaching of Psychomotor Skills (Minnesota Baccalaureate Skills Faculty Group, 1998)**
>
> - *Knowledge of instruction in all three domains of learning: cognitive, affective, and psychomotor*
> - *Clinical competence*
> - *Facilitation skills to progress the student from a beginning level of socialization*
> - *Awareness of students' unique learning styles*
> - *Knowledge about general principles in nursing in addition to specific procedures*
> - *Facilitation skills to promote critical thinking and adaptability in the clinical area*
> - *Empowerment skills to help students provide safe, competent nursing care*

The experience of opening conversations regarding practice within a community of baccalaureate faculty who teach psychomotor skills was valuable. Participants were able to extend their thinking as well as provide support and resource systems for each other. As Tanner (1993), Diekelmann (1993), and Maeve (1994) have described, the outcomes of the teaching experience are consistent with the rewards reflecting on nursing practice.

Tarnow and King (2004) describe another faculty approach to teaching psychomotor skills that has to do with "questioning." In order to keep their knowledge base current, nurses need to continually question the traditional ways of performing nursing skills or various tasks. The traditional methods for performing such skills as parenteral injections, tracheostomy care, urinary catheter insertion, and management of phlebotomy needs to be questioned. It is suggested that nurses need to refrain from making statements like, "That's how I was taught" or "It's always been done that way." Tarnow and King believe that if educators fail to question traditional practices, then this mindset can lead to stagnation in practice. It is in the questioning that nurses are continually seeking to ascertain the best practice methods for various technical skills or techniques. It is the role of the faculty to seek evidence-based practice in each and every skill taught. As an example of applying this philosophy, Tarnow and King did a study using quantitative and qualitative methods to examine differences regarding the traditional needle bevel-up versus the bevel-down method of giving intradermal injections. This study revealed there were no differences in technique with regard to accuracy of placement, bleeding or comfort. Using the best practice current techniques means that, for now, nurses can continue to use the bevel-up method for intradermal injections.

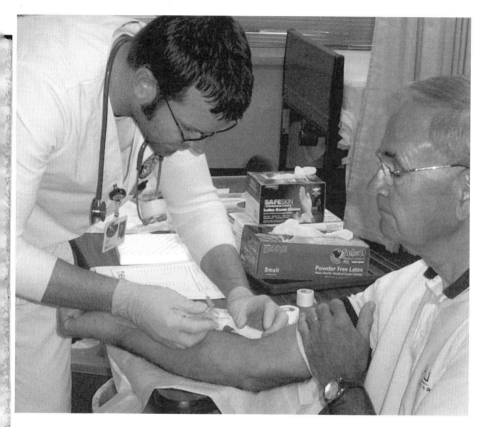

Although the list of teacher abilities generated by the 1998 Minnesota cohort of baccalaureate faculty teaching psychomotor skills to undergraduate students and Tarnow and King's (2004) concept of questioning are helpful, these are not lists of faculty qualities and strategies for teaching psychomotor skills generated through research. In fact, no research reports were found about defining and evaluating the faculty role when teaching psychomotor skills in nursing. Clearly, more research is needed in this area.

## INSTRUCTIONAL STRATEGIES USED

This section reviews the literature that addressed different teaching strategies used to help students learn psychomotor skills. Although a variety of strategies have been studied, there is virtually no replication of these studies and their generalizability is very limited.

*Lecture.* Lecture is probably one of the most common and traditional instructional strategies for relaying information to students. One research-based article (Le, Reed, Weinstein, Matthew, & Brown, 2001) discussed this strategy in relation to the instruction of placing a Flexguide in patients to facilitate difficult intubations. Thirty-five paramedic students enrolled in a New York State paramedic recertification course were taught how to do the skill using only a 5-minute lecture on the principles and use of the endotracheal tube intubation (ETTI) to facilitate difficult intubations. The lecture included verbal instructions on the procedure. Results showed 97% of the paramedics were able to successfully intubate the mannequin in less than 30 seconds using the ETTI, which was the criterion for "success" used. However, the study also found that, following a brief introduction to the device, paramedics were able to master the skill of ETTI intubation and perform the skill with equal success rates without the lecture. It is difficult to conclude much from one study, but from this one finding, lecture seemed to serve as a modality to teach a psychomotor skill when principles and the instructional procedure were delivered in a lecture modality.

***Work-Based Learning Approach.*** Education often is conducted "on-the-job" as opportunities for experiences present themselves. Given this reality, educators in England (Thorne & Hackwood, 2002) chose to teach clinical skills to nursing students using an approach called "work-based learning." These educators found that the usual classroom-based approach to teaching these skills was inflexible and inappropriate at times, but work-based learning avoids these limitations. This approach blends practice and education, fosters the integration of theory with practice as the drive to explore related knowledge is initiated by events occurring in the practice, and is thought to increase knowledge and confidence of the learner, as well as motivation and empowerment of the clinician who is doing the teaching on site. Researchers found that students could learn knowledge and skills from using a work-based learning approach. Today this concept is replicated in the nursing apprentice programs and summer preceptor offerings provided by educators in clinical agencies to students where the learner is paid for working, yet at the same time, is learning and being instructed on important clinical knowledge and skills for that specific unit assigned.

***Simulations/Simulators.*** Another approach to teaching psychomotor skills is through the use of simulation. Unlike the traditional classroom setting, a simulation allows the learner to function in an environment that is close to a real-life situation and provides the opportunity for the learner to think spontaneously and actively, rather than be passive. Simulations are most effective when they are well designed, present realistic situations, require active involvement in problem-solving, provide feedback to the learner, require the learner to manage the effects of the harmful actions, and are followed by a thorough debriefing session.

Several studies (Agazio, Pavlides, Lasome, Flaherty, & Torrance 2002; Alinier 2003; Engum & Jeffries, 2003; Khattab & Rawlings, 2001; Nicol & Freeth, 1998; Wilson, Shepherd, Kelly, & Pitzner 2005.) have evaluated the impact of using this strategy to teach and to assess the performance of skills by health professionals. Findings from these studies

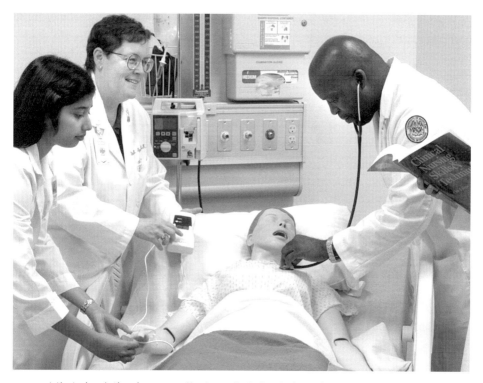

suggest that simulation is an excellent way to help students learn psychomotor (as well as cognitive) skills. The use of clinical simulations in nursing education is exploding, but few studies have been reported regarding their impact on helping students develop or refine psychomotor skills; instead, most studies reported regarding the use of simulation focus on cognitive thinking, problem-solving, and the development of clinical reasoning skills.

Two studies, Agazio et. al. (2002) and Engum and Jeffries (2003), used a commercial virtual reality (VR) simulator to teach students how to perform a venipuncture. Both studies examined user satisfaction and skill competence in IV insertion after learning this skill with a) the Cath Sim Intravenous Training System or b) the traditional IV arm. Agazio et al. (2002) randomly assigned participants to the VR training (N = 25) or the standard model of instruction (N = 26), with each participant being tested on both models with and without MOPP (Mission Oriented Protective Posture) gear (protective equipment worn by the military). The computer program produced an evaluation score for each step, calculated the time it took a leaner to complete a procedure, recorded errors, and evaluated the actual insertion procedure. The insertion procedure was rated as successful or unsuccessful based upon the accuracy of placement of the IV cannula. For all participants tested at baseline with the IV arm test without MOPP gear, 50 of the 52 cases were successful in starting the

IV in the IV arm and 25 of the 26 in the Cath Sim group were similarly successful. While in MOPP gear, 88% in the IV arm group were successful and 89% in the Cath Sim group were successful. Performing venipunctures while in MOPP gear is important since many times required skills are performed wearing protective gear, yet without practice functioning while wearing protective gear, the skill set may be a challenge to perform. Overall the participants rated both models positively. The results of the project demonstrated no significant differences in success rate or performance time needed between the use of the current arm model and the Cath Sim IV insertion.

Engum and Jeffries (2003) tested 93 third-year medical students and 70 sophomore baccalaureate nursing students using the same VR cath simulator (the "technology group") and IV arm model (the "traditional group"). Results indicated the traditional group was more satisfied with their learning than the technology group, although, there were no significant differences in the IV start accuracy or self-efficacy of the learners by group. Using the computer-based method was recommended as more of a supplemental strategy to instruction than a stand-alone instructional method to teach venipuncture, something we may find is pertinent to teaching other skills when research related to such skills is undertaken.

Effective educators attempt to make learning meaningful so students can make connections, problem-solve and think critically, and simulations appear to be effective in promoting problem-solving, as well as the recall and connection of information. When deciding whether to develop and incorporate simulation in the learning environment, faculty should consider the advantages and challenges of this strategy. Advantages include providing standardized learning experiences for all students, allowing students to practice in a safe, non-threatening, and more realistic environment, and engaging students in active learning and practice of a skill, rather than merely talking about or verbalizing the procedural steps required for it. Disadvantages include lack of resources, equipment, or adequate preparation of faculty related to using the simulator and/or simulations to learn and then teach the skill set to students.

Wilson, Shepherd, Kelly, and Pitzner (2005) assessed a low-fidelity human patient simulator (Nursing Annie Complete™) for realism, and compared this simulator's use to other traditional teaching tools. A questionnaire was given to 70 Australian nurses and/ or nursing students (61% of the participants were Division I Registered Nurses, 23% were completing their training at the university, and 16% were undergraduate students completing clinical placements) to assess a low-fidelity human patient simulator for realism and comparison with traditional methods using task trainers and plastic models to teach psychomotor skills.

The researchers from this small research study stated that a low-fidelity mannequin, such as Nursing Annie Complete™, was found to be sufficiently realistic for improving clinical performance, superior to existing training products, and suitable for teaching purposes. Given the limited sample size, results need to be interpreted with caution, but this finding helps educators know that low-fidelity mannequins can be used effectively to teach clinical skills and, perhaps, to improve overall clinical performance.

***Objective Structured Clinical Examinations (OSCEs).*** The OSCE is another approach to simulated learning using a multiple station performance examination where students are expected to demonstrate skill competency in a clinical simulation with a specified time at each station (Hannadeh, Lancaster, & Johnson, 1993). The OSCE was developed and has been used for more than 20 years in medical schools as a way to make clinical exams more valid, reliable, and practical. Although this type of instruction and testing is now being incorporated in many nursing programs in and outside the United States, its use in the nursing discipline is still limited.

The Royal College of Nursing (RCN) in England uses an OSCE (at Bournemouth University) as a measure of clinical competence for student nurse practitioners and as a certification tool at the end of the first year of a two-year course. In this exploratory study, two nursing faculty at this university (Khattab & Rawlings, 2001) used the OSCE as a formative and summative evaluation tool. In the teaching sessions, knowledge and understanding were built through lectures about the anatomy and physiology of the body system under consideration, students then observed demonstrations of proper technique by the teaching staff, and finally students spent "hands-on" time acquiring and practicing the technique. They then participated in an OSCE as a way to assess their ability, an approach that received positive evaluations from teachers and participants. During the formative evaluation using the OSCE, immediate feedback was provided to each student about her/his performance. Feedback on the summative OSCE was given a few weeks following the assessment because of the possibility of disrupting test reliability. Providing specific feedback following an OSCE is an important step, because it helps students learn what they did correctly and incorrectly, and it guides them to reflect on the skill and procedure just performed.

Nicol and Freeth (1998) also used a modified OSCE to assess selected clinical skills. The researchers assessed 140 nursing students, all in one day, at each of the 10 stations (6 hospital and 4 community). The OSCE was designed to test clinical skills through the observation of simulated practice in the realistic setting of the Skills Center. With their modified OSCE, the students remained at one station to demonstrate their competency in only a sample of skills assessed within the scenarios. Students did not know their allocated station in advance and did not know the particular skills they would be asked to perform. Although specific measurement instruments for the study were not discussed, the authors concluded that the use of the OSCE approach where students demonstrate their psychomotor skills in front of faculty members is a valuable approach for assessing psychomotor skill development and skill performance of nursing students.

Alinier (2003) completed a study using hybrid formative OSCEs to assess both nursing students and lecturers to determine the usefulness and favorability of this assessment method. To gather information regarding the students' (N=86) and lecturers' (N=39) perception of these OSCE sessions and the favorability of the OSCEs as an assessment method, a separate questionnaire was designed for each group. Alinier concluded that the OSCE sessions were "generally appreciated by students and examiners," since 96.5% of the students and 94.9% of the examiners believed OSCE sessions should be incorporated into the nursing curriculum as an assessment methodology.

**Problem-Based Learning (PBL).** Like the OSCE, PBL had its origins in medical education, but is now used by a variety of disciplines, including nursing. The concept of PBL emphasizes knowledge acquisition embedded within a contextual framework using the deductive format (Barrows & Tamblyn, 1980; Feletti & Bond, 1997). PBL is designed to facilitate the development of clinical reasoning skills and safe, holistic practice. Using a PBL teaching format, the educator can focus on, for example, psychomotor skill development, particularly in relation to professional/ethical practice, teamwork, and reflective practice as well as provide problem-solving opportunities. Using the PBL approach with students to practice and learn psychomotor skills on their own has been tested by few researchers. Candy, Crebert, and O'Leary (1994) used the PBL approach to teaching skills and found that students lacked confidence in performing technical skills, were unable to differentiate what was normal and important, and expressed feelings of "stumbling in the dark" when using the PBL approach to learning psychomotor skills. Its value to this domain of learning, therefore, was questioned.

Candy et al. asked clinical educators from the first two years of a new curriculum to evaluate the extent to which the use of PBL helped students bridge the theory-practice gap. Using open-ended questions, interviews conducted with 14 educators in focus groups were used to evaluate the curriculum with such questions as "Would you like to comment on the student self-directed learning?"

Findings showed that clinical educators found group dynamics to be better with PBL and students less likely to be "sitting at their desk" under the PBL curriculum since they used more initiative to seek more learning opportunities. Students appreciated any type of feedback and support, since PBL is self-directed in nature and student learning in the laboratory was often unsupervised. One student commented, "We've got to teach ourselves — we're not sure whether we are holding the syringes and ampules correctly." Once in the clinical setting, the student received immediate feedback from performing "real" nursing skills on "real" patients, but not in the laboratory setting. Candy et al. (1994) concluded that the theory-practice gap may have decreased in some areas by using PBL, but clinical preparedness of the student was worse. The major conclusion of this study was that students require supervision and demonstrations in the laboratory that a purely self-directed PBL curriculum does not accommodate. However, further research is needed to correlate student variables such as learning styles, prior work experience, and other factors with their ability to learn in a self-directed manner using PBL.

PBL is a helpful teaching strategy in the classroom, but as an instructional strategy to teach psychomotor skills, more research needs to be conducted and reported as to whether this method is an effective one. More guidance and instruction were needed, as reported by the students in this one study, in order to achieve the expected competencies of the skill course; we need to understand if this is a common phenomenon.

***Student-Centered Approaches to Learning Skills.*** As part of a curriculum revision being undertaken at a major university, the second semester sophomore skills course was redesigned to address the most required clinical nursing skills, not just a selected few of them (Jeffries, 2002). Using a student-centered approach, 15 self-paced study modules that incorporated Chickering and Gamson's (1987) *Principles of Best Practices in Undergraduate Education* were designed. Each module had four dimensions of learning (general principles, process, patient teaching, and critical thinking), and students were able to "test out" on any skills with which they already had experience or for which they had completed the cognitive learning activities. Interactive stations were established in the laboratory where students could work with a facilitator to receive guided practice in performing each skill, and guidelines at each station explained how to perform that skill safely and accurately. Students could, and often did, work in dyads to practice selected skills, learn content from multimedia products, and discuss focused study questions. In essence, the instructors served as facilitators of learning, and the students were responsible for their own learning.

Jeffries et al (2002) compared the experiences of 70 BSN students enrolled in this new, student-centered learning laboratory with 50 sophomore students enrolled in the teacher-centered laboratory course that was running parallel to the new curriculum course. During the sixth week of the semester, when surgical asepsis was introduced, a study was conducted to assess student satisfaction with their learning methods, self-efficacy in learning, cognitive gains, skill acquisition, and self-reliance in learning. The researcher-developed questionnaire used to evaluate student satisfaction with the teaching methods (student- or teacher-centered), had a Cronbach's alpha of 0.989 for the sample and showed that students in the student-centered group were significantly more satisfied ($p < .01$) than students in the traditional group. No significant differences were found in learning self-efficacy, self-reliance, or cognitive gains. The study was a beginning step in program/course evaluation to assess new teaching methodologies and their effects on learning outcomes and behaviors, including transfer of laboratory learning to the clinical setting.

Using yet another student-centered learning strategy, Darr (2000) used a self-directed mastery, scenario-based course format to teach Advanced Cardiac Life Support (ACLS) incorporating principles of adult learning (Knowles, 1978), and meeting the newest curriculum guidelines of the American Heart Association (AHA). In accordance with the new AHA philosophy, participants were to be offered remediation until they were successful in passing the ACLS course, and the researchers were to study the effect of this strategy on self-directed, mastery learning.

A convenience sample of 26 RNs and one physician participated in the course. Eighteen (67%) of the participants had taken ACLS previously, and many had attended two or more courses. The instructional strategies used in this course were a traditional lecture, the ACLS video series, and an interactive, computer-assisted instruction (CAI) program. Learners could use these resources whenever and however often they wished, and they signed up for testing whenever they believed they were sufficiently prepared. Written exams were scheduled by appointment.

Findings indicated that 37% of those who returned the surveys used the video series, and 22.2% reported using the interactive computer programs. The majority (96.3%) of the respondents said they attended one or more teaching laboratories and attended as many as five teaching labs during the study period. Fifty-nine percent of the respondents reported less stress and anxiety with the flexible, self-directed course design, and 29% noted appreciation for the "flexibility in scheduling." Overall, the findings suggested the self-directed ACLS course format resulted in a desirable learning environment for the ACLS participants. It also provided a cost savings of $149.27 per participant. This cost-effective format created an optimal learning environment that fostered development of the complex cognitive and psychomotor skills required to perform ACLS.

Goldsmith, Stewart, and Ferguson (2005) initiated a *peer learning strategy* that involved partnering 125 first-year and 115 third-year students for clinical skill practice sessions. The aims of this peer learning approach were to increase first-year student's self-confidence and optimize the learning of psychomotor skills. For the third-year students, the aim was to encourage leadership development through peer mentoring. Initially, the first-year students, in a didactic format, were given a demonstration of the skill in an hour-long teaching session. To ensure that the third-year students were competent, each of them was given a program tutorial session on the skills being taught. By week three, both the first- and third-year students were participating in joint practice sessions.

The evaluation of this teaching strategy was done by questionnaires given to both groups during the final week of the semester. Findings revealed that both first- and third-year nursing students commented about their interaction with each other, noting they "felt comfortable in the learning relationship" and that the peer learning experience gave them an opportunity "to review their skills" and "evaluate their knowledge base" (Goldsmith, Stewart, & Ferguson, 2005). Seventy-five percent of first-year and 97% of third-year nursing students agreed that their learning was enhanced by the peer learning partnership, with third-year students' responses being more positive than those of the first-year students. Students identified that one of the biggest problems using this learning strategy was synchronizing their schedules so that they could come together on campus to practice. Both groups of students reported that this learning strategy was beneficial and should be continued.

***Use of Multimedia and Computer-Based Learning.*** Through the years, labs for learning nursing skills have become the norm, as the value of learning psychomotor skills in a safe, controlled, nonthreatening laboratory environment before performing such skills on patients in the clinical setting is well documented (Cook & Hill, 1985). Students are better prepared and less apprehensive when they move to the clinical setting after having lab experiences (Baldwin, Hill, & Hanson, 1991). However, while the focus of such lab-based learning is well known, there is a little research to guide instructors in selecting the most appropriate types of media, computer programs, or other teaching strategies for teaching basic psychomotor skills (Baldwin, Hill & Hanson).

The literature search for this review yielded five studies on the use of computer-based learning to teach psychomotor skills, with each study focusing on different skills: administering medications, performing a 12-lead ECG, taking blood pressure, conducting a physical assessment, and completing a comprehensive psychomotor skill examination. Jeffries (2001) studied 58 baccalaureate nursing students enrolled in a junior-level fundamentals course. These students were divided into two groups: one using a computer CD-ROM and the other using more traditional methods to learn oral medication administration. The study was designed to compare the two approaches in relation to cognitive learning, satisfaction with the learning experience, skills in performing medication administration, and length of instructional time to learn the skill. Results indicated that both groups had cognitive gains from pre-test to post-test scores, and there were no significant differences found in this area between the two groups. Overall students' satisfaction with their learning was high for both groups, but the computer group had a significantly higher ($p \leq .01$) satisfaction with their learning experience than did the traditional group. There were no significant differences found between groups on skill competency for administration of medications, but mean time on task for the computer group was 31% less than the traditional group. In essence, the CD-ROM format — when used to teach oral medication administration to beginning nursing students — was more efficient (as measured by time); but it was found to be equally effective for cognitive knowledge gains, skill performance, and student satisfaction.

In a similar study, Jeffries, Woolf, and Linde (2003) compared two groups of senior students, each of which received a different instructional strategy (computer or traditional), to learn how to perform a 12-lead ECG. Using the same research design as the medication study, the study was conducted with 77 senior baccalaureate nursing students in a required critical care course. The study found no significant group differences in learner satisfaction with their instructional method, cognitive gains, or competency in demonstrating the skill of performing a 12-lead ECG.

In an effort to minimize demands on faculty time, but still provide students with a valuable learning experience, many laboratory instructors moved to the auto-tutorial model of using CAI. Interactive CAI requires the learner to participate actively in the learning process in order for instruction to continue. This instructional strategy to teach blood pressure measurement was used for the 104 sophomore nursing students enrolled in an assessment course. Beeson and Kring (2003) found that factual knowledge did not significantly differ between the two groups of students, and there were no significant differences on performance of blood pressure measurement between the traditional and computer-based groups.

Anderson, Skillen, and Knight (2001) designed a study of RN case managers to identify their perceived learning needs in physical assessment skills, barriers to their learning these skills, and the supports they needed to enhance the skills. Using a sample of 150 case managers and 39 nurse administrators from 19 continuing care facilities in Alberta, Canada, these researchers found that 44% of the sample reported having no previous course work in physical assessment. Furthermore, 80% of those surveyed expressed excitement about learning through computer technology. Barriers to using this mode of instruction included no opportunities at the worksite to acquire and practice the physical assessment skills previously learned. Learning outcomes included information and skills on how to conduct a physical assessment via the CAI platform. The CAI teaching modality was seen as a viable mode of instruction to target priority learning needs, such as physical assessment skills, as a means to help nurse case managers enhance their skills.

In a quasi-experimental study, Salyers (2007) asked the question, "Would students receiving web-enhanced instruction perform better on the final psychomotor skills examination than students receiving traditional instruction?" A sample of 36 students enrolled in a fundamental skills course was divided into two groups. The control group consisted of 14 students who received traditional instruction in a three-hour session consisting of a lecture, skill demonstration and limited practice time. The experimental group consisted of 22 students who also received a three-hour session that included demonstration of the skills and practice time with increased opportunity for feedback from the instructor; these students, however, received the lecture content using a web-enhanced format.

The findings from this study showed that the experimental group performed better on the final psychomotor skill examination than the control group, although not significantly better, a finding Salyers (2007) could not explain. Another finding showed that the control group was significantly more satisfied with the course, which the researcher concluded may be due to software and computer support problems the experimental group encountered. Overall, findings were inconclusive, and using this technology to facilitate learning of psychomotor skills needs further investigation.

In essence, the research summarized here shows that computer-based and web-based learning can be a viable strategy for learning psychomotor skills, depending on the quality, comprehensiveness, and content of the computer-based program. If this strategy is used, barriers will need to be removed and resources (e.g., computers) made available for students to access content and the teaching programs. Clearly, more research is needed on the use of technology to enhance learning in the psychomotor domain.

# EVALUATION OF PSYCHOMOTOR SKILL PERFORMANCE

Clinical instructors observe behaviors and psychomotor skills to determine whether students have the skill sets assumed necessary for safe, effective delivery of nursing care. Several researchers (Bishop et al., 2001; Devlin, 1999; Drevenhorn, Hakansson, Peterssen, 2003; Miller, Nichols & Beeken, 2000) have conducted studies to validate and evaluate *skill performance* using a variety of measures.

Devlin (1999) assessed basic life support (BLS) skills of nurses in the United Kingdom. Thirty trained nurses from a population of 150 were tested over a three-day period to evaluate whether they could perform these skills correctly. The practical assessment of BLS skills took place in a clinical teaching room using the Skillmeter Resusci-Anne Manikin (Laerdal Medical). On entry into the test room, each subject was told that the manikin represented a collapsed patient, that they were on their own, and they should respond appropriately. The performed skills were assessed using (a) observational data to record "calls for help" and (b) information from printed data sheets obtained from the manikins' recording equipment to record all other aspects of the performance. One mark was awarded for successful performance of each skill and, in order to achieve an overall pass score, a score of 10 (100%) was required.

Results showed none of the subjects was able to perform all BLS skills satisfactorily. Scores for individual subjects ranged from 10% to 90%, and the overall level of competence for this skill was low. Chest compression was the worst performed skill, with not one nurse being able to compress the chest to the correct depth of 4-5 cm. consistently. The fact that none of the subjects was able to perform chest compression adequately is worrisome and may indicate an inherent contradiction in the methodologies used to teach resuscitation skills. Much resuscitation training relies on rote learning of treatment algorithms, concentrating on "what to do" and "when to do it." Nurses, however, not only need to be able to perform individual skills competently and in the right order, but also to modify their performance in response to a change or absence of change in the patient's condition. Cooper and Libby (1997) advocate the need for a greater awareness of the educational and psychological aspects of planning and delivering resuscitation training.

Drevenhorn et al. (2003) used checklists to assess the basic skill of taking blood pressure among 21 randomly selected public health nurses from Skane County in Sweden while they performed three blood pressure measurements. The checklist was found to be easy to complete while observing the three performances of each nurse. After each nurse finished taking the three readings, she was asked whether the equipment was calibrated, whether she had made a note in the patient's record about which arm was used for the measurement, and whether the reading was performed in the morning or afternoon. Overall, the public health nurses used a correct method for performing blood pressure measurement, but they needed more information about how to choose the right width of cuff. In addition, the checklist was reported to be adequate as a standardized measure to assess the blood pressure skill, but the report of this study did not discuss how the scale was developed or how its validity and reliability were determined.

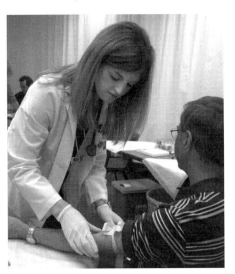

Also using *skill checklists* to evaluate the mode of instruction and effectiveness of skill performance were Bishop et al. (2001), who assessed the retention of tracheal intubation skills one year after initial training of 11 respiratory therapists on staff at a 253-bed hospital. Prior to returning to the operating room for skills assessment and recertification, each respiratory therapist (RT) took a 21-question written exam and then went to the operating room with a trained observer, who monitored the intubation performance to see whether critical steps were followed. A second trained observer, an anesthesiologist, monitored the skills checklist as the intubation was performed. Findings included a poor correlation ($r = -.25$, $p \geq .01$) between the number of intubations performed by the therapists for emergencies in the previous year and the number of intubations needed by the respiratory therapists for RT recertification. There was a negative correlation ($r = -.08$, $p \leq .05$) between the score on the written test and the number of intubations required for recertification; a higher score meant fewer intubations were needed to achieve recertification. In other words, occasional performance of the skill did not ensure skill maintenance. Cognitive and procedural abilities were correlated with each other, suggesting benefits to didactic learning as well as to practical training; and two specific mistakes were identified that need to be emphasized more in the teaching and recertification education.

Miller, Nichols, and Beeken (2000) did a quasi-experimental study with a post-test only design comparing videotaped and faculty-present return demonstrations of clinical skills. Students were divided into two evaluation groups at the beginning of the semester. Thirteen skills were evaluated throughout the semester. One group of students completed return demonstrations using the videotaped method and the other group performed return demonstrations using the faculty-present method. In summary, this study revealed that students and faculty reported that the faculty-present method was more conducive to learning; however, the study results demonstrated that student learning did not vary between the two groups. In addition, neither faculty nor students indicated any difference in the perception of the level of stress between the two methods.

## CONCLUSIONS

Through the efforts of researchers in the United States, the United Kingdom, Sweden, and Australia, a small body of research has begun to emerge regarding strategies used to teach and evaluate psychomotor skill performance. The studies reviewed here indicate that learning outcomes using nontraditional psychomotor instructional strategies are typically equivalent to those of traditional classroom instruction on skills. Cognitive or knowledge gains have not been shown to be different as measured by pre-/post-test scores and course grades. Other learner outcomes, such as learner self-efficacy, student satisfaction, more efficient use of time, and cost-effectiveness also are positive. One approach to teaching psychomotor skills that did not seem to be effective was PBL, where students were "on their own" to learn without teacher facilitation until they entered the clinical setting. In contrast, the two student-centered studies, where the teacher served as a facilitator who guided students' learning activities, showed very promising results in terms of student learning and skill performance.

Only one study reviewed specifically evaluated costs of instruction: the self-directed method showed a cost saving of $149.27 per learner compared with the traditional method of teaching ACLS. Clearly, costs of teaching psychomotor skills are not well understood or regularly reported.

Students learning psychomotor skills in various nontraditional settings and immersed in different teaching strategies require considerable instruction, explanation, support, and facilitation about the process. They must be oriented to the instructional process and encouraged to learn and practice the skills in the environment provided.

Educators can use a variety of strategies to provide instruction as well as "hands-on" practice, even though the content can be delivered using a variety of approaches. For example, faculty can provide actual props and equipment in the computer environment as students learn skills via multimedia, computer-based methods. Laboratory kits with equipment can be provided for the learner to practice at home or in another convenient setting as the skill is learned via CD-ROM, self-instructional modules, or a recorded lecture.

Other instructional strategies include periodic review of skills content throughout the semester or year, even if the instruction is only content-based. Simulations with paid actors/actresses or volunteer senior students as used in the OSCEs could be utilized more as a teaching method in addition to its much-discussed role in assessment and evaluation. However, very few studies comprehensively address these settings and teaching strategies.

The role of the educator in helping students learn in the psychomotor domain is evolving, and only one narrative research study addressing the talents needed by instructors teaching psychomotor skills was found, despite the fact that an increasing variety of approaches to teach psychomotor skills are being used. Traditional faculty activities such as student/faculty interaction and feedback continue to be essential to validate learning, stimulate problem-solving and critical thinking, and validate correct procedures in performing the skill. In addition, it seems that the physical presence of the educator is essential when students are learning psychomotor skills, but the role must be reexamined and perhaps modified to ensure that learning outcomes are positive and competencies are attained.

## RECOMMENDATIONS FOR FURTHER RESEARCH

As nurse educators revisit methods of teaching, modify nursing curricula to meet the needs of diverse learners and deal with the nurse educator shortage, innovative teaching strategies used to teach psychomotor skills will need to be examined to ensure positive learning outcomes and effective use of resources, including the instructor's time. Building on previous research, which has addressed learner outcomes and satisfaction, additional questions can be raised to understand the role and the best method of teaching psychomotor skills in nursing education. The following questions arise after conducting the literature review:

1. **The educator.** With new and innovative instructional methods to teach skills, how does the educator role change? Should the educator demonstrate the psychomotor skill first? How much instructor feedback is needed? When is the feedback best given? What type of faculty development offerings and education are most effective in helping faculty learn how to teach psychomotor skills? What pre-laboratory preparation by the teacher makes for a more effective lab experience?

2. **The learners.** What student-centered approach is most effective in helping students learn psychomotor skills? Is collaborative learning among students

effective for psychomotor skill development? What skill sets brought to the first clinical laboratory experience by the student enhance the learning of fundamental nursing skills? What learner support systems need to be in place to promote optimum learning of skills? What pre-laboratory preparation by the learner makes for a more effective lab experience? What should be the nature of peer feedback on skills performance?

3. **Instructional models.** What instructional approach is most effective in facilitating psychomotor domain learning? For example, should the instruction always be given in a lecture format, followed by a demonstration mechanism? And should that demonstration be via face-to-face instruction with the instructor, on video, or through a web-based program? What learning experiences in skill development are most helpful to students as they move into the clinical setting? What teaching strategies best promote naturalization of skills?

4. **Learning outcomes.** How can critical-thinking and problem-solving skills be enhanced when teaching psychomotor skills? Can outcome measurement tools be standardized for each fundamental skill that is taught? How can skill retention be enhanced and measured? When is it appropriate to assess only skill performance, and when should psychomotor skills be assessed in conjunction with cognitive and affective domain learning?

## SUMMARY

This review of the current literature on teaching and learning in the psychomotor domain shows that many studies have not used a theoretical/conceptual framework to design the mode of instruction delivered to the student, and more research is needed on best practices for teaching/learning psychomotor skills. Many reports provide only brief discussions of the research designs used, and the instruments used to measure learning outcomes and skill acquisition often lack clarity. Two studies provide guidance to nurse educators in selecting appropriate teaching strategies for student psychomotor skill development, but no studies were found on mastery learning or competency learning of psychomotor skills. Researchers need to describe the learning environment, teaching strategies, and equipment used when conducting their studies, and valid and reliable instruments need to be developed for, and then used across, settings in order to standardize the measurement.

Future research must continue to measure, describe, and answer questions about course and program outcomes. Many studies measured cognitive outcomes and learner satisfaction, but there has not been consistency in measuring performance outcomes. How to enhance learning in the psychomotor domain clearly is an area where more evidence is needed to help faculty provide optimal, quality instruction.

**Table 5.2. Literature Review for Research-Based Articles on Teaching Psychomotor Skills (1998-2008)**

| Author | Title | Type of Skill | Sample | Purpose | Findings |
|--------|-------|---------------|--------|---------|----------|
| Agazio, Pavlides, Lasome, Flaherty, & Torrance (2002) | Evaluation of a virtual reality (VR) simulator in sustainment training | Venipuncture | Two groups: N=25 in VR training; standard IV arm N=26; Army medical personnel | To compare the effectiveness and user satisfaction of the Cath-Sim Intravenous Training System to the traditional IV arm for teaching and achieving competence at IV insertion while in mission-oriented protective posture (MOPP) level 4 for Army Medical personnel. | The results demonstrated no significant difference in success rate or time to be successful between the use of the current IV arm model and the Cath-Sim in IV insertion. Both advantages and disadvantages were noted with each model. |
| Alinier (2003) | Nursing students' and lecturers' perspectives of objective structured clinical examination (OSCE) incorporating simulation | Psychomotor skills | N=86 nursing students and N=39 lecturers | To assess the students' and lecturers' perception of OSCE using a Likert scale. | According to the information collected, the "mixed mode" OSCE sessions were generally appreciated by students and examiners, who rated them, respectively, with means of 1.58 and 1.82 on a five-point Likert scale ( 1, very useful; 5, not useful at all). 96.5% of the students and 94.4% of the examiners also think that those sessions should be incorporated in the nursing curriculum. Students think that the OSCE sessions should take place 3-4 times per year. |

**Table 5.2. Literature Review for Research-Based Articles on Teaching Psychomotor Skills (1998-2008) (continued)**

| Author | Title | Type of Skill | Sample | Purpose | Findings |
|---|---|---|---|---|---|
| Anderson, Skillen, & Knight (2001) | Continuing care nurses' perception of need for physical assessment skills | Physical assessment skills | N=19 continuing care facilities in one Alberta Health Region, two independent groups; case managers N=150, and nurse administrators N=39 | To identify the perceived learning needs of RN case managers for physical assessment skills, their use of computers and business supports to enhance application of physical assessment skills by the caregivers. | 44% of the sample reported no course work in physical assessment; 80% expressed excitement about learning through computer technology. This sample found their greatest learning needs were in assessing the thorax and lungs, and secondly assessing the cardiovascular system. Barriers included no opportunities to acquire or practice the physical assessment skill at the worksite. |
| Angona, Searles, Nasrallah, Darling (2001) | Status of pediatric perfusion education: 2000 survey | Pediatric perfusion skills | Three groups: program directors N=22; recent nursing graduates N=61; pediatric cardiac anesthesiologists N=16 | A survey questionnaire designed to assess current pediatric perfusion education was administered to three groups: program directors, recent graduates of perfusion programs, and pediatric anesthesiologists, asking three core questions pertaining to the core perfusion skills. | There are limitations to pediatric perfusion education. A postgraduate program in infant perfusion is one possible solution to the identifier and perfusion problems. |

**Table 5.2. Literature Review for Research-Based Articles on Teaching Psychomotor Skills (1998-2008) (continued)**

| Author | Title | Type of Skill | Sample | Purpose | Findings |
|---|---|---|---|---|---|
| Beeson & Kring (2003) | The effects of two teaching methods on nursing students' factual knowledge and performance of psychomotor skills | Measuring blood pressure | N=104 sophomore students | To compare the effects of two teaching methods (interactive video and traditional lecture/linear video) on students' factual knowledge about BP and their ability to measure blood pressure. | The mean pretest score did not significantly differ between the two groups of students: lecture group and interactive video group. ANCOVA on knowledge gains with the knowledge pretest as the covariate indicated that both groups (p<.0001) showed significant gains in knowledge at the posttest. There was a significant group effect (p<.01) for the teaching method. Students taught by the traditional lecture/linear video method gained significantly more knowledge than students taught by interactive video. |
| Bishop, Piotr, Hussey, , Massey, & Lakshmina-rayan (2001) | Recertification of respiratory therapists' intubation skills one year after training: An analysis of skill and retention and retraining | Tracheal intubation | N=11 respiratory therapists on staff at a 253-bed hospital | To assess retention of skills one year after initial training and identify specific areas of knowledge critical to successful performance of intubation. | Findings of the study were: 1. occasional performance of intubation did not ensure skill maintenance; 2. cognitive and procedural abilities correlated, suggesting benefits to practical training; and 3. two specific mistakes were associated with a high incidence of failure. |

**Table 5.2. Literature Review for Research-Based Articles on Teaching Psychomotor Skills (1998-2008) (continued)**

| Author | Title | Type of Skill | Sample | Purpose | Findings |
|--------|-------|---------------|--------|---------|----------|
| **Darr (2000)** | Advanced Cardiac Life Support education: A self-directed, scenario-based approach | Psychomotor skills required to perform ACLS | N=26 RNs and one physician | To evaluate whether a self-directed, scenario-based course format, developed to incorporate principles of adult learning and to meet the newest AHA guidelines, met expected learning outcomes. | The self-directed, scenario-based format created an optimal environment that fostered the complex psychomotor skills learning required to perform ACLS. A cost savings resulted when ACLS participants utilized the self-directed scenario-based course format; 59% reported lower stress levels and 29% appreciate the flexible schedule. |
| **Devlin (1999)** | An evaluative study of the basic life support skills (BLS) of nurses in an independent hospital | Basic life support | N=30 trained nurses from a population of 150 | A research study was conducted to assess the BLS skills of nurses in independent hospitals vs. public institutions in south east of England. | None of the subjects were able to perform all the BLS skills satisfactorily. Individual scores ranged from 10% to 90%, with a mean score of 13.17 that represents an overall low level of competence. Chest compression was the worst performed skill. This fact may be indicative of an inherent contraindication in the methodologies used to teach resuscitation skills. |

**Table 5.2. Literature Review for Research-Based Articles on Teaching Psychomotor Skills (1998-2008) (continued)**

| Author | Title | Type of Skill | Sample | Purpose | Findings |
|---|---|---|---|---|---|
| Drevenhorn, Hakansson, & Petersson (2003) | Blood pressure measurement — an observational study of 21 public health nurses | Blood pressure measurements | N=21 randomly selected public health nurses | To observe how public health nurses perform blood pressure measurement. | The public health nurses used an overall correct method for blood pressure measurement. Five nurses out of 21 used the Tri-cuff, but the soft cuff was used most frequently. To ensure a completely correct method, additional information is needed by the nurses. |
| Effken & Doyle (2001) | Interface design and cognitive style in learning an instructional computer simulation | 3 physiological problems using 3 interface designs to solve problems by administering drugs targeted at different aspects of the simulated hemodynamic system | N=18 nursing students | To investigate how cognitive style interacts with interface design to affect users' abilities to learn to use a computer simulation. | The visual group outperformed the verbal group on the percent of scenarios solved and percentage of trials in the target range. Time to initiate treatment and number of drugs used did not differ significantly by cognitive style. |
| Engum & Jeffries (2003) | Intravenous cath training system: Computer-based education versus traditional learning methods | Venipuncture | Two groups: N=93 third-year medical students<br><br>N=72 sophomore baccalaureate nursing students | To compare the effectiveness, user satisfaction and self-efficiency of the Cath-Sim IV training system with the traditional laboratory method (lecture, video, and demonstration) for teaching health professionals how to perform venipuncture. | Results indicated the traditional groups were more satisfied with their learning than the technological group; however, there were no significant differences in IV start accuracy or self-efficiency of the learners in both groups. The computer-based methods would be a supplemental teaching strategy rather than stand-alone instruction. |

**Table 5.2. Literature Review for Research-Based Articles on Teaching Psychomotor Skills (1998-2008) (continued)**

| Author | Title | Type of Skill | Sample | Purpose | Findings |
|---|---|---|---|---|---|
| Goldsmith, Stewart, & Ferguson (2005) | Peer learning partnership: An innovative strategy to enhance skill acquisition in nursing students | Psychomotor skill acquisition | First- and third-year nursing students | To assess if participation in a peer learning experience increases skill performance and confidence, and provides for an opportunity for personal growth. | Both groups (75% of first years and 97% of the third years) agreed that their learning was enhanced by the experience. Confidence improved. |
| Holloway (1999) | Developing an evidence base for teaching nursing practice skills in an undergraduate nursing program | Ten most important clinical skills | N=33 clinicians in med-surg setting with hospitals that were used for students' clinical experiences | To determine research that provides evidence to teach clinical skills and to determine the ten most important skills needed by new registered nurses. | Newly registered nurses performed best in the category of "fundamental" skills. Levels of competency that were selected most often were that of "advanced beginner" and competent learner. |
| Jeffries (2001) | Computer vs. lecture: A comparison of two methods of teaching oral medication administration in a nursing skills laboratory | Medication administration | N=42 baccalaureate junior students placed in 2 groups | To compare the effectiveness of both an interactive, multimedia CD-ROM and a traditional lecture for teaching oral medication administration to nursing students. | Results showed significant differences between the two groups in cognitive gains and student satisfaction (p=.01), with the computer group demonstrating higher student satisfaction and more cognitive gains than the lecture group. |

**Table 5.2. Literature Review for Research-Based Articles on Teaching Psychomotor Skills (1998-2008) (continued)**

| Author | Title | Type of Skill | Sample | Purpose | Findings |
|---|---|---|---|---|---|
| Jeffries, Rew, & Cramer (2002) | A comparison of student-centered vs. traditional methods of teaching basic skills in a learning lab | Surgical asepsis | Two groups: N=70 sophomore baccalaureate students in the student centered group; N=50 junior baccalaureate students in the traditional group | To compare effectiveness of two instructional methods in teaching basic nursing skills in the learning lab. One method used an interactive student-centered focus, the other used a traditional focus with lectures and demonstrations. | There were no significant differences between the group pretest to posttest cognitive score gains, although there were cognitive gains for both groups. The groups were similar in their ability to perform skills. There were significant differences in students learning satisfaction with the student-centered group being more satisfied. |
| Jeffries, Woolf, & Linde (2003) | A comparison of two methods for teaching the skill of performing a 12-lead ECG | Performing a 12-lead ECG | N=77 baccalaureate senior nursing students | To compare the effectiveness of an interactive, multimedia CD-ROM with traditional methods of teaching the skill of performing a 12-lead ECG. | There were no significant baseline differences (p< .05) in pretest scores between the two groups. Overall results indicated that both groups were satisfied with the conventional method and were similar in their ability to demonstrate the skill correctly on a live simulated patient. This study is a beginning step to assess new and potentially more cost-effective methods to teach skills. |

**Table 5.2. Literature Review for Research-Based Articles on Teaching Psychomotor Skills (1998-2008) (continued)**

| Author | Title | Type of Skill | Sample | Purpose | Findings |
|---|---|---|---|---|---|
| **Khattab & Rawlings (2001)** | Assessing nurse practitioner students using a modified objective structured clinical exam (OSCE) | Clinical skills for nurse practitioners | Nurse practitioner students | The article describes and analyzes a modified OSCE, which is currently being used at Bournemouth University, as a measure of clinical competency for student nurse practitioners, and as a certification tool at the end of year 1 in a two-year course. | The modified OSCE was found to be helpful as an assessment tool for formative and summative assessment, as a resource for learning, as a basis for abbreviated versions of physical exam assessment, and to identify gaps and weaknesses in clinical skills. |
| **Le, Reed, Weinstein, Matthew, & Brown (2001)** | Paramedic use of endotracheal tube introducers for the difficult airway | Intubation with a flex guide endotracheal tube introducers | N=35 students enrolled in a New York state paramedic recertification course | To evaluate the ability of paramedics to learn and apply the skill of introducers-aided oral intubation in the setting of the simulated difficult airway after a five-minute lecture on the principles and use of the eTTi. | The use of the eTTi was mastered by the participants after only a brief didactic introduction to the device. Their ability to intubate an immobilized mannequin using the eTTi was observed. |

**Table 5.2. Literature Review for Research-Based Articles on Teaching Psychomotor Skills (1998-2008) (continued)**

| Author | Title | Type of Skill | Sample | Purpose | Findings |
|---|---|---|---|---|---|
| Menix (2003) | Domains of learning: Interdependent components of achievable learning outcomes | Not Applicable | Not Applicable | To define the cognitive, affective and psychomotor domains and accompanying levels of complexity, show relatedness to the three, discuss their value and provide examples of their use. | The educational taxonomies of the cognitive, affective and psychomotor domains and their levels of complexity provide educators with tools useful for developing learning objectives. These objectives give the teaching-learning process and outcomes, particularly planning, implementing, and evaluating learning situations, a means to improve competency. |
| Miller, Nichols, & Beeken (2000) | Comparing videotaped and faculty-present return demonstrations of clinical skills | Clinical psychomotor skills | N=48 junior nursing students in a intermountain west baccalaureate nursing program | To assess if there are differences in student performance levels and student and faculty satisfaction when return demonstrations of clinical skills were done with faculty present or with videotape. | Scores on only one skill differed at a statistically significant level between the two student groups. (One group did a return demonstration in front of a faculty person and the other group did a return demonstration in front of a videotape.) The videotaping group had more overall satisfaction ratings than the faculty present group. However, when comparisons were made for each skill, this difference was statistically significant only for the skill of administering oral medications. |

**Table 5.2. Literature Review for Research-Based Articles on Teaching Psychomotor Skills (1998-2008) (continued)**

| Author | Title | Type of Skill | Sample | Purpose | Findings |
|---|---|---|---|---|---|
| Minnesota Bacca-laureate Psychomotor Skills Fac-ulty Group (1998) | Conversations: An experience of psycho-motor skills faculty | Psychomotor skills educa-tors coming together to "tell teacher tales" | A community of baccalau-reate fac-ulty teaching psychomotor skills in a large set-ting from 8 baccalaure-ate nursing programs | The community's reason for com-ing together was to share ideas and experiences regarding any topic, specific or broad. Discussions revolved around: psychomotor skill content, teaching methodologies, laboratory manage-ment, education resources, and issues on how to teach critical care skills, and to an-swer the question: How can we best teach psychomotor skills? | One of the outcomes of the sharing com-munity was support for one another in the role as teacher of psychomotor skills. Talents re-quired to teach psy-chomotor skills were identified: teaching cognitive and affec-tive skills along with the psychomotor do-main; demonstrating clinical competence; facilitating student progression from be-ginning to applica-tion level; teaching general principles of nursing practice; and recognizing the uniqueness of students' learning. |
| Nicol & Freeth (1998) | Assessment of clinical skills: A new ap-proach to an old problem | Clinical skill assessment using the "Barts" Nurs-ing OSCE | N=140 students examined in one day (20 per hour in a seven-hour day) | To assess the use of Bart's Nursing OSCE (10 stations: 6 hospitals/4 com-munities). | The Bart's Nursing OSCE has been well-evaluated by students, staff and external stakehold-ers. The construct validity of the as-sessment was done through a discussion with a panel of expert teachers. The development of this Nursing OSCE raised the profile of clinical and communica-tion skills, and influenced student learning. |

**Table 5.2. Literature Review for Research-Based Articles on Teaching Psychomotor Skills (1998-2008) (continued)**

| Author | Title | Type of Skill | Sample | Purpose | Findings |
|---|---|---|---|---|---|
| **Salyers (2007)** | Teaching psychomotor skills to beginning nursing students using a web-enhanced format | Psychomotor skills | N=36 nursing students enrolled in a beginning nursing skills laboratory course | To determine if<br><br>1. students receiving web-enhanced instruction perform better on a final comprehensive cognitive examination than students receiving traditional instruction?<br><br>2. students receiving web-enhanced instruction perform better on a final psychomotor skills examination than students receiving traditional instruction?<br><br>3. students receiving web-enhanced instruction indicate a greater level of satisfaction with the course than students receiving traditional instruction? | 1. The experimental web-enhanced group performed significantly better on the comprehensive cognitive final examination than the control group.<br><br>2. The experimental group performed better on the final psychomotor skills examination than the control group, although not significantly better.<br><br>3. The experimental group was somewhat dissatisfied to neutral about their overall satisfaction with the course. In contrast, the control group was somewhat satisfied with the course. |
| **Sorrento & Pichichero (2001)** | Assessing diagnostic accuracy and tympanocentesis skills by nurse practitioners in management of otitis media | Physical exam to assess for otitis media | Two groups: N=1271 pediatricians, N=206 nurse practitioners, who viewed nine different video-recorded pneumatic otoscopic exams of tympanic membranes (TMs) | To assess health care provider accuracy in recognizing the physical examination finding of acute otitis media and otitis media with diffusion and technical competence in performing tympanocentesis using a simulated model. | Overall the average correct diagnosis by all health care providers was 46%, by pediatricians 50% and by NPs 42%. Interactive continuing medical education with simulation technology may enhance skills and lead to a willingness to change and improve diagnostic accuracy and treatment paradigms. |

**Table 5.2. Literature Review for Research-Based Articles on Teaching Psychomotor Skills (1998-2008) (continued)**

| Author | Title | Type of Skill | Sample | Purpose | Findings |
|--------|-------|---------------|--------|---------|----------|
| Tarnow & King (2004) | Intradermal injections: Traditional bevel up versus bevel down | Correct placement of injection, leaking or bleeding, time to administer injection, and comfort of persons administering and receiving an intradermal injection | N=98 nursing students | To assess the difference in correct placement of the injectate between the bevel-up and bevel-down technique for intradermal injections; to assess the time required for administering an intradermal injection between the bevel-up and bevel-down technique; to assess if there is a difference in the comfort level of the person receiving an intradermal injection between the bevel-up and bevel-down technique; and to assess if there is a difference in the comfort level of the person administering an intradermal injection between the bevel-up and bevel-down technique. | After second injection, each student reported which was better. 82% of the time a wheal was produced. Leaking or bleeding occurred a fourth of the time. Subjects rated the first injection better with no preference regarding technique. Subjects administering injections reported bevel up more comfortable. Bevel up was found to be significantly faster. |

**Table 5.2. Literature Review for Research-Based Articles on Teaching Psychomotor Skills (1998-2008) (continued)**

| Author | Title | Type of Skill | Sample | Purpose | Findings |
|---|---|---|---|---|---|
| Thorne & Hackwood (2002) | Developing critical care skills for nurses in the ward environment: A work-based learning approach | Critical care skills | Participating nurses on the assigned critical care wards /units | To implement a new approach to developing the care of critically ill patients from two perspectives: an in-house educational program as an introduction to critical care skills for ward-based nurses, and involvement of the patient at-risk team as supporters of work-based learning. | Results indicated the practitioners involved provided evidence of expanded skills in caring for sick patients, an increased ability to recognize the clinical urgency when a patient is deteriorating, and greater confidence to refer appropriately. The experience of developing and delivering the course provided insight into the diversity of skills of the practitioners involved and opportunities to nurture potential among the ward nurses. |

**Table 5.2. Literature Review for Research-Based Articles on Teaching Psychomotor Skills (1998-2008) (continued)**

| Author | Title | Type of Skill | Sample | Purpose | Findings |
|---|---|---|---|---|---|
| Williams (1999) | An antipodean evaluation of problem-based learning by clinical educators | Clinical skills in a learning laboratory using a Problem Based Learning approach to learn | N=8 sections of clinical educators for year one; N=14 focus group clinical educators for year two of a nursing program | To evaluate whether student learning through a problem-based learning curriculum has a positive impact on bridging the reported theory-practice gap. | Clinical education is complex. The ability of each student varied between each group, clinical educator, and clinical placement. The motivated or mature student tended to do well, whereas the younger student was overwhelmed and less confident. Group dynamics were up with PBL. Student learning in the lab was unsurpassed. Foundational knowledge and skills are necessary prior to using PBL to enhance a theory-practice link. Students need more supervision in the lab than a purely self-directed PBL curriculum can accommodate. |
| Wilson, Shepherd, Kelly, & Pitzner (2005) | Assessment of a low-fidelity human patient simulator for the acquisition of nursing skills | Health assessment knowledge and skills | N=70 registered nurses | To assess a low-fidelity human patient simulator as a precursor to developing and evaluating nurses' health assessment knowledge and skills. | Most of the components and functions of a low-fidelity simulator were realistic, better than existing training products, and suitable for teaching purposes. |

# REFERENCES

Agazio, J., Pavlides, C., Lasome, C., Flaherty, N., & Torrance, R. (2002). Evaluation of a virtual reality simulator in sustainment training. _Military Medicine_, 167, 893-897.

Alinier, G. (2003). Nursing students' and lecturers' perspectives of objective structured clinical examination incorporating simulation. _Nurse Educator Today_, 23, 419-426.

Anderson, M., Skillen, L., & Knight, C. (2001). Continuing care nurses' perceptions of need for physical assessment skills. _Journal of Gerontological Nursing_, 27(7) 23-29.

Angona, R., Searles, B., Nasrallah, F., & Darling, E. (2001). Status of pediatric perfusion education: 2000 survey. _Journal of ExtraCorporeal Technology_, 33(4), 233-238.

Baldwin, D., Hill, P., & Hanson, G. (1991). Performance of psychomotor skills: A comparison of two teaching strategies. _Journal of Nursing Education_, 30(8), 367-370.

Barrows, H., & Tamblyn, R. (1980). _Problem-based learning: An approach to medical education_. New York: Springer.

Beeson, S. & Kring, D. (2003). The effects of two teaching methods on nursing students' factual knowledge and performance of psychomotor skills. _Journal of Nursing Education_, 38, 357-359.

Bishop, M., Piotr, M., Hussey, J., Massey, L., & Lakshminarayan, S. (2001). Recertification of respiratory therapists' intubation skills one year after initial training: An analysis of skill retention and retraining. _Respiratory Care_, 46(3), 234-237.

Bloom, B. S. (1953). Thought-processes in lectures and discussion. _Journal of General Education_, I, 160-169.

Candy, P., Crebert, G., & O'Leary, J. (1994). _Developing lifelong learners through undergraduate education_ (National Board of Employment Education and Training Commissioned Report No. 28). Canberra, Australia: Australian Government Publishing Service.

Chickering, A. W. & Gamson, Z. F. (1987). Seven principles for good practice in undergraduate education. _American Association for Higher Education Bulletin_, 45(8), 3-7.

Cook, J. W., & Hill, P. M. (1985). The impact of successful laboratory systems and the teaching of nursing skills. _Journal of Nursing Skills_, 24(8), 344-346.

Cooper, S., & Libby, J. (1997). A review of educational issues in resuscitation training. _Journal of Clinical Nursing, 6_, 5-10.

Darr, L. R. (2000). Advanced cardiac life support education: A self-directed, scenario-based approach. _The Journal of Continuing Education in Nursing, 31(3)_, 116-120.

Dave, R. (1970). _Psychomotor levels in developing and writing objectives._ Tucson, AZ: Educational Innovators Press.

Devlin, M. (1999). An evaluative study of the basic life support skills of nurses in an independent hospital. _Journal of Clinical Nursing, 8(2)_, 201-205.

Diekelmann, N. (1993). Interpretive research and narratives of teaching. _Journal of Nursing Education, 32_, 5-6.

Drevenhorn, E., Hakansson, A., & Petersson, K. (2003). Blood pressure measurement: An observational study of 21 public health nurses. _Journal of Clinical Nursing, 10(2)_, 189-194.

Effken, J., & Doyle, M. (2001). Interface design and cognitive style in learning an instructional computer simulation. _Computers in Nursing, 19(4)_, 164-171.

Engum, S., & Jeffries, P. R. (2003). Intravenous catheter training system: Computer-based education versus traditional learning methods. _American Journal of Surgery, 186(1)_, 67-74.

Feletti, G., & Bond, D. (Eds.). (1997). _The challenge of problem-based learning_ (2ⁿᵈ ed.). Sterling, VA: Stylus Publishing.

Goldsmith, M., Stewart, L., & Ferguson, L. (2005). Peer learning partnership: An innovative strategy to enhance skill acquisition in nursing students. _Nurse Educator Today, 26_, 123-130.

Hannadeh, G., Lancaster, C., & Johnson, A. (1993). Introducing the objective structure clinical examination to a family practice residing program. _Family Medicine, 25(4)_, 237-241.

Harrow, A. J. (1972). _A taxonomy of the psychomotor domain: A guide for developing behavioral objectives._ New York: Pearson Longman.

Holloway, K. (1999). Developing an evidence base for teaching nursing practice skills in an undergraduate nursing program. _Nursing Praxis in New Zealand, 14(1)_, 22-32.

Jeffries, P. R. (2001). Computer versus lecture: A comparison of two methods of teaching oral medication administration in a nursing skills laboratory. _Journal of Nursing Education,_ 40, 323-329.

Jeffries, P. R., Rew, S., & Cramer, J. M. (2002). A comparison of student-centered versus traditional methods of teaching basic nursing skills in a learning laboratory. _Nursing Education Perspectives,_ 23(1), 14-19.

Jeffries, P. R., Woolf, S., & Linde, B. (2003). A comparison of two methods for teaching the skill of performing a 12-lead ECG. _Nursing Education Perspectives,_ 24(2), 70-74.

Khattab, A., & Rawlings, B. (2001). Assessing nurse practitioner students using a modified objective structured clinical examination (OSCE). _Nurse Education Today,_ 21, 541-550.

Knowles, M. S. (1978). _The adult learner: A neglected species_ (2nd ed.). Houston: Gulf Publishing.

Le, D. H., Reed, D., Weinstein, G., Matthew, G., & Brown, L. (2001). Paramedic use of endotracheal tube introducers for the difficult airway. _Prehospital Emergency Care,_ 5(2), 155-158.

Maeve, M. K. (1994). The carrier bag theory of nursing practice. _Advances in Nursing Science,_ 16(4), 9-22.

Menix, K. (2003). Domains of learning: Interdependent components of achievable learning outcomes. _Journal of Continuing Education in Nursing,_ 27, 200-208.

Miller, H., Nichols, E., & Beeken, J. (2000). Comparing videotaped and faculty-present return demonstrations of clinical skills. _Journal of Nursing Education,_ 39, 237-239.

Minnesota Baccalaureate Psychomotor Skills Faculty Group. (1998). Conversations: An experience of psychomotor skills faculty. _Journal of Nursing Education,_ 37, 324-325.

Nicol, M., & Freeth, D. (1998). Assessment of clinical skills: A new approach to an old problem. _Nurse Education Today,_ 18, 601-609.

PageWise, Inc. (2002). Psychomotor development and learning. [Online]. Available: http://utut.essortment.com/psychomotordeve_pqs.htm.

Reilly, D. E., & Oermann, M. H. (1999). _Behavioral objectives: Evaluation in nursing_ (3rd ed.). New York: National League for Nursing.

Salyers, V. (2007). Teaching psychomotor skills to beginning nursing students using a web-enhanced approach. *International Journal of Nursing Education Scholarship*, 4(1), 3-12.

Sorrento, A., & Pichichero, M. (2001). Assessing diagnostic accuracy and tympanocentesis skills by nurse practitioners in management of otitls media. *Journal of the American Academy of Nurse Practitioners*, 13(11), 524-529.

Tanner, C. A. (1993). Conversations on teaching. *Journal of Nursing Education*, 32(7), 291-292.

Tarnow, K., & King, N. (2004). Intradermal injections: Traditional bevel up versus bevel down. *Applied Nursing Research*, 17(4), 275-282.

Thorne, L., & Hackwood, H. (2002). Developing critical care skills for nurses in the ward environment: A work-based learning approach. *Nursing in Critical Care*, 7(3), 121-125.

Williams, A. (1999). An antipodean evaluation of problem-based learning by clinical educators. *Nurse Education Today*, 19, 659-667.

Wilson, M., Shepherd, I., Kelly, C., & Pitzner, J. (2005). Assessment of a low-fidelity human patient simulator for the acquisition of nursing skills. *Nurse Educator Today*, 25, 56-67.

Yoder, M.E. (1993). Computer use and nursing research: Transfer of cognitive learning to a clinical skill - Linear versus interactive video. *Western Journal of Nursing Research*, 15, 115-117.

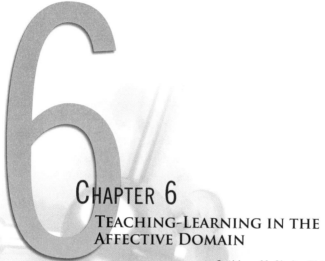

# CHAPTER 6
## TEACHING-LEARNING IN THE AFFECTIVE DOMAIN

*Cathleen M. Shultz, PhD, RN, CNE, FAAN*

"The 'who' that any of us is ethically is in large part a function of the 'what' that any of us knows intellectually. The circulatory systems of our intellect and our ethos merge with each other all the time, and the living blood of influence flows in both directions. Change what I know and you change who I am. Change what your students know and you change who they are as well."

Gregory, 2004, p. 3

## OVERVIEW

Since the mid-1980s, the influence of cognitive psychology and an emphasis on student learning has gained favor in nursing programs primarily due to the curriculum revolution conferences sponsored by the National League for Nursing and the outcomes movement led in nursing by the National League for Nursing through its accreditation requirements. By focusing on outcomes of the educational experience, faculty realized that our curricula, teaching practices, and relationships with students needed to change.

While much of education and educational research has emphasized and continues to emphasize cognitive learning, educators are increasingly realizing that learning must address more than knowing or understanding if graduates are to function effectively in today's complex, chaotic environments. One of the most significant outcomes of this realization is the increased recognition of the importance of affective domain learning. Nursing educators have a societal responsibility to address the development of students' values, and they accomplish this through learning activities such as service-learning initiatives, social justice projects, cultural competence discussions, and ethics education.

The notion of integration of and overlap among the three domains of learning was addressed long ago by Harrow (1972) and Simpson (1972). They noted that while the three domains offer a discrete classification system, learning outcomes often overlap two or more domains. For example, cognitive outcomes often have some affective components, and motor skills typically include both cognitive and affective elements. Thus, the domains are not discrete, independent categories...a concept that presents challenges when examining research in teaching and learning in any particular domain. But what is meant by the affective domain, and what implications does it have for nursing education?

The affective domain was initially described by Krathwohl, Bloom, and Masia (1964), whose work focused on learning about interests, attitudes, values, and appreciation. These higher education scholars outlined stages of affective growth from listening to responding, participating, seeking, demonstrating, relating, and finally valuing. To illustrate, once exposed to a value through learning, the student "responds" by studying the material, "participates" in activities where the value is evident, actively "demonstrates" how actions are guided by the value, "relates" the value to actions in other situations, and ultimately "values" the value by integrating it into the fabric of her/his thinking, acting, and being. The approach is developmental and evolves as the student matures and is challenged to engage with ideas that call values into question. Although such development is time-intensive, faculty must devote efforts to help students carefully consider and then integrate their own set of values, which will guide their thinking and actions as nurses and as members of society.

Krathwohl, Bloom, and Masia (1964) defined affective competencies as those that "emphasize a feeling tone, an emotion, or a degree of acceptance or rejection, interests, attitudes, appreciations, values, and emotional sets or biases" (p. 7). According to these authors, the ultimate aim of learning in this domain is internalization, where values become an integral part of an individual. While affective learning may be discussed in isolation, it is, in reality, closely tied to cognitive learning and psychomotor learning. In essence, the affective domain is a "Pandora's Box" that contains "the forces that determine the nature of an individual's life" (Krathwohl et al., 1964, p. 91), and learning in this domain is best demonstrated by changes in behavior rather than by scores on objective tests.

Affect also has been defined as a feeling or emotion separate from cognition, thought, or discipline. Emotions and feelings are considered essential attributes of affective learning across disciplines (Anderson & Phelps, 2002; Bechara, Damasio, & Damasio, 2000; Diaz & De la Casa, 2002; Everhart & Demaree, 2003; Everhart, Demaree, & Wuensch, 2003; Hamm & Vaitl, 1996; Kahn, Lass, Hurtley, & Kornreich, 1981; Kraiger, Ford, & Salas, 1993; Kritzer & Phillips, 1966; Lipp, Neumann, & Mason, 2001; Morris, Ohman, & Dolan, 1998; Myers, 2002; Ross & Stanley, 1985; Rychalak, 1975; Simpson et al., 2000; Stancato & Hamachek, 1990; Woods, 1993; Zimmerman & Phillips, 2000). While Krathwohl et al. recognized feelings and emotions as essential to affective development, no recent studies were found in nursing that explored emotions as a concept central to learning in our field. Attitudes are often conceptualized as affect, and feeling is a component of both affect and attitude, the latter of which has a behavioral component. Therefore, affect may be thought of as the behavioral outcome of attitude. Figure 6.1 depicts the relationships among attitude, affect, feelings, and behaviors.

Beliefs, values, and attitudes also are discussed as affective learning, but they are more accurately thought of as outcomes of affective learning (Lamude & Chow, 1993; Maier-Lorentz, 1999; Martin, Myers, & Mottet, 2000; Neidt & Hedlund, 1969; Rodriguez, Plax, & Kearney, 1996; Snider, 2001). Despite different perspectives and definitions, most scholars writing on the topic note that some cognitive or conscious processing of affect is needed to achieve such outcomes. The nature of this relationship between affective learning and affective learning outcomes is unknown, but it is clear that something happens to the learner's processing of emotions and feelings that result in beliefs, values and attitudes. Figure 6.2, which has been developed by the author based on a careful review of the literature, presents a visual representation of the complexity of the affective domain as it relates to nursing.

**Figure 6.1. Realtionships among Attitude, Affect, Feelings and Behaviors**

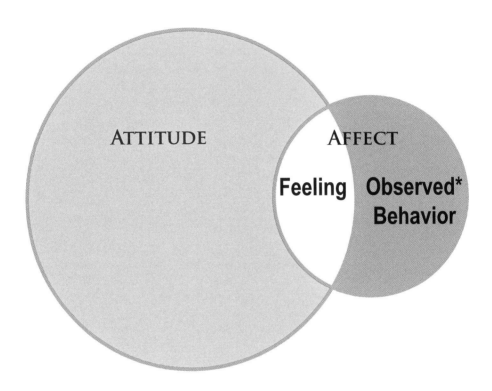

**\*Behavior Outcome of Attitude**

**Figure 6.2 Shultz Model of Affective Teaching-Learning in Nursing Education**

# NURSING CURRICULUM

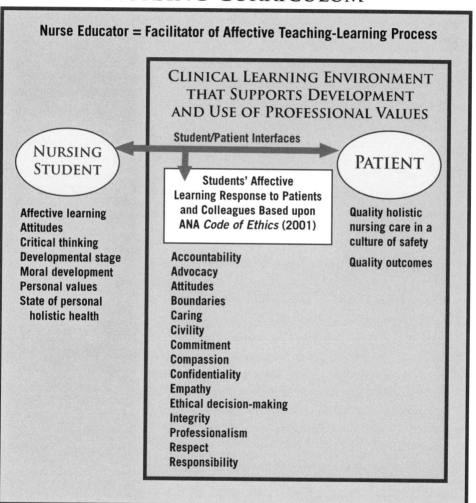

**Nurse Educator = Facilitator of Affective Teaching-Learning Process**

## CLINICAL LEARNING ENVIRONMENT THAT SUPPORTS DEVELOPMENT AND USE OF PROFESSIONAL VALUES

**Student/Patient Interfaces**

NURSING STUDENT

PATIENT

Students' Affective Learning Response to Patients and Colleagues Based upon ANA *Code of Ethics* (2001)

Affective learning
Attitudes
Critical thinking
Developmental stage
Moral development
Personal values
State of personal
  holistic health

Accountability
Advocacy
Attitudes
Boundaries
Caring
Civility
Commitment
Compassion
Confidentiality
Empathy
Ethical decision-making
Integrity
Professionalism
Respect
Responsibility

Quality holistic
nursing care in a
culture of safety

Quality outcomes

© 2008 by Cathleen M. Shultz.

Permission to reproduce granted by copyright owner.

The Shultz Model of Affective Teaching-Learning in Nursing Education is student-centered in the learning environment. The predominant document for identifying current nursing values is the American Nurses Association's *Code of Ethics* (2001), which is embedded in the nursing curriculum. (See Chapter 3 for detailed information concerning the learning environment and student characteristics.) Additional studies are summarized in this chapter, including the affective learning outcomes. The teaching-learning process, depicted as linear for the written page, is highly interactive and complex. The ultimate measure of affective learning occurs in the clinical setting, depicted as the students' behavioral responses to patients and colleagues. These concepts are used to organize the chapter's findings and stimulate areas for further nursing education studies.

Research findings support the need for delineation and teaching of affective domain professional values across all program types. The model proposes combining the ANA *Code of Ethics* (2001) values plus values expanded upon by Fowler (2008) as a place to initiate national affective domain learning expectations. The nurse educator, as a facilitator of professional values development, implements teaching strategies that mature the learner's cognitive and affective development, ability to assess the patient's status and affective responses, and overall affective skill attainment to produce therapeutic nursing interventions and quality patient outcomes. In each learning environment, values development and use is fostered and emphasized as essential to practice and healthy patient outcomes.

## Literature Search Process

Searching the literature regarding affective domain learning was a challenge, as specific descriptors were limited, making extraction of resources difficult. "Affective domain" does not exist as a search term in electronic retrieval databases, various disciplines use different terms to address this domain, and affective concepts and search terms have changed over time. For example, the phrase "values clarification" was a dominant method of identifying and developing values from the 1960s through the 1980s, but the phrase is rarely seen in current research literature. As a result, the literature for the affective domain was reviewed for concepts matching existing search descriptors, such as caring and empathy.

The literature search was limited to the period between 1995 and 2008, and included varying, nondiscrete terms from electronic databases such as Qwest (MEDLINE and CINAHL, etc.), ArticleFirst, WorldCat, ProQuest, and Dissertation Abstracts, as well as hand searches of specific journals (e.g., *Nursing Education Perspectives* and *Journal of Nursing Education*) that are known to publish nursing education research. The search terms used are noted in Table 6.1. This exercise led the author to conclude that present electronic databases are limited regarding affective domain concepts, and hand searches are recommended.

**Table 6.1. Search Terms Used to Conduct the Literature Review**

| Affective | Ethics | Socio-Emotional Maturity |
|---|---|---|
| Attitudes | Moral Judgment | Suffering |
| Caring | Professional Identity | Uncertainty |
| Civility | Professional Values | Values |
| Cultural Sensitivity | Psychosocial Dimensions | Valuing |
| Educational Aspirations | Self-Confidence | |
| Empathy | Self-Efficacy | |

The *Journal of Cognitive Affective Learning* contains many valuable resources about the affective domain, but none of its research articles appeared in the searched databases. The *Annual Review of Nursing Education* (Oermann & Heinrich, 2003-2007) summarizes trends and research in nursing education, but none of the relevant articles found through a hand search of these five volumes appeared in the electronic database searches.

## LITERATURE REVIEW

Of the articles generated by electronic and hand searches, most focused on nursing education, with a selected few focusing on other disciplines. Several doctoral dissertations about affective learning completed by nurses were identified, and most of the early research studies on this topic appeared in two nursing journals, the *Journal of Nursing Education* and the *Journal of Continuing Education in Nursing.* More recent studies about affective domain learning in nursing appeared primarily in the *Journal of Nursing Education* and *Nursing Education Perspectives,* but other journals publish such research as well (see Appendix C). The majority of studies were completed in associate degree or baccalaureate nursing programs, several involved students enrolled in online programs, and only one focused on students in a graduate nursing program. Most reported studies were done in the United States, but there were reports about affective learning studies completed in Australia, Israel, Canada, Taiwan, and the United Kingdom. Only one study addressed affective learning specific to minority students, and few studies have been reported that address affective teaching and learning in the clinical setting. As recognition of the importance of affective domain development in achieving positive patient care outcomes gains attention in education and practice arenas, research on this topic is expected to increase.

Although nursing publications about teaching and measuring affective learning have been reported for decades, the total number of studies found through this search was limited, and all those found are cited in this chapter. Most early studies used quantitative designs to describe students' affective learning, but more recent studies use qualitative designs to enhance our understanding of how students learn in this domain and what that learning is like for them. (A list of current educational databases for literature searches is provided in Appendix D.)

Table 6.2 summarizes how research on learning in the affective domain has changed from the 1940s to the present, and documents the broad scope and meaning of this concept in higher education and nursing education. Such meanings include attitudes, values, caring, empathy and spirituality. No comprehensive programs of research on affective education seemed evident in the literature reviewed, but some trends were noted over time. The table presents dominant research foci in educational research studies.

## THEMES IN THE RESEARCH LITERATURE

Content analysis of the studies yielded nine general categories into which research concerning affective learning can be grouped. Each of the following categories is explained below:

1.  The concept or meaning of "affective," particularly in an education context.

2.  Affective domain competencies.

3.  Professional values and professional identity.

4.  Affective concepts of nursing practice.

5.  Instructional strategies for affective domain learning.

6.  Non-instructional strategies that promote affective development.

7.  Faculty behaviors or characteristics that enhance affective learning.

8.  Research on the affective domain from other professional disciplines.

9.  Emerging affective domain initiatives and technology.

Affective learning theories emerged from developmental models such as Bloom's (1956). All affective learning theories are student-focused. No affective learning theories that provide guidance to educators in developing teaching methodologies that facilitate values development or moral reasoning were located.

Table 6.2. Dominant Research Trends in Affective Domain Learner Development

| Dominant Trend | Development of Learner | Learner Outcomes |
|---|---|---|
| **Earlier Research (1940s to 1970s)**<br><br>*Developmental*<br><br>Progresses from simple to complex | Sequential Stages of Affective Growth<br><br>• Listening<br>• Responding<br>• Participating<br>• Seeking<br>• Demonstrating biases<br>• Relating<br>• Valuing | • Interests<br>• Attitudes<br>• Values<br>• Appreciation<br>• Emotional sets<br>• Behavior changes |
| **Later Research (1970s to 1980s)**<br><br>*Values Development*<br><br>Includes a cognitive process recognized as essential to values development<br><br>*Cognitive Psychology* | • Process of internalization<br>• Valuing is internalized | • Behavior changes that are consistent and stable<br>• Skills in moral reasoning<br>• Career choices<br>• Professional values are demonstrated |
| **Current Research (1990s to present)**<br><br>*Emerging — Eclectic*<br><br>Feelings and emotions are separate from cognition<br>Progression is not a linear process<br>Neuroscience | • Cognitive or conscious processing of affect<br>• Linked to critical thinking and clinical reasoning<br>• Limbic system involvement<br>• Emotions found to affect learning | • Affect<br>• Beliefs<br>• Values<br>• Attitudes<br>• Retention of knowledge<br>• Dominant professional values<br>  • *Integrity*<br>  • *Accountability*<br>  • *Caring*<br>  • *Civility*<br>  • *Empathy* |

## The Concept or Meaning of "Affective"

Numerous researchers used the basic framework developed by Krathwohl, Bloom, and Masia (1964) to study affective domain learning (Astin, 1977; Beane, 1990; Ewell, 1987; Reilly, 1978; Reilly & Oermann, 1992; Vogler, 1991); but some researchers modified the framework for their own interest areas. Beane, for example, believed that affective thought and behavior are exclusively related to preferences and choices, and his work emphasized these elements. Ewell focused on the outcomes of affective learning and was a strong advocate for assessing attitudes and values as "results" of postsecondary education, a concept that was not readily embraced. Later, Vogler asserted that the affective domain is measured through behaviors and may be labeled succinctly as beliefs; he therefore collapsed Krathwohl's six areas to three: awareness, distinction, and integration.

In higher education, Astin (1977) created a taxonomy for outcomes of postsecondary education. Using a matrix with affective-psychological outcomes (personality characteristics, values, attitudes, beliefs, self-concept and satisfaction with college) on one axis and affective-behavioral outcomes (choice of major and educational aspirations) on the other, this scholar helped faculty understand the variety of outcomes to be achieved, given the multiple intersections of these two dimensions. This research also connected affective content with cognitive and psychomotor content and emphasized the importance of all domains in outcome studies. This work is foundational to the current educational outcomes movement.

It seems clear from this literature review that the conceptual meaning of "affective" in an educational context remains consistent with Krathwohl's original thinking, but modifications have been made for specific areas of interest that enhanced our understanding of the concept. The affective domain continues to evolve as educational practices move from teacher-centered approaches to ones that are concerned with student perceptions and acknowledge the relationships of affective domain learning to cognitive and psychomotor domain learning.

### Affective Domain Competencies

Given findings that support the positive impact of a college education on students' affective competency development, subsequent researchers sought to examine the impact of various aspects of a college environment on growth in students' affective domain competence. Several studies (Astin, 1977; Pascarella, 1985; Pascarella & Terenzini, 1991) found that affective growth was enhanced by residential living, attending a private institution, and involvement in campus activities; no recent studies were located on these topics. Felton and Parsons (1987), Kimball (1993), and Mentkowski (1991) reported that addressing, teaching and assessing values were related to increased affective growth during college. Also, Astin (1977) found that non-instructional activities, such as living on campus, might have contributed indirectly to increased student interactions with faculty and peers, factors that he thought accelerated or enhanced affective domain learning.

In an effort to study the link between course work and the formation of professional attitudes in business students, Kimball (1993) used standardized and self-developed instruments to assess the perception of "professionalism" in 35 business careers among 121 students at three different stages of their business program (beginning, mid-point, and end). Results suggested that there were different attitudes about particular careers among students at different points in their program, leading this researcher to conclude that course work itself plays an important role in the formation of attitudes and perceptions among business students. The study also noted the importance of student interaction with faculty as having an impact on affective development. Results were obtained through standardized and author-developed survey instruments. No study was found that addressed use of online or computer technologies that shaped professional development values.

In nursing, Reilly (1978) and Reilly and Oermann (1992) defined affective competencies as moral reasoning. They emphasized that affective competencies relate to "the individual's ability to use moral reasoning in the decisions for the management of moral and ethical dilemmas and to the development of a value system that guides decisions and activities compatible with the individual's and society's notion of what is good and what is right" (p. 292). These researchers identified that affective domain content pertains to ethics; moral judgment; value indicators such as attitudes, interests, beliefs and goals; and values themselves. Mentkowski (1991) found that growth in affective domain learning occurred during college as the result of a specifically planned values development component in the curriculum, with "growth" being defined as "increasingly sophisticated moral and intellectual mind-sets as well as integrated performance of interpersonal and intellectual abilities in situations" (p. 26). She concluded, therefore, that experiencing an education specifically designed to do more than deliver content seemed to make a difference in the development of students' affective competencies as well as promote their cognitive learning.

There are numerous studies on the development of affective competencies in college students, and these studies vary in the way in which affective has been described and assessed. Despite these differences, however, there are several conclusions that can be drawn from these studies: there is a positive correlation between attaining a college education and affective development; college environmental factors impact affective development, even indirectly; the primary environmental factor facilitating the development of affective learning is student involvement with faculty and peers; and, the identification, teaching, and assessment of specific affective content in the educational program positively influences growth in this domain of learning. Thus, faculty could enhance their students' holistic development by attending to affective domain learning as part of the academic program.

No studies were identified that addressed affective program outcomes in a total online learning environment. Most nursing articles about the affective domain are not research studies, but are anecdotal, in which teaching and curriculum ideas and experiences are shared. However, nursing authors have long supported the need for affective competencies in nursing practice (Bucher, 1991; Fosbinder & Vos, 1989; King, 1984; Raya, 1990;

Reilly & Oermann, 1992; Tanner, 1990). Such competencies, however, often are vague, difficult to teach, and even more difficult to evaluate.

Cullen (1994) believed that nurse educators and employers must work in tandem to clarify the affective competencies needed by the nurse in practice. In an effort to reduce dissonance between what nursing graduates were taught about affective behavior and employer affective competency expectations, a three-group (faculty, students, employers) descriptive design compiled affective expectations of teachers and employers. Mentkowski's (1991) descriptive research used five hospitals' employer performance appraisals and professional organizations' printed materials, such as the ANA's *Code for Conduct* (2002), educational outcomes developed by the National League for Nursing, and accreditation criteria to develop behavioral indicators of affective competencies. From this, an affective checklist was formulated to improve the planning, delivery, and evaluation of content for affective domain maturing in associate degree nursing students. This multistage study also sought congruence in affective behavioral indicators between nurse employers, nurse educators, and nursing students. This study was the first in nursing education literature to define affective competencies with an extensive list of affective behavioral indicators. No mention was made to validate the competencies with national curriculum guidelines and program outcome expectations. However, an affective competency checklist was created as an initial effort to identify workplace affective competency expectations and behaviors that students could learn and refine in clinical courses.

A more recent study (Mallory, Konradi, Campbell, & Redding, 2003) partnered nurse educators from a public university with nurse colleagues of employed graduates to collaborate in creating teaching strategies for a baccalaureate curriculum. Built upon the belief that educators have a responsibility to construct evidence-based curricula to achieve desired program outcomes, the authors used professional and academic standards to design student learning experiences. Using a qualitative design and purposive sampling, focus and interview group sessions (which were co-moderated by a staff nurse and a faculty member) were held in three regional medical centers. Data from these focus groups developed "The Ideal Graduate" as a model for learning outcomes. Among the characteristics of the ideal graduate was the ability to prioritize, adapt, continuously learn, connect with people, be accountable, express positive attitudes, and apply the nursing process. But they also identified affective domain characteristics such as "self-awareness, integrity, humility, honesty, a strong work ethic, a thick skin, critical thinking, motivation, willingness to jump in, the ability to have fun at the job, a sense of excitement about their work, strength of character, appearance of being in control, passion for nursing and confidence" (p. 105). Thus, both cognitive and affective learning are critical to the practice of nursing. (See Appendix E for additional information about guidelines to recognize and develop learner outcomes in affective learning.)

## *Professional Values and Professional Identity*

Core values of the nursing profession, identified first by the ANA in 1893, are expectations of all nursing graduates, and the ANA's *Code of Ethics* (2001) serves as a social contract with the public it serves. Fowler (2008) identified professional values within the *Code* and its interpretive statements of commitment, integrity, professional boundaries, moral self-respect, ethical decision-making, ethical concepts such as confidentiality and social reform, articulating nursing values and wholeness of character. The American Association of Colleges of Nursing (AACN) (1998, 2008) defined five core professional nursing values: human dignity, integrity, autonomy, altruism, and social justice. In addition, the National Council of State Boards of Nursing (1997) speaks to "professional boundaries," advocacy, and civility as part of the affective behaviors expected of a professional nurse. In essence, nurses are expected to consistently demonstrate these core and professional values when caring for patients and families and when working with other professionals to achieve optimal health and wellness. Values like altruism, excellence, caring, ethics, respect, communication and accountability give voice to who we are as individuals and as the nursing profession.

While the literature search conducted for this analysis yielded several studies about professional values, not all values (e.g., "altruism" and "professional boundaries") were found, indicating there are research gaps about professional values and perhaps in students educational exposure to them. Except for the concept of caring, limited studies were found that addressed many of the other identified professional values. One case study (Fahrenwald et al., 2005) described the school's conceptual framework, examples of teaching strategies, value-based learning, and resources and methods of embedding professional core values into their baccalaureate curriculum, and noted that students were expected to apply those abstract values into their clinical practice. They believed that caring, as a multidimensional concept, is actualized through "purposeful teaching and student-centered learning of core values" (p. 46), but no formative or summative values measurements or results were described.

Professional identity and professional values are highly regarded by nurses and are incorporated into the profession's code of conduct, various practice standards, and curriculum documents. No one study examined all components of professional identity and values within nursing, and some disagreement exists as to what these are (Bixler & Bixler, 1945; Moloney, 1992). Ohlen and Segesten (1998) did report that professional identity is foundational to assuming diverse nursing roles, and they noted that nurse educators are charged by legal mandate through nurse practice acts to foster and maintain professionalism in nursing students.

Professional values are seen as an essential element in the formation of a nursing identity, and students are introduced to those values throughout nursing courses. They

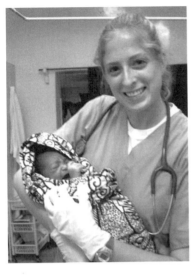

also are expectations evident in various documents published by nursing's major organizations (i.e., ANA, NLN, and AACN).

Peer mentoring has been found to facilitate the transition of students from the learner role to the nursing practice role. Peer-partnered learning during senior undergraduate nursing education experiences (McAllister & Osborne, 1997) was found to foster the movement of students from dependent to independent (autonomous) learners.

Duchscher (2001) developed a student-student teaching/learning project where students were helped to strengthen existing reflective abilities, develop a sense of responsibility and accountability (professional values), and advance personal leadership and facilitation skills in the clinical setting. Participants described their practice as increasing in precision, diligence, confidence, clinical decision-making, and accepting accountability for their decisions.

Competence, which has been identified as a precursor to autonomy in practice (Grinnell, 1989; Kramer & Schmalenberg, 1993), was found to be directly affected by students' self-esteem and perceived instructor caring (Kosowski, 1995; Wade, 2004). Such studies emphasize the significance of attitudes, autonomy, competence, and caring in nursing students and the need for faculty to foster the maturation of each.

Additional studies examined the connection between personal and professional identity and nursing students' perceptions of professional identity (Glen, 1998; Manninen, 1998), as well as conceptualizations of nursing and factors that influence its development (Ohlen & Segesten, 1998; Watson, Deary, & Lea, 1999). Beck (2000) found that early conceptualization of a nursing identity may foster student academic success. Spouse (2000) reported that when British students were helped to view themselves as practicing nursing (professional identity) from early on in the program, retention was enhanced. Maturation of professional identity development was demonstrated in another British study (Buckenham, 1988), and nursing identity experiences were found to mold Swedish nursing students' professional development (Fagerberg & Ekman, 1998).

Qualitative studies have emphasized the importance of instructor caring behaviors to the development of caring professional nurses (Halldorsdottir, 1990; Hanson & Smith, 1996; Kosowski, 1995; Miller, Haber, & Bryne, 1990; Nelms, Jones, & Gray, 1993). The theme of caring has been studied as an attribute of nursing identity in nursing students from Ireland (Ryan & McKenna, 1994), Scotland (Watson et al., 1999) and Australia (du Toit, 1995).

Cook, Gilmer, and Bess (2003) asked all incoming students, on the first day of class, an open-ended question about their definitions of nursing. Three major themes of nursing as a noun, verb, and transaction emerged from the responses of the 109 students. These three themes were further defined to include caring, nurturing, advocating, and professional identity, all of which are affective domain concerns. Although participants gave rich descriptions of nursing, very few addressed the concepts of ethics, culture, legal parameters or economics, and few identified nursing as a distinct discipline. Such findings give direction to how nurse educators can facilitate student professional identity development.

For at least six decades, researchers in various disciplines have focused on life and work values. In the values field, Super (1957) was the predominant researcher until his death in 1994; he defined values as "objectives that one seeks to attain to satisfy a need" (1973, p. 190). Values do affect vocational choice, and, building on Super's (1970) empirical work, the Work Importance Study (WIS), under Super's guidance, was initiated as an international effort with psychologists from seventeen countries. Major outcomes were the Values Scale and the revised Life Roles Inventory-Values Scale (LRI-VS) (Macnab, Fitzsimmons, & Casserly, 1985, 1987), which represented societal changes since 1970. The LRI-VS has been used with various adult populations.

Thorpe and Loo (2003) wanted to establish a profile of values essential to nursing practice using the work of Super (1973), the findings from his Work Importance study (Super & Sverko, 1995), and insights from other studies that addressed altruism or caring (Boughn & Lentini, 1999; Fagermoen, 1997), autonomy (Ballou, 1998; Boughn, 1995; Schutzenhofer, 1987, 1988; Schutzenhofer & Musser, 1994; Tompkins, 1992; Wade, 1999; Webb, Price, & Coeling, 1996), achievement (Saarmann, Freitas, Rapps, & Riegel, 1992), and authority (Webb et al., 1996), values used to select nursing as a career and the developmental processes of being socialized into a profession (Holland, 1999; Magnussen, 1998; Reutter, Field, Campbell, & Day, 1997). Thorpe and Loo compared 152 nursing and 111 management students enrolled at a small, liberal education Canadian university regarding the values each saw as most important. For all students, personal development and altruism were found to be the most important values identified, followed by social relations, ability utilization, and achievement. Nursing students had significantly higher mean scores on the altruism value and significantly lower mean scores on life style, advancement, autonomy, authority, creativity, economics and risk values than did management students, findings that support the occupational stereotype and sex-type norms associated with nursing (Batson, 1991; Bem, 1974; Fagermoen, 1997; Rushton, 1980; Super & Sverko, 1995; Wood, Christensen, Hebl, & Rothgerber, 1997). Recommendations to nurse educators include providing opportunities for students to discover their values, discuss the role of values in nursing, explore how values change, and providing experiences to improve skills in those values rated lower in importance, such as risk and creativity.

## Affective Concepts of Nursing Practice

Concepts with affective (and cognitive) components are identified with the practice of nursing and health care. Affective domain studies include student attitudes, professional identity, values and responses to emotional states such as poverty, suffering, caring, empathy and civility experienced during learning situations. Cultural competency was identified as essential to effective nursing practice and a challenge to foster in the educational environment. These affective concepts have been studied for at least the last two decades. The research results indicate diverse teaching methods, with most studies being or partly including a qualitative design. Authors urge continuing exploration of the concepts and the teaching methodologies to produce graduates with affective capabilities to work within a difficult health care environment.

*Poverty.* Most nursing students have limited understanding of poverty's impact on physical, psychological, social and spiritual well-being. Nurse educators are challenged to expose students' affective learning to impoverished clients, as poverty is a major determinant of health. Personal experience with an issue such as poverty has a significant influence on understanding of attitudes about that issue (Mayo, 2000; Sword, Reutter, Meagher-Stewart, & Rideout, 2004; Zrinyi & Balogh, 2004). DeLashmutt and Rankin (2005) created a seminar-driven clinical experience at a crisis center to address this challenge. Students explored political aspects of poverty, advocacy, and social responsibility, which are concepts found in early writings of Nightingale (1980). They worked holistically with and on behalf of mentally ill, homeless and single parent mothers. After working with the poor, 61% of the students stated that their initial responses changed, and 33% indicated that they no longer believed that they could recognize a poor person by physical appearance. Responses shifted from believing that poverty has an equal impact on all poor to believing that "the brunt of the impact of poverty is borne by single mothers with children" (p. 146), and changes in attitudes and beliefs (34%) were primarily made due to exposure to poverty, interactions with the poor and the acquired knowledge. The nurse educators believed that, with direction and encouragement, teaching strategies could nurture students' social responsibility through the advocacy role.

Nursing presence can be a connectedness that enhances the spiritual growth of both parties as esteem and respect thrive and trust comes into being. Students developed an interactive advocacy relationship with impoverished mothers, most of whom were single (DeLashmutt, 2007). The concepts of spirituality and presence were embedded throughout seminar discussions and writing assignments, which encouraged critical thinking and self-discovery. On the last clinical day, students achieved their preclinical understanding of poverty and spirituality. Of the 188 students who took the clinical course between 2000 and 2004, all but one spoke positively of the course. They identified their own spirituality as they practiced nursing presence and gained understanding of the essential interplay between the two concepts. Nursing presence is a skill that can be both role modeled as well as taught (DeLashmutt & Rankin, 2006).

In coping with poverty, DeLashmutt (2007) explored the role of spirituality through the student nurses' presence with impoverished women. Spiritual health fosters love, faith, hope, inner strength, a purpose for living, and healthy coping mechanisms (DeLashmutt, 2000; Frankl, 1946; Herth, 1996; Meraviglia, 1999). Spirituality consists of a religious, outwardly expressed component (beliefs, values, codes of conduct, and practical rituals) and an internal spiritual dimension giving meaning to one's life and relationships (DeLashmutt, 2000; Emblem, 1992). In their ongoing struggle against poverty, poor homeless women consistently discuss the sustaining motivation of their faith and spirituality (Banyard, 1994; Banyard & Graham-Bermann, 1995; DeLashmutt, 2000; Herth, 1996; Thrasher & Mowbray, 1995) as they try to find meaning in their suffering and circumstances (DeLashmutt, 2000; Meisenhelder, 2006).

Because no studies existed about nursing students attitudes toward people living in poverty and a significant portion of people in poverty interface with nurses, Sword et al. (2004) examined attitudes toward poverty among baccalaureate nursing students (N = 740) at three Canadian universities. A semi-structured interview guide was used for focus group interviews. Information about experiences with and attitudes toward poverty as well as beliefs about the relationship between poverty and health were obtained. Personal and more diverse experiences with those in poverty significantly affected the students' attitudes toward poverty. Students' attitudes were not affected by course content, but during interviews students emphasized the need for more experiential learning and direct contact with people living in poverty. Small group discussions using problem-based or context-based learning were encouraged as teaching strategies to explore the topic in depth (Wolff & Rideout, 2001). Through systematic processing of information (Wood, 2000) and reexamination of specific attitudes (Clarke, 1999; Wood, 2000), students may modify or reject existing attitudes toward poverty and consider adopting new ones, which alter holistic care of those in poverty.

*Empathy.* Empathy is considered foundational to nursing practice and was documented as linked to improved health outcomes. Empathy is affected by stress. Nursing students report high levels of stress due to academic, financial, work-related, and interpersonal circumstances (Beck, Hackett, Srivastava, McKim, & Rockwell, 1997; Jones & Johnston, 1997; Kendrick, 2000). Multidimensional stress management, which addresses cognitive, physiological and behavioral components, is effective with nursing students; however, stress management is not routinely taught in nursing programs (Grossman & Wheeler, 1999; Heaman, 1995; Mahat, 1996; Manderino, Ganong, & Darnell, 1988; Meisenhelder, 1987). Stress has been documented to decrease effective communication, interpersonal relationships and empathy expression (Kendrick, 2000; Marcus, 1999; Motowidlo, Packard, & Manning, 1986).

Several definitions of empathy reflect its multidimensional nature. Social psychologists regard empathy as having two main strands: cognitive empathy and emotional empathy. Recently, the latter was relabeled affective empathy (Lawrence, Shaw, Baker, Baron-Cohen, & David, 2004). Some studies use the phrases interchangeably, making comparisons of research designs and results a challenge.

Empathy, in the context of health care, is the capacity to understand and respond to clients' emotions and their experiences of illness; empathy is considered a multidimensional construct. Expressions of empathy have been linked to increased patient satisfaction and decreased distress, significant decreases in emergency room visits by homeless people, and a reduced risk of physician malpractice litigation (La Monica, Wolf, Madea, & Oberst, 1987; Levinson, Roter, Mullooly, Dull, & Frankel, 1997; Olson, 1995; Redelmeier, Molin, & Tibshirani, 1995).

Alligood (1992) conceptualized two forms of empathy: basic empathy, which is a universal human trait, and trained empathy, which is a skill developed through learning experiences. Morse, Bottorff, Anderson, O'Brien, and Solberg (1992) found four components of empathy: emotive, moral, cognitive and behavioral. Empathy has relational components (Bennett, 1995) and has been described as a feedback loop between providers and patients proceeding from active listening to cognitive understanding, with a behavioral response of communication.

Recognizing the importance of empathy development in medical students, Shapiro, Morrison, and Boker (2004) designed a quantitative/qualitative study to assess whether the humanities, through the teaching strategies of reading and discussing poetry and prose relating to patients and doctors, could increase medical-student empathy. First-year students in a literature and medicine elective course completed two quantitative measures of empathy and an attitude toward humanities scale and participated in pre- and postintervention group interviews. Empathy and attitudes toward the humanities improved significantly ($p < 0.01$) after class participation. Also, medical student understanding of the patient's perspective became more detailed and comprehensive following the course.

McAllister and Irvine (2002) described 34 practicing teachers' beliefs regarding empathy as an attribute of their effectiveness with culturally diverse students. All participants took a professional development program designed to foster culturally responsive practices; the program included cross-cultural simulations, cultural immersion trips, and their own experiences as minorities. Findings support creating context to use and nurture empathetic dispositions and behaviors.

Attempts have been made to encourage empathy development among nurses by combining cognitive and interpersonal strategies; results have been mixed (Cutcliffe & Cassedy, 1999; LaMonica et al., 1987; Oz, 2001; Reynolds & Presly, 1988; Wheeler, Barrett, & Lahey, 1996). Researchers consistently found that empathetic responses creating helping behaviors are more effective than cognitive responses. Also, trained empathy may deteriorate over time (Baillie, 1996; Davis, 1983; Dzurec, Allchin, & Engler, 2007; Evans, Wilt, Alligood, & O'Neil, 1998; Oswald, 2002). As a result, there has been a shift from the behavioral/communication approach toward strategies that foster empathy through an intrapersonal approach.

Regan (2000) completed a quasi-experimental study using Rogers' Theory of Learning, which supports development of affective (as well as cognitive and psychomotor) learning. Through a researcher-developed Nurse-Patient Relationship Game, associate degree nursing students were taught empathetic communication during a psychiatric nursing course; data was collected using the LaMonica Empathy Profile (LEP) (LaMonica, 1986). The LEP measures empathetic communication and affective (and cognitive) empathy. Results found that gaming increased empathetic communication, but not cognitive or affective empathy. The study was a one-time intervention. It was recommended that more than one gaming experience over time may be needed to produce lasting effects. The author acknowledged the study's limitations of lack of generalizability and possible methodological issues like using only three samples, and the limited testing of the LEP instrument.

Until Kohlberg (1972) began researching moral development, morality was considered an affective quality. Since then, the interaction between cognitive and affective factors was studied, and empathy is now considered the interconnection of the affective and cognitive domains in moral reasoning. Empathy is defined as an emotional response that stems from another's emotional state and condition that is congruent with the other's emotional state or situation. Empathy is an affective response requiring the cognitive processes of role-taking and the recognition of one's own emotions (Arangie-Harrell, 1998).

When teaching empathy, distinguishing between emotional contagion and empathetic concern is important. The former, referring to taking on the emotions of another, is ultimately harmful to nurses, who experienced emotional exhaustion and were more prone to burnout. Nurses with empathetic concern were more likely to act altruistically and without aggression, less prone to burnout, less likely to depersonalize patients, and less likely to report diminished personal accomplishment (Miller, Stiff, & Ellis, 1988; Omdahl & O'Donnell, 1999; Williams, 1989). Fostering flexible boundaries during empathy development encourages self-awareness, which may foster empathy by providing insight into what others feel (Baillie, 1996; Levenson & Ruef, 1992; Shapiro, Schwartz, & Bonner,

1998). Future studies were recommended to determine strategies to prevent emotional contagion and strengthen the kind of empathetic concern that benefits both students and patients.

Nursing education provides ample opportunities for empathy development. Fostering empathy could have positive long-term results in students' educational, professional, and personal lives. Research identified prerequisite qualities to empathy development as receptivity to being empathetic, freeing the mind from distractions, attention to cues, suspending judgment of others, active attending and listening, and remaining in the here and now while interacting with others (Barrett-Lennard, 1993; Forsyth, 1980; Wiseman, 1996).

A teaching intervention, mindfulness meditation, similar to empathy development, can transform one's perceptions and enhance insight; the practice is based on the ancient contemplative tradition called *vipassana,* which means seeing clearly.

Mindfulness-based stress reduction (MBSR), developed by Kabat-Zinn (1990) and colleagues, is a wellness program based on mindfulness meditation. The intervention has been widely used and is linked with improved physical, emotional, social, and mental health (Shapiro et al., 1998; Williams, Kolar, Roger, & Pearson, 2001; Young, Bruce, Turner, & Linden, 2001); two studies included nursing students (Roth, 2001; Young et al., 2001). One correlated the practice of medical students with increased empathy (Shapiro et al., 1998).

Mindfulness training, in a pilot study of first-semester nursing students (N=16), was used to foster empathy and mitigate experienced stress. Beddoe and Murphy (2004) explored the effects of an MBSR course on stress and empathy. Using a pretest-posttest design with no control group, the participants agreed to maintain journals and to take the Derogatis Stress Profile and Interpersonal Reactivity Index (IRI), which measures four dimensions of empathy. In addition, participants were to attend eight two-hour sessions followed by thirty-minute guided meditation audiotapes at home, five days per week. Mindfulness techniques included progressive relaxation, sitting meditation, hatha yoga, and walking meditation.

Participants' pretest mean scores in all four IRI dimensions were 40% to 50% higher than mean scores of non-nursing female students of the same age in other studies (Atkins & Steitz, 2000; Davis, 1983). Meditation compliance varied and only 44% practiced three or more times per week. Participants who meditated more often reported greater benefits. IRI scores did not significantly increase, but this may be due to the unusually high pretest scores or due to indirectly addressing empathy via mindfulness techniques rather than using a direct intervention. The study results are not generalizable due to the sample size, and the intervention emphasized self-care to decrease anxiety but did not directly encourage empathy for others. The researchers recommend that the results support adding a cognitive component to the course to directly enhance empathy development.

Empathy can be altered by narrative teaching strategies. Propositional reasoning and narrative thinking have been compared for results of teaching tolerance. Narratives prompted more affective responses, resulting in greater attitudes of tolerance toward differences. While reasoning is helpful in teaching students to determine choice of action based on principles, fairness or rationality, the use of narrative further promotes empathetic understanding (Colesante & Biggs, 1999). Initiating self-awareness through storied events can assist in reconstructing beliefs, biases and discriminations. Findings reinforce that skill in expressing empathy is important for nurse educators to encourage in students in order to help them develop empathy.

***Suffering.*** Learning, for the nursing student, involves clinical experiences that challenge students as they see and respond to difficult patient circumstances. One dominant affective response to these circumstances that crosses clinical specialties is suffering. No studies were located that focused on a curriculum approach to teaching related to suffering. However, researchers acknowledge the concept of suffering and have studied teaching strategies to promote students' ability to recognize and respond therapeutically to suffering. Also, studies address students' vulnerability to the suffering experience, teaching strategies to prevent personal damage to them and enhancing their coping abilities when encountering suffering in the clinical setting (Lashley, 1994).

Using interpretive phenomenology, Eifried (2003) studied the lived experience of nursing students as they cared for patients who were suffering. Participants were drawn from a convenience sample of 13 baccalaureate nursing students studying an advanced medical-surgical nursing course. During one semester, students participated in individual and group conversational interviews, shared journal entries discussing their experiences in caring for suffering patients, and visited with the researcher, a non-course teacher, on site.

Students were requested to tell a story about a time they could not forget when they cared for a suffering patient. All students told stories that brought a rich history and unique lived experience to the study. "Bearing witness" to suffering emerged as a metatheme; students see, hear, and feel suffering in clinical settings and "bear witness" to it. These subthemes "captured the essence of bearing witness to suffering: 1) grappling with suffering; 2) struggling with the ineffable; 3) getting through; 4) being with patients who are suffering; 5) embodying the experience of suffering; and 6) seeing possibilities in suffering" (Eifried, 2003, p. 60). Students become acutely aware of their own vulnerability and struggle to be authentically present to patients.

Empathy and suffering are interrelated in nursing practice. In grappling with suffering experiences, students expressed feeling powerless, alone while giving their best care, and awareness of discomfort, vulnerability, helplessness, and loneliness (Eifried, 2003). Students struggled with the ineffable. They were compelled to ask questions; many of those questions had no answers. Situations seemed surreal and caused some students to question their moral beliefs.

Students described many ways of responding to their feelings of helplessness, sadness, and loneliness from clinical experiences involving suffering. They reported "getting through" by confiding in each other and finding comfort during the process, forming a sharing and supporting circle that rarely included faculty, seeking places to escape when feeling overwhelmed and helpless, seeking safe places that were familiar to them, seeking their own or other sources of strength, responding to the patient's need for them, and praying. When people pray, they expose inner feelings, hope, and the need for help (Bolen, 1996). "Praying can heal our isolation, strengthen our ability to keep on keeping on, and nourish our spirit" (p. 129).

Students wanted to share feelings about these clinical experiences, but seldom risked sharing with faculty or shedding tears. Students' vulnerability experienced with suffering patients is compounded by their fear of appearing inadequate to a teacher. They were unsure when to share their woundedness. They were, however, able to sense their responsibilities to patients and respond. "They also learned how to recognize suffering at a new level…in the patient's eyes, when tears ran but there was no voice, and in the gaze of another, which initiates self-reflection" (Leder, 1990, p. 60). Patients expressed suffering with their words and through their bodies. Students sensed their patients' suffering through their own bodies. All students described learning "possibilities" through the suffering that they witnessed; these included observing patients' courage and strength, finding peace and meaning, learning about love, patients touching their lives, and experiencing the grace of relationships between patients and loved ones.

Students described feeling abandoned in the clinical setting. When asked what would help them, they responded with two things: 1) "having instructors who say it is OK to cry, make students feel important, foster closeness and accessibility to the clinical group as a support group, allow time in the clinical setting to talk about experiences and feelings surrounding the suffering experience, and 2) knowing how to prepare patients with terminal illnesses for death" (Leder, 1990, p. 65). This study reinforced the need for students to have supportive teachers when disheartened, feeling there is nowhere else to turn for comfort, needing to express what they are going through and acknowledging their struggles. Students expressed the need to have instructor feedback.

Students also experienced the relationships (Bolen, 1996) found within a circle of people who gather in a safe place to talk about important matters and are committed to listening compassionately. These relationships are bonds that keep members who "falter from plummeting into despair by the heart and hand of another" (p. 112). The study

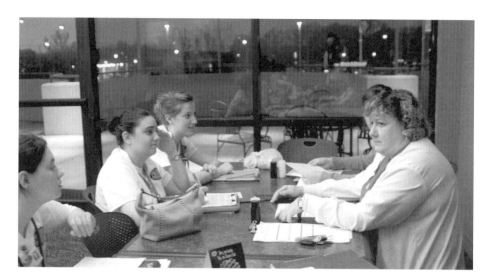

supports the value of having a circle of support in difficult clinical learning situations that stir strong emotions in nursing students.

In summary, pedagogical implications have relevance to other learning environments in nursing that evoke strong emotions such as suffereing and empathy. Attending to the pedagogy of suffering is essential as is creating support that recognizes students' vulnerability and fosters their courage. Teachers enhance the development of caring by expressing caring in a manner that promotes student development through difficult clinical circumstances such as the suffering experience. Further recommendations involved the design of clinical experiences to teach and learn about caring, to develop teaching methods that facilitate writing and thinking about emotions during clinical experiences, and helping students find a turning point in their ability to cope with their feelings and respond to the suffering they witness and experience. Also, faculty could introduce students to narrative pedagogy for sharing personal stories, facilitating peer bonding, and healing their "broken hearts" perceptions so that a more present caring heart is developed.

***Cultural Competency.*** For two decades, cultural competency has been part of the nursing literature (Rew, Becker, Cookston, Khosropour, & Martinez, 2003). The American Academy of Nursing (Lenburg, 1995) defined it as "a complex integration of knowledge, attitudes, and skills that enhances cross-cultural communication and appropriate effective interaction with others" (p. 35). Culturally competent health professionals have awareness of and respect for people differences along with a valuing of diversity (Sodowsky, Taffe, Gutkin, & Wise, 1994). Cultural competence has been determined to be an essential component of nursing research efforts (Campinha-Bacote & Padgett, 1995), counseling (Pope-Davis, Eliason, & Ottavi, 1994) and continuing nursing education (Campinha-

Bacote, 1999). The development of culturally competent nurses is, to faculty, essential to meeting needs of multicultural populations (Capper, 1993; Chrisman, 1998; Marchesani & Adams, 1992; Schmitz, Paul, & Greenberg, 1992).

Teaching cultural competence, like all affective domain concepts, is complex. Various approaches were studied, ranging from offering entire courses focusing on cultural issues (Lockhart & Resick, 1997) to the development of a virtual classroom (Jackson, Yorker, & Mitchem, 1996). Effective approaches are Internet assignments (Kirkpatrick, Brown, & Atkins, 1998), using non-nursing literature (Bartol & Richardson, 1998), and measuring amounts and types of competency by surveys (Alpers & Zoucha, 1996; Motwani, Hodge, & Crampton, 1995; Pope-Davis et al., 1994; Rew et al., 2003; Warda, 1997). Survey results often determined that simply raising students' cultural awareness levels do not culturally competent practitioners make.

Seeking a valid and reliable method to measure results of a program to promote multicultural awareness, Rew developed a Cultural Awareness Scale (CAS) (Rew, 1996; Rew et al., 2003), and established beginning validity and reliability of the instrument with 120 nursing students at one university. The CAS is a tangible instrument to monitor progress of students in developing cultural competence. Few studies exist that address teaching and measuring cultural competency, although nursing literature strongly advocates culturally competent nursing interventions in practice.

*Caring.* Caring is a value embraced by nurses. Numerous publications focus on caring student-teacher interactions (Beck, 2001; Sanford, 2000; Woodward, 1997), effective teaching and learning strategies incorporated into a curriculum that purposely teaches and influences caring (Cook & Cullen, 2003; Katims, 1995; Sadler, 1997), and indicators of caring (Watson 1990). In addition, many nursing organizations address caring in the practice of nurses and its effect, or lack thereof, on patient outcomes.

Over time, prominent nursing values such as caring, empathy and integrity were studied (Altun, 2002; Fahrenwald, 2003; Gormley, 1996; Jacobs, 2001; Kneipp & Snider, 2001; Liaschenko, 1999). Numerous authors identify caring as the essence and core of nursing (Benner & Wrubel, 1989; Watson, 1988a, 1988b). Although caring and professional were terms found to be in opposition (Gardner, 1992; Woodward, 1997), they are often positively intertwined in publications. Caring is emphasized in the ANA *Code for Conduct* (2002). Accordingly, caring is valued by nurses and those they serve in a society that undervalues caring. Maturing as an expert nurse could be described as personal and professional caring, which produces moral development. Behaviors that represent the ANA values compose the caring, professional nurse (AACN, 1998).

Nursing education is designed to prepare nurses for professional practice, and the foundation of nursing practice is caring (Bevis & Watson, 1989; Leininger, 1991). Wide variations in the measurement of caring are possibly due to numerous definitions of the caring phenomenon; 35 definitions were documented in one analysis (Morse, Solberg, Neander, Bottorff, & Johnson, 1990).

Brown (2005) attempted a preliminary exploration to identify and describe ADN faculty beliefs and attitudes about caring, their experiences with curriculum design that creates caring outcomes, and with curriculum elements that best exemplify the integration of caring attitudes. At the time, most ADN education was limited to a behaviorist approach. Watson's theory of caring (1990) was infused throughout the curriculum and organized by hierarchical levels of affective development (receiving, responding, valuing, organization, and characterization by a value or value complex) (Krathwohl et al., 1964). Built on Boykin and Schoenhofer's (2001) caring theory, which describes the caring perspective of nursing education, nursing practice and nursing administration, a convenience sample of 110 ADN faculty in Florida was surveyed. This theory supports inculcating nurse caring attitudes that differ from those the students have prior to entering the nursing profession. Faculty's description of caring were consistent with descriptions found in the literature. Faculty perceived including caring learning objectives important in curriculum design. However, when affective objectives were present in courses, affective objectives that specifically focused on developing caring student attitudes were less likely to be used. "An equally significant finding was the infrequent use of caring affective learning objectives designed hierarchically in the nursing curriculum to facilitate nursing students' internalization of caring..." (p. 96).

Brubaker (2005), based upon Noddings' (1984, 1992, 1995, 2002) ethics of caring, constructed the Caring Actions and Responses with Encounters Survey (CARES) tool to measure caring. One part describes student action statements representing how student nurses demonstrate conceptual components of the ethics of caring. The second part provides possible patient responses to the action statements. Initial validity and reliability were established. The survey requests the frequency of each action statement and patient response experienced during interactions between students and patients. Using a descriptive approach, 131 BSN students and 20 clinical nursing instructors completed separate versions of the tool. Brubaker concluded that an ethic of caring can be assessed using student-patient encounters and recommended validating student self-reports with clinical nursing instructor findings. Although results are limited to this sample, replication of the study should be considered with larger sample sizes and various types of nursing educational preparation.

Benner (1999) acknowledged that caring is required for developing critical thinking and outcome activities. This three-year observational pilot study involved interventions accessing two traditional domains and control groups using convenience samples. A short essay prompt addressed the student's view of knowledge, teacher, and self as learner. Trained raters scored the essays using the Perry scheme of intellectual and ethical development

(Perry, 1970; 1981). Additional instruments were the Measure of Intellectual Development (MID) (Moore, 1988) and the California Critical Thinking Disposition Inventory (CCTDI). The latter assesses the constellation of attitudes, or habits of the mind, necessary for critical thinking (Facione, Facione, & Giancarlo, 1998). The context of community was a caring community in which various teaching methods were used, such as music, poetry, art and storying, which accesses the affective domain. Due to design flaws related to curriculum constraints on the student population, this study's findings could "not pinpoint Narrative Pedagogy as a 'best practice' in nursing education (p. 194)." Facione et al. urge that this does not mean the teaching strategy is ineffective, but rather, in this instance, its worth

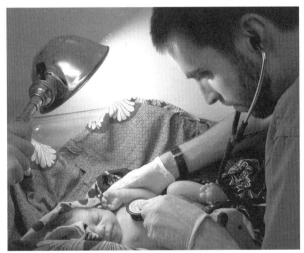

could not be demonstrated. The study is complex and well thought out; it is useful for additional study. A more detailed review of this research is recommended for nurse educator researchers.

Numerous studies exist over time about the ways of knowing in nursing. Nurses (Benner, 1984; Carper, 1978; Watson, 1988b, 1990) and non-nurses (Belenky, Clinchy, Goldberger, & Tarule, 1986; Bruner, 1963; Gilligan, 1982; Schön, 1987, 1991) have added to an understanding of the complex process of becoming a nurse. Carper (1978) first identified four foundational and interconnected patterns of know-ing in nursing that relate to the affective (and cognitive) domain; these are nursing science, nursing art, knowledge of self, and ethical knowledge. Wagner (1998) explored aesthetic reflection as a needed partnership between cognitive and affective knowing that underpins caring, described as the essence of nursing. Her descriptive, qualitative, multiple-case study investigated three baccalaureate nursing students' experiences reflecting on practice through story, artistic expression, and sharing. Data were collected through the participants' written stories, poetry, art, and journals as well as the researcher's observation of each class.

Data analysis found that artistic expression of story and sharing challenged students to different levels of reflection, which changed their sense of caring. Story writing about a caring moment with a patient represented a cognitive-level exercise that prompted recall of factual detail. Through the creative process of translating their stories into poetry and art, students reported a deeper affective level of reflection that increased their awareness of self, suppressed feelings, and fostered relationships. Class sharing of artwork and evolving stories promoted collective reflection through dialogue, support and affirmation that expanded students' perspective of self and their nursing practice. New meaning was found in their day-to-day caring. The findings supported existing research, and contributed to Watson's Transpersonal Theory of Human Caring (1988a) and models of reflective practice.

Another pilot study examined the measurement of the caring efficacy of baccalaureate nursing students (Sadler, 2003). Caring is frequently identified as the very essence of nursing. Characteristically, it is created by intentionally developed relationships and abilities acquired over time through self-reflection, role model observations, and experiences (Sadler, 1997). A cross section of students from prenursing through graduation semesters reported their caring competency using the Coates Caring Efficacy Scale (CES) (Coates, 1997). The nursing program was established in the 1990s using a caring curriculum model. Comparing Coates mean scores with the students' responses, mean scores were higher for prenursing students and lower than those reported for final semester students. The study does provide beginning evaluative data about nursing students' self-reported caring competencies and descriptors of events or people that most influenced development of their caring. Further, Beck (2001) completed a meta-analysis of qualitative studies about caring covering a 24-year time period; 14 studies were found in nursing education. She found five metaphors, or themes, included in these studies: presencing, sharing, uplifting effects, supporting and competence. Possibly, these are additional descriptors that could be used to further retrieve affective domain research in nursing education and shape future research initiatives.

*Civility.* Civil behaviors are expected of nursing students in all learning situations and ultimately in nursing practice, as described in the ANA *Code of Ethics* (2001). Incivility is defined as speech or action that is discourteous, rude, or impolite; in academe, incivility may range from insulting remarks and verbal abuse to explosive and even violent behavior (Tiberius & Flak, 1999). On American campuses, evidence suggests that incivility is a serious and growing concern. In nursing education, there have been attempts to document incidences of student incivility (Luparell, 2003; 2004), faculty (intentional and unintentional) incivility (Amada, 1994; Clark, 2006, 2008) and both faculty and student incivility (Clark, in press a, in press b; Clark & Springer, 2007a, 2007b; Hanson, 2001). While the answers to promoting civil behavior in the educational environment are not easy, research findings suggest that faculty being a positive role model (Richmond & McCroskey, 1992), exhibiting civil behavior toward peers and students (Kuhlenschmidt & Layne, 1999), developing conflict resolution skills and addressing uncivil classroom and clinical behaviors rather than tolerating the behaviors (Hanson, 2001; Luparell, 2005) are key to promoting civil student responses in learning situations.

Exposure to uncivil student behavior is highly likely for the nurse educator. Hanson (2001) found that higher education is relatively silent on the topic and few research studies exist that explore the professional value of civil behavior even though ANA promotes civil behavior to create a healthy workplace and a safer patient environement. She explored incidents of incivility, as did Clark and Springer (2007a, 2007b); they documented specific lists of uncivil behaviors and identified behaviors that were beyond uncivil. Students (43.5%) believed that a faculty member disparaging another faculty member's abilities was beyond uncivil while 60.1% of both faculty and students believed that students challenging a faculty member's knowledge or credibility was the highest rated "beyond uncivil" behavior. General taunts or disrespect of faculty or students were given the second highest rating by both groups (25.3% of students and 49.6% of faculty).

Luparell (2007) researched the effect of student incivility on nursing faculty. Using a snowballing sampling technique, 21 faculty members from six states were interviewed. Thirty-six critical incidents of incivility were described and most were precipitated by a period of escalating tensions and unsuccessful faculty efforts to resolve and defuse the situation. Often faculty were surprised and did not anticipate the uncivil behavior. Faculty reported perceived immediate or delayed threat to their own and their loved ones well-being, job security or possessions. The aftermath of the encounters varied and faculty reported loss of sleep and interrupted sleep patterns, altered self-esteem and self-confidence, posttraumatic stress responses, significant time and effort expenditures, financial costs including attorney fees, changes in pedagogy and grading criteria to avoid conflict, and withdrawing from the teaching position. Morale and job satisfaction were negatively impacted. Luparell (2005) suggested several strategies nurse educators could use, including being prepared for the possibility of uncivil encounters with students and being proactive in responses to such encounters, developing competency for handling uncivil encounters, holding students accountable for their behavior, and developing course objectives that address the need for appropriate conduct in all aspects of professional education. Programs should have policies that are enforced and consider critical incident debriefing for faculty following uncivil encounters. More research was advocated by all researchers on the topic of incivility, because of its complex consequences in the learning situation and ultimately in practice.

## Instructional Strategies for Affective Domain Learning

Instructional strategies, methods, or interventions to enhance affective domain learning and development were varied among the nursing research studies reviewed. Teaching strategies that engaged emotions in concert with the strategy indicate promise in enhancing memorization, knowledge acquisition, skill acquisition, and behavioral changes such as demonstrating caring and compassion. Student attitudes were studied often, primarily to change attitudes toward a topic such as research, those with mental health disorders, elders and euthanasia, with the expectation that the student and ultimately society would benefit from developing professional behaviors associated with the attitude.

*Nursing Education.* The affective domain has been studied less than the psychomotor and cognitive domains. These trends followed the dominant positivist societal view that emotions are not rational and therefore are suppressed as a way of knowing. Although enmeshed in a discipline that markets "caring," an affective domain concept, most nurses are educated with teaching strategies that foster psychomotor and cognitive domain development. Some of the affective domain nursing research studies did not lend themselves to placement in previous categories. These studies are summarized here.

Developmental processes that promote the maturity of learners who become RNs occurs from one (LPN-to-RN, accelerated or second degree programs) to four years; most students are exposed to a nursing curriculum of two to three years in length. Benner's (1984) research on clinical competence development begins following graduation; she acknowledges that two to three years must pass before clinical competence has been attained. There are no affective learning development models in nursing that incorporate the nursing student. Such an undertaking would be a challenging task.

Most nursing education research has not designed nor utilized teaching interventions to elicit affective responses as a variable. Most studies examine components of affect, such as empathy, caring, humor, or cultural sensitivity, and define it as a part of affect. Although Bloom (1956) and later theorists' work on the developmental theory of values attainment has been evident for decades, there is no consistent definition of affect in nursing education. Also, nursing education is not targeting the affective domain, which could facilitate learning and improve patient outcomes (Ulloth, 2003). This extremely limits serious consideration of what affective learning and development means to nurses, whose practice affects the birth, health, illness recovery, and dying of humans. The human experience is predominantly affective, and, as such, deserves nurses who are developing increasingly complex affective competencies.

All nursing education research studies were descriptive; none measured affective learning as an outcome. Traditionally, nursing has based affective learning on cognitive and behavioral descriptors (Maier-Lorentz, 1999; Reilly & Oermann, 1992; Woods, 1993). Several studies operationalized instructional methods to foster affective learning (Letizia, 1996, 1998; McCausland, 2002; Ritchie, 2003; Ulloth, 2002); these were humor, journaling, clinical experience and clinical post-conference. Other instructional strategies are discussed earlier in this chapter and in Chapter 3.

Self-efficacy, "beliefs in one's capabilities to organize and execute the courses of action required to produce given attainments" (Bandura, 1997, p. 3), influences the student's motivation and volume of persistence to accomplish difficult tasks (Tompson & Dass, 2000). Personal triumphs foster transformational experiences and when used in simulations can be transferred to enhance self-efficacy in other domains. Clinical scenarios can provide contexts for building self-efficacy (Dearman, 2003). These may include diverse approaches, such as photographs, video- and audio-taped scenarios, case studies, and simulations in formats such as interactive video and virtual reality. The common element is active student participation and faculty facilitation. Ideally, these are in controlled environments with no endangerment to patients (Johnson, Zerwic, & Theis, 1999). Jeffreys and Smodlaka (1999) developed a transcultural self-efficacy instrument containing three subscales; one subscale measured the affective domain of self-efficacy. The scale was limited to values, attitudes and beliefs that are cognitive and behavioral manifestations of affect (L. Taylor, personal communication, February 20, 2004).

Evans and Bendel (2004) studied the effect of narrative pedagogy on nursing students' ability to mature ethically, an affective concept, and cognitively, to ultimately achieve autonomous practice. Valiga (1983) believed that autonomy is a function of cognitive and ethical development.

Writing-to-learn, described as a wide variety of teaching approaches that include writing activities that are consistent with course objectives and students' concerns and interests (Cowles, Strickland, & Rodgers, 2001), requires teacher coaching and feedback. These activities are also useful for online environments and are designed to encourage student internalization of beliefs and values because applications hold personal meaning. They purported to support teaching and evaluation of the development of the affective domain (and critical thinking) in clinical settings. Using the Faciones' critical thinking dispositions, faculty and students explored mutual understanding of the dispositions to cultivate learning in the affective domain. The task of writing was found to assist students in developing the affective domain.

Creative writing that encourages deep exploration of a life experience is suited to complex situations such as application of multiple concepts, personal knowing, ethical understanding, the ability to empathize, and caring and compassion in nursing (Evans & Severtsen, 2001; Severtsen & Evans, 2000; Smith, 2000). In contrast, reflective writing focuses on something that the student has read or experienced. It includes a description of the experience or reading (Smith, 2000). Journaling is not the same as reflective writing, because it is not shared and is a powerful personal growth and self-care tool. Journaling nurtures deep inner experience (Chinn & Kramer, 1999). Reflective writing is similar to journaling, but is planned to be shared in a teaching-learning context; the purpose is to obtain insight into professional experiences and become a reflective practitioner (Schön, 1987).

One study (Hanna, 1997) sought to determine the effectiveness of a total curriculum methodology identified as self-paced mastery learning. With a sample of 478 consisting of current students, program graduates, program withdrawals and faculty, the study found the self-pacing format fostered affective attributes of personal growth, individual responsibility, self-awareness, self-confidence and self-discipline. Although not fully described, all attributes were mentioned in other research as possible outcomes of affective learning. The report did not provide specific methodological procedures nor address rigor.

Why assess nebulous, ineffable phenomena? Nursing education has numerous rational-empirical evaluation tools such as competency checklists, NCLEX pass rates, and Likert-scale summative course and program evaluation tools. However, these tools limit learning assessment to narrowly defined, didactic learning outcomes (Krechevsky & Stork, 2000). Acknowledging the ineffable encourages teachers to attend to process, embed learning in context (Eisner, 1997; Krechevsky & Stork) and add richness in meaning (Starr-Glass, 2002).

Recently, nursing scholars explored the ineffable of nursing with interpretive, inductive processes (Heinrich, Chiffer, McKelvey & Zraunig, 2002; Heinrich & Neese, 2004; Miller & Morgan, 2000). In its infancy to nurse educator researchers, the process is being explored through assessment dialogs producing "productive ambiguity" (Eisner, 1997, p. 8). Addressing complexities, reductionistic thinking is avoided and new insights are generated (Eisner, 1997; Starr-Glass, 2002). Some ineffable assessment examples are the use of metaphor (Akin & Palmer, 2000; Kemp, 1999), narrative or storytelling (Harrison, 1999; Sims & Swenson, 2001), dialogue (Bilinski, 2002; Heinrich, 1992; Hodges, 1996), dialogue to create a scholarly identity (Diekelmann & Ironside, 1998; Hofmeyer, 2002), focus groups (Heinrich & Witt, 1998; Maki, 2002), drawings (Krueger & Irvine, 2001), experiential collages (Keddy, 2002), role play (Kennedy, 2001) and caveats (Harrison, 1999; Kemp; Brooker & MacDonald, 1999). These qualitative studies were designed to enhance affective learning, expand existing assessment methodologies and encourage faculty scholars to explore the invisible, an affective component of nursing student learning (Heinrich, Bona, McKelvey, & Solernou, 2001. Additional studies are summarized in Chapters 3 and 5 and in Appendix F.

Storytelling was recommended as a method to enhance the development of affective (as well as psychomotor) domain achievement (Festa, 1987). Although it may be thought of as a cognitive process, Festa believed storytelling is a valid affective teaching method because a story contains vivid images; the story could be an experience story, a fantasy, or a combination of both. For example, a story could present a nurse faced with a situation that leads her to think carefully about her own values, those of the patient, and those of the health care system. Festa found that reflection on and discussion of stories such as this enhanced students' development of attitudes and values as professionals.

Pullen, Murray and McGee (2001) created Care Groups to enhance the development of novice students' in a skill acquisition clinical course. The teachers guided students, using caring relationships, to also address the affective (and cognitive) domains of learning. Within a learning environment that encouraged relationship building, students also reported developing strategies for academic success and learning to value caring in practice. Findings from teacher-developed survey instruments indicated that students, through Care

Groups, developed professional values and socialization skills and experienced less stress and more confidence in their first clinical nursing course.

The move toward online education spurred research on technology's effect on attitudes toward the teaching strategy. Russo and Benson (2005) discussed the relational effect of learning with invisible others on affective (and cognitive) learning outcomes. Collected from student survey responses, results indicated significant positive correlations between student perceptions of the "presence" of other students in the class (even virtually) and scores on an attitude scale and satisfaction with their own learning. Perceptions of the instructor's "presence" (even virtually) were significantly correlated with both attaining affective learning and with student learning satisfaction.

***Nursing Student Attitudes.*** Attitudes influence students' learning, career choices, and delivery of care (Gething et al., 2002a; 2002b), thus influencing professional and personal behavior. Attitudes toward topics such as research were explored to foster research utilization in practice. Various nursing specialty groups have explored how students' attitudes toward vulnerable populations — for example, the aged and those with mental illness — could be changed. The intent was to foster positive attitudes toward vulnerable populations that then encouraged students to pursue nursing careers in mental illness and gerontology, thus improving care delivery in those areas.

Baccalaureate nursing graduates are expected to be consumers of nursing research findings (American Academy of Nursing, 1998; National League for Nursing Accrediting Commission, 2005). Often, they begin undergraduate nursing research courses with negative attitudes toward research (Laschinger, Johnson & Kohr, 1990; Schlapman, 1989; Swenson & Kleinbaum, 1984). Nurse faculty have reported several innovative teaching practices to help undergraduates learn and value nursing research. These included the use of crossword puzzles (Beck, 1986), student participant observations (Dean, 1986), field trips (Kessenich, 1996), oral histories (Duggleby, 1998), small group work (Halloran, 1996), patient chart reviews (Neidich, 1990) and poster sessions (Beal, Lynch & Moore, 1989).

Writing a research proposal enhanced students' knowledge and understanding of research concepts, thus improving their attitudes (Slimmer, 1992). Student attitudes were more positive at the end of a program than at the beginning of a research course when faculty incorporated the use of research article critiques and examinations and required small groups to develop research proposals (Harrison, Lowery, & Bailey, 1991). Also, actively including students in data collection improved students' attitudes and behaviors regarding research, compared to lecture approaches (Pond & Bradshaw, 1996). Pugsley and Clayton (2003) compared attitudes toward research of baccalaureate nursing students exposed to traditional lectures and experiential model approaches of teaching. The former consisted of lecture, article critiques and examinations. The latter consisted of a hands-on problem-solving activity, a mini-research project, and a critique; the first two were group activities. Faculty facilitated learning and guided each group's mini-research project. The experiential model group demonstrated a more positive attitude toward research.

Recognizing that students share the same attitudes as the general public toward people with mental illness, nurse educators have studied strategies to improve those attitudes, especially those that view the mentally ill as "dangerous, prone to violence, unpredictable, and in some measure responsible for their own illnesses" (Emrich, Thompson, & Moore, 2003, p. 18). Increases in interpersonal contact between students and people with psychiatric disorders (Esters, Cooker, & Ittenbach, 1998; Halter, 2004; Murray & Steffen, 1999), classroom instruction, fear-reduction strategies, and length of mental health practicum (Esters et al.) positively changed attitudes that influenced quality of care. Also, Emrich et al. sought to embed psychiatric nursing principles in a course focused on care of people with chronic illnesses and to use fear-reduction strategies to improve students' attitudes toward people with mental illnesses. Using a modified attitude scale (Yuker, Block & Campbell, 1966) for pre-post measurement comparisons, the students' attitudes were significantly more positive at the course's completion. Designing a curriculum that actively seeks to change negative attitudes toward population groups has merit to enhance learning and ultimately patient outcomes.

A major education effort to prepare registered nurses for the aging U.S. population has been under way for over a decade. Few nurses are adequately prepared for older adults' unique needs (Mezey & Fulmer, 2002) due, in part, to limited attention of nurse educators to incorporating the basics of gerontology nursing into pre-licensure programs (Rosenfeld, Bottrell, Fulmer, & Mezey, 1999). Increasing the geriatric content prepares nurses for the growing older population (Bednash, Fagin, & Mezey, 2003; Kovner, Mezey, & Harrington, 2002) and minimizing ageism among nursing students impacts their nursing career choices and their quality of care to older adults (Gething et al., 2002a; 2002b).

The John A. Hartford Foundation (JHF) has been a major influence for over a decade in funding national initiatives to prepare nurses to care for older adults' unique needs. Readily available evidence-based teaching and learning materials are accessible at the John A. Hartford Institute for Geriatric Nursing (www.hartfordign.org). Through JHF efforts, three universities introduced innovative educational strategies designed to increase knowledge and improve attitudes of nursing students who care for older adults. Using Kolb's (1984) experiential learning theory, the three baccalaureate nursing programs used different approaches (Burbank, Dowling-Castronovo, Crowther, & Capezuti, 2006) to promote attitudinal (and knowledge) changes toward the elderly.

New York University nursing students included accelerated second-degree and traditional baccalaureate students. Two courses, one at each end of the curriculum, exposed students to geriatric nursing experiences. Faculty development occurred to increase geriatric nursing competence. Following placement in long-term care (LTC) facilities during a fundamentals nursing course, a nondescribed survey was distributed to 124 students to measure their interest in seeking LTC employment; 22.5% reported yes and 9.6% reported maybe. Graduates reported an improved ability to deal with common geriatric syndromes. In addition, a Senior Mentor Project connected students with community dwelling older adult volunteers. Students explore their experiences, attitudes, and communication styles within these student-elder relationships. This one-on-one project, due to increased enrollment, evolved into a focus group of five students per volunteer; the group explored healthy aging issues. After the group event, the authors report focus groups and surveys indicated improvement in students' attitudes toward older adults. No description of the focus groups or surveys was provided.

At Tuskegee University School of Nursing and Allied Health, a psychologist taught primarily traditional undergraduate students a holistic approach toward promoting successful aging and risk reduction. This course is an elective for junior and senior nursing students. Through a course evaluation, students evaluated their ability and understanding of the holistic approach toward successful aging. Seventy percent of the students rated their ability to meet six of the nine course objectives as good or excellent. In holistically promoting successful aging, students rated their ability as improved following the course.

The third university was the University of Rhode Island. Geriatric content was integrated into the undergraduate nursing program and two new sophomore nursing courses in foundations of nursing care of older adults were required. Students provide nursing care to a variety of older patients. Critical reflective inquiry (CRI) was used in weekly journaling to analyze provision of nursing care. CRI fosters learning and change in nursing practice. The two student groups rated their satisfaction with the gerontology courses as excellent or very good. A pre-post design was used to assess student attitudes toward older adults. By completing a statement "Older people are…" with 10 words, the frequency of positive and negative adjectives were counted. For both semesters, the number of positive adjectives doubled and the number of negative adjectives decreased between 18% and 29%. Together, the three nursing programs' research found that the following promote success in gerontological nursing education: indentifying a "geriatric nurse educator champion," faculty development in geriatric nursing, and a strong administration infrastructure that supports innovation.

Additional studies identified successful teaching innovations that also positively impacted student attitudes toward elders. Puentes and Cayer (2001) modified Feeley's (1991) research on campus wellness vacation intervention. The modified vacation had two parts. The first was a weeklong 15-hour theory class about basic gerontological nursing for the students. The second was a 42-hour, weeklong series of seminars on elders maintaining a healthy lifestyle; the same students and community-invited well elders participated.

Teaching-learning activities involved interaction between the groups during class and in social settings. Students documented learning through a structured diary format and changes in elder knowledge were evaluated using Palmore's (1998) Facts on Aging Quiz. Attitudes toward elders were evaluated using Kogan's (1961) Attitudes Toward Old People Scale. The study used Knowles' (1980) framework. Results found that the teaching intervention significantly positively impacted knowledge of and attitudes toward elders (p = .000 and p = .001, respectively) of senior baccalaureate RN students. Using the same measurement instruments, Sheffler (1995) found attitudes toward elders improved whether students were exposed to them during clinical experiences in hospitals or long-term care facilities.

Within the last two decades, a number of studies have focused upon the effects of teaching-learning activities on health providers' knowledge of and attitudes toward elders. Results have been mixed. Several studies found that participation with elders could have a positive effect (Donovan, 2002; Feeley, 1991; Harrison & Novak, 1988; Hoffman, Brand, Beatty & Hamill, 1985; Masters, 2005; Puentes, 1995). Southall (2002) determined that all of the attitudes improved actual delivery of nursing care to elders. Other studies found that there was no significant improvement in knowledge or attitudes (Haight & Olson, 1989; Treharne, 1990; Williams, Lusk, & Kline, 1986).

According to Margalith, Musgrave and Goldschmidt (2003), two major variables identified in the literature on nursing students' values regarding ethical behavior are nursing education (Cassells & Redman, 1989; Dierckx de Casterle, Janssen & Grypdonck, 1996; Duckett et al., 1992; Gaul, 1989) and religious beliefs (Sorbye, Sorbye, & Sorbye, 1995; Weiss, 1996). Margalith et al. (2003) examined the two variables for a relationship with nursing students' attitudes toward physician-assisted dying (PAD). A convenience sample of 192 nursing students from three Israeli nursing schools was used; two were secular, one was a religious diploma school. All three schools were required by the Israeli Ministry of Health to teach the same core curriculum.

Attitudes toward PAD were measured by responses to the Nurses' Attitudes Regarding Physician Assisted Dying (NARPAD) questionnaire, which consisted of four situational vignettes; a patient requested PAD and a choice of four responses that required various levels of nurse involvement with PAD (Young, Volker, Rieger, & Thorpe, 1993). A Hebrew translation was used. Content validity and readability of NARPAD was established (Young et al., 1993). The authors also addressed test-retest reliability and stability over time using a Kappa measure. Religious beliefs were measured by students' religious affiliation and degree of religiosity, based upon a rating scale of perceptions.

Study results found that prior exposure to euthanasia theory or clinical experience in oncology had a small role in shaping students' attitudes toward PAD. The greatest determinant of their attitudes was their religious beliefs. The more religious they were, the less likely they were to support PAD. Theoretical knowledge of euthanasia did not affect students' attitudes toward PAD; this contradicted earlier findings (Cassells & Redman, 1989; Dierckx de Casterle et al., 1996; Duckett et al., 1992; Gaul, 1989). In prior studies, Jewish nursing students generally were more supportive of PAD than non-Jewish students (Kinsella & Verhoef, 1993; Young et al., 1993). Larger samples were recommended for future studies of the same topic.

Nursing is a demanding program and an increase in the incidence of student depression has been recognized (Cress & Ikeda, 2003; Sax, Bryant, & Gilmartin, 2002; Young, 2003). Dzurec et al. (2007) implemented a longitudinal study to investigate the academic experiences of nursing students to support evidence-based teaching. Early findings of 119 first-year baccalaureate students found that 29 (34%) were at risk for developing depression. When describing causes of feeling down or depressed, the most frequently reported themes were "overload, or sense of feeling overwhelmed," "loneliness and isolation," and "sense of inadequacy." Intervention strategies to foster coping (e.g., face stressors with optimism) are under study to develop teaching methods that minimize and prevent depression reactions to a course of study.

Case studies, clinical decision-making, group work, practice experiences, and writing also were methods of instruction employed to enhance learning in the affective domain. They demonstrate that educators continue to use a variety of strategies to teach aspects of the affective domain. Most of the research results are described in this chapter; additional results are found in Chapters 3 and 5. Also, some teaching strategies are explained under other headings in this chapter, which organizes these findings under professional values such as caring. Table 6.3 summarizes the numerous teaching strategies studied in educational research of the affective domain.

### Non-Instructional Strategies That Promote Affective Development

A research legacy has existed about affective learning outcomes in the education literature since the 1940s. Despite the fact that these studies have focused on different concepts and used different instruments, all have concluded that a positive correlation exists between attaining a college education and affective development. Early research focused on different affective learning development outcomes more than contemporary research studies do. These are discussed further using studies representative of these outcomes.

**Table 6.3. Teaching Strategies and Interventions Found in Educational Research Studies of the Affective Domain**

| Art | Motivation | Simulation |
|---|---|---|
| Case Studies | Movies/Videos | Storytelling |
| Clinical Decision-Making | Narrative Pedagogy | Stress Management |
| Clinical Experiences | Online Presence | Teacher Behaviors |
| Clinical Immersion | Plays | Teacher Immediacy |
| Clinical Postconferences | Poetry | Technology |
| Conditioning | Practice Experiences | Uncertainty |
| Drawings | Presencing | Verbal Anecdotes |
| Group Work | Reflective Journaling | Visual Imaging |
| Humor | Role-Playing | Visual Procedures |
| Meditation | Role-Reversal | Writing |
| Memory Prompts | Self-Reflection | Written Tests |
| Mindfulness | Short Stories | |

**Values and Attitudes Development.** Most measures concerning attitudes and values are self-report instruments and surveys. These are the most common measures used to evaluate the attitudinal and values development of students. They do not evidence cognitive learning, but the yielded information is useful in determining change and growth in what students perceive or others perceive that students have learned or done. Examples of these measures are student satisfaction and attitude surveys, alumni surveys, and employer surveys.

Student values have been the object of most studies about affective domain learning of college students (Astin, 1977; Feldman & Newcomb, 1969; Pascarella & Terenzini, 1991), and the instrument used most often in these and other studies was the Allport-Vernon-Lindzey Study of Values (Sciortino, 1970). The instrument profiles a student's values through prominence of six basic interests or personality motives: theoretical, economic, aesthetic, social, political, and religious. Other studies used an instrument created by the Cooperative Institutional Research Program (Astin, 1997) that was similar to the Study of Values, but used six different value factors: altruism, artistic, athletic, business, and musical interests, as well as status needs.

Two studies used the Study of Values to measure changes in student values during college. May and Ilardi (1970) studied 41 female students at four different times during their final two years of a baccalaureate nursing program; they reported that religious and social values were stronger than initially determined, that there was a significant decrease in religious values over time, and that many students experienced an increase in aesthetic values during their college years. Kirchner and Hogan (1972) found changes in student values by comparing students at one institution in 1964-65 with values of seniors majoring in the same field in 1970-71. The latter students were more drawn to social values and less inclined toward religious values. Astin's (1977) lengthy study of more than 200,000 students at 300 institutions reported more liberal attitudes toward social issues and a decline in traditional religious affiliation over time.

Feldman and Newcomb (1969) analyzed four decades of values research. They reported prominent forms of change including: "Declining authoritarianism, dogmatism, and prejudice, together with decreasingly conservative attitudes toward public issues and growing sensitivity to aesthetic experiences....They add up to something like openness to multiple aspects of the contemporary world...increased intellectual interests and capacities and decreased commitment to religion" (p. 326). No studies were found that comprehensively analyzed similar concepts over the almost four decades.

Pascarella and Terenzini (1991) synthesized twenty years of research from the 1960s through the 1980s to document how values and attitudes of groups of undergraduates changed over time. They reported "...shifts toward openness and a tolerance for diversity, a stronger 'other-person' orientation and concern for individual rights and human welfare... combined with an increase in liberal political and social values and a decline in religious beliefs" (p. 559).

Most studies about students' values and attitudes found movement toward greater individual freedom over the course of the educational experience. Each also noted that values must be studied in the context of dominant societal forces and trends, so care must be taken about conclusions drawn from the findings. In essence, however, taking college courses was found to consistently influence values and attitudes regardless of societal trends, and changes in values occurred regardless of the type of institution or student. One would conclude, then, that post-high school academic experiences affect the values and attitudes of students and those affective components are not "set in stone" by that point in a student's life.

**Psychosocial Affective Changes.** Another affective change relates to interpersonal relations (i.e., psychosocial), and is best exemplified by the early work of Chickering (1969). Using 13 private colleges in the Northeast, he found that a college education made a difference in human development along seven major dimensions or vectors of change: developing competence, managing emotions, developing autonomy, establishing identity, freeing interpersonal relationships, finding purpose, and developing integrity. Others (Astin, 1977; Feldman & Newcomb, 1969; Pascarella & Terenzini, 1991) also reported psychosocial growth due to the college experience. These changes included a more positive self-image, more independence, increased self-confidence and improved self-esteem, which are components of the affective domain.

Solomon, Bisconti, and Ochsner (1977) documented that the development of values and attitudes by college graduates was of more importance to employers than the acquisition of specific knowledge. They also found that college provided worthwhile values not necessarily related directly to one's work, such as political awareness, enjoyment of the college experience, and development of specific interests and appreciations.

Mentkowski (1991) studied student outcomes in relation to 12 measures. Two outcomes related more specifically to the affective domain. While performance at the beginning of college tended to cluster around two separate developmental factors (logical or analytical thought and socio-emotional maturity or interpersonal ability), the two clusters had merged by graduation. Student interview data confirmed that students' commitment to personal, career, and professional values developed during college. Mentkowski found that education made a difference in the development of personal growth and integrated performance in preparation for practice as professionals in management or nursing.

*Moral Development.* Another aspect of affective development studied during college was moral development. The dominant theorist in this area is Kohlberg (1972), who described six stages of development ranging from preconventional moral reasoning to a postconventional view of morality as a set of universal principles. Pascarella and Terenzini (1991) stated that there was "...clear and consistent evidence that students make significant gains during college in the use of principled reasoning to judge moral issues. These finding hold across different measurement instruments and even different cultures" (p. 562). Also, they noted that growth in moral development was correlated positively to growth in cognitive development, values, and psychosocial changes. It was concluded, therefore, that obtaining a college education could cause changes in a holistic manner in students' affective (also, cognitive and psychomotor) domain.

In nursing education, Felton and Parsons (1987) conducted a study of 227 baccalaureate and 111 master's nursing students to determine the influence of the level of formal education on three selected factors: ethical/moral reasoning, attribution of responsibility, and ethical/moral dilemma resolution. Kohlberg's theory of moral development and Heider's attribution of responsibility construct were the reported theories. The study found that graduate students reasoned at a higher level than undergraduate students. Cassidy (1991) reviewed the literature from 1970 to 1987 to determine recognition of ethical responsibilities for nurses and level of ethical decision-making. This researcher found a positive correlation between attaining a college education and a higher level of ethical decision-making. The results of both studies supported other findings in the literature that students with more formal education reason morally at higher levels.

*Impact of College Environment on Affective Domain.* Given that findings of studies from the previous section support the positive impact of a college education on students' affective competency development, subsequent researchers sought to examine the impact of various aspects of a college environment on student growth. Several studies (Astin, 1977; Pascarella, 1985; Pascarella & Terenzini, 1991) found that affective changes were enhanced by residential living, attending a private institution, and student involvement in campus activities. Felton and Parsons (1987), Kimball (1993), and Mentkowski (1991) reported that the identification, teaching and assessment of specific competencies led to increased affective growth during college. Astin (1977) reported that a high level of student involvement, whether interpersonal, academic or athletic, led to "...increased chances of completing college, implementing career objectives, and satisfaction with the undergraduate experience" (p. 241). Also, Astin found that living on campus and attending a private college may have contributed indirectly to increased student interactions with faculty and peers, factors he believed to accelerate or enhance affective domain learning. No similar studies were located that focused on the college impact on nontraditional students such as those over age 25 or in the online college environment.

## *Faculty Behaviors or Characteristics That Enhance Affective Learning*

Limited studies exist to document specific faculty characteristics that enhance affective learning or how such influence occurs. While many studies have examined student perceptions of effective and ineffective teachers, predominantly clinical teachers, few address teacher behaviors that specifically impact affective learning.

It is acknowledged that nursing faculty significantly influence students' feelings of success or failure in nursing practice (Davidhizar & McBride, 1985) and that student perceptions of teacher effectiveness develop early in their programs. The most successful student-teacher relationships consist of the affective domain concepts of mutual respect and admiration. Both groups report experiencing troublesome relationships identified with anxiety and tension; these relationships often result in failed learning experiences and frustrating teaching and learning experiences (Griffith & Bakanauskas, 1983; Kirschling et al., 1995; Kleehammer, Hart, & Keck, 1990; Krichbaum, 1994; Kushnir, 1986; Meisenhelder, 1987).

Saltzberg (2002) explored the use of uncertainty experiences in nursing education. She traced the evolution of the assumptions of the concept of certainty along a continuum from certain to uncertain and its relevance to changing expectations in nursing education. She found that faculty members who explore uncertainty as a given of nursing practice and significant component of education are more likely to help students successfully manage today's uncertain world and facilitate progression of their affective learning. Shor (1992) recognized that learning is not a purely intellectual activity and suggested that the traditional curriculum, with its competitive practices and resulting emotions, may actually interfere with student development by placing cognitive and affective learning in conflict.

Teacher immediacy behaviors have been positively linked to affective learning outcomes. Immediacy behaviors are defined as communication that serves to reduce the psychological distance between people (Anderson, 1979; Mehrabian, 1969). Comstock, Rowell and Bowers (1995) noted that teachers could use immediacy to communicate positive regard, an affective concept that stimulates learning by their students. Several researchers provided evidence of a link between teacher immediacy leading to higher affective (and cognitive) learning outcomes (Frymier, 1994; Frymier & Thompson, 1995; Kelley & Gorman, 1988; Rodriguez et al., 1996). These findings appear consistent across ethnic groups (Sanders & Wiseman, 1990).

Regan (2000) discussed teacher behaviors that fostered empathic communication, which is composed of affective empathy as well as cognitive empathy. These include teacher modeling of empathic communication, demonstrating unconditional positive regard, providing congruence in relational behaviors, and teaching effective use of learning resources and simulation techniques.

### Research on the Affective Domain from Other Professional Disciplines

Disciplines other than nursing have shown a growing interest in studying the affective domain. Again, lack of operational definitions across disciplines, the variance in search terms over time, and the method of storing and retrieval of electronic holdings made these findings difficult to locate and interrelate. Six disciplines were searched to determine research trends regarding affective teaching and learning; these included social work, communication, behavioral neurosciences, psychology, education, and medicine. Additional nursing education studies that did not correspond with previous chapter categories have been included under nursing education.

***Social Work.*** Social work affective learning studies focused on the following topics: cultural sensitivity to differing health beliefs and promoting values that are highly prized in the field, such as those of client self-determination (Biestek, 1957) and autonomy. Congress and Lyons (1992) explored the cultural and subcultural diversity in health care beliefs of Blacks, Hispanics, and Asians. While many immigrants do assimilate health beliefs over time, a large proportion has beliefs of both the prevailing and their own cultures; this duality of beliefs may occur through generations of immigrants who are now considered citizens. Socioeconomic status is a dominant factor in cultural beliefs about health and treatment, including the ability to use health care services. The more economically deprived, the more likely the group retains beliefs and values of the country of origin than their middle class counterparts from the same cultures. Although the social worker may experience conflict while advocating for quality client care and negotiating for client autonomy, Congress and Lyons identified educational and clinical strategies to improve services to clients with culturally conditioned values and reactions to the dominant health care system:

1. increase sensitivity to culturally diverse beliefs.

2. learn more about clients' beliefs about health, disease and treatment.

3. avoid stereotyping and emphasize individual differences in diagnostic assessments.

4. increase the ability of culturally diverse clients to make choices.

5. enlarge other health care professionals' understanding of cultural differences in the health beliefs of clients.

6. advocate for understanding and acceptance of differing health beliefs in the health care facility and in the larger community (adapted from pp. 90-92).

Social workers coined the term "cultural mediator" to describe their role in asserting that cultural beliefs be incorporated into treatment plans (Fandetti & Goldmeier, 1988). Using this framework in the educational process assures the likelihood of social workers basing practice on the application of cultural sensitivity.

**Communication.** Intercultural sensitivity research is foundational to practice in the communication field. Effective teaching strategies exist for the presentation of basic intercultural concepts (Bennett, 1986; Paige & Martin, 1983; Pusch, 1981). Experiential classroom techniques were reviewed by several authors (Asuncion-Lande, 1975; Gudykunst & Kim, 1984; Hoopes & Ventura, 1979; Kohls & Ax, 1979) and intercultural group development processes were identified. The basic learning areas of intercultural communication are generally agreed-upon and are categorized as cultural self-awareness, other-culture awareness, and various approaches to intercultural communication and perception (Gudykunst & Hammer, 1983; Paige & Martin, 1983).

Bennett (1986) proposed a developmental model to training, or educating, for intercultural sensitivity. He believed that this model fosters successful intercultural training as more than acquiring a new set of skills; the model heightens the possibility of awareness and changed attitudes. The model is based on the participants' immediate subjective experience, which he designated as the "phenomenology of training." People do not respond directly to events, rather, they respond to the meaning they attach to events (Kelly, 1963). Using the developmental model provides one with the ability to diagnose the individual's or group's level of intercultural sensitivity, to select strategies that would likely move them in a new direction, and to sequence interactions and material to facilitate movement toward greater cultural sensitivity.

The developmental model is ideally based upon a key organizing concept that must be internalized for development, or progression, to occur. This concept is difference – that cultures differ fundamentally in the way they create and maintain worldviews. The model describes a learner's subjective experience of difference, not just the objective behavior of either learner or educator.

As it is impossible to incorporate all the variables relevant to cross-cultural adaptation, the large number of variables is reduced to a few theoretically meaningful constructs, while others are treated as situational or intervening variables. Like all constructs, intercultural effectiveness is not amenable to direct observation and, therefore, is identified through a series of measurable variables. Intercultural effectiveness includes affective (cognitive and behavioral) competencies (Gudykunst & Kim, 1984; Kealey & Ruben, 1983; Kim, 1988). These are specified in Table 6.4.

**Table 6.4. Competencies of Intercultural Effectiveness**

| Dimension | Competencies |
|---|---|
| **Cognitive** | • Knowledge of language<br>• Nonverbal behavior<br>• Communication rules of the host country |
| **Affective** | • Set of perceptions toward host culture that enables cultural strangers to position themselves in a psychological orientation that is favorable or compatible with that of the host culture<br>• Ability to acknowledge cultural differences, to empathize with the host country's cultural norms and working styles |
| **Behavioral** | • Requires demonstration of cognitive and affective qualities in social interaction with the host people |

The dimensions are interdependent upon each other and competency is required in each area. One dimension cannot function effectively without the other two. For example, cognitive competence, such as in language and interpersonal skills, provides the tools for intercultural communication. Without the affective components of competence, such as empathy and tolerance, one may not be able to establish positive and meaningful communication with the host people. It is the integration that enables people to be fully engaged in their encounters with the host people.

**Behavioral Neuroscience.** Although the behavioral neuroscience field studied aspects of learning for decades, very few of those findings were documented and tested in other fields. The field has much to offer for successful teaching and learning. Neuroanatomical structures are involved with affect. Specifically, the memory of facts improves when connected with emotions; in contrast, extensive stress can impair memory (Bechara et al., 2000; Cahill, Babinsky, Markowitsch, & McGaugh, 1995). Abnormal brain interactions result in affective disorders, inadequate regulation of affective behaviors and affective symptoms (Rosenkranz, Moore & Grace, 2003).

The anatomical structures associated with emotion are the midline limbic structures, such as the cingulate gyrus, thalamus, hypothalamus, hippocampus, and the amygdala (Anderson & Phelps, 2002; Bechara et al., 2000; Cahill et al., 1995; Mayberg et al., 1999). The amygdala modulates the hippocampus and is implicated in memory for emotional events. Also, the amygdala assigns emotive responses to sensory stimuli (Simpson et al., 2000). Behavioral neuroscientists are seeking the biologic markers for affect and are interested in locating the anatomical foci for affect.

Using the Affective Auditory Verbal Learning Test (AAVLT), which elicits emotional stimuli, Everhart, Demaree and Wuensch (2003) examined the variance on learning and believed that the AAVLT could be a measurement tool for inducing mood within clinical populations. Cahill, Babinsky, Markowitsch and McGaugh (1995) used short stories to influence affect.

Education began integrating affect with emotional links to enhance learning. For example, Sywester (1994) described the application of brain function and emotions in the classroom. Role-playing and simulation were learning activities that evoked emotions that provided memory prompts. The science demonstrates that an instructor can mediate affect to facilitate knowledge acquisition. Affective learning is not subject to extinction, and learning, when facilitated by this method, is permanent (Lipp et al., 2001).

*Psychology.* Psychology has always focused on affect and affective disorders as components of this behavioral field. Diaz and De la Casa (2002) described affective learning as changing participants' affective rating of a neutral stimulus. Using affective conditioning, they found that affective learning is highly resistant to extinction. Once developed, affective learning is difficult to forget.

In other studies (Hamm & Vaitl, 1996; Hamm et al., 2003), attempts were made to alter affect through stimuli interventions. Negative stimuli like shock, loud noise, or startle effects were used. Also, motivation as a concept of the affective domain was measured through several standardized and author-developed measurement tools. There are numerous standardized tests available in the discipline to further explore this concept. Some of these are articulated in the interconnected educational psychology fields.

*Education.* Much has already been discussed about the origins of 20th century studies of the affective domain that were generated through the work of Krathwohl et al. (1964). Education, as a discipline, retains an ongoing interest in this domain. Most research, however, is with the K-12 populations, and practical application dominates the research findings. For example, Rodriguez et al. (1996) created a causal model relating teacher immediacy to student learning. Findings support that teacher immediacy influences student affective learning that, in turn, influences student affective (and cognitive) learning. This model supports the idea that teachers can affect students' affective development.

Snider (2001), in the learning environment of a ninth grade poetry class, explored the interrelatedness of affective (and cognitive) learning. Using the taxonomy developed by Krathwohl et al. (1964), the study found that values developed when studying and learning poetry. Through testing evaluative learning theory, which posits that affective learning is not subject to blocking by negative stimuli, Lipp et al. (2001) found that inhibitory stimuli will interfere with affective learning. Education holds a practical science worldview that reinforces facilitation of student learning. Additional educational studies are included in Chapters 3 and 5 of this book and are therefore not repeated in this chapter.

**Medicine.** Physicians are studying affective learning in areas such as empathy. These studies began in the mid-1980s. Hojat et al. (2004), in an empirical study, found that empathy declined in students of medicine during their medical education. Results were not statistically significant, but do indicate a downward trend along with the values of humanitarianism, enthusiasm, and idealism (Maheux & Beland, 1986; Wolf, Balson, Faucett & Randall, 1989). The research used the newly developed Jefferson Scale of Physician Empathy (JSPE), which was created through a grant from the Medical Humanities Initiative of Pfizer, Inc.

As previously discussed, empathy is widely accepted as an essential component of therapeutic, supportive, and caring relationships. However, professional roles and expectations influence the degree to which empathy is expressed in a clinical setting. Caring, a nursing expectation, and curing, a physician expectation, may actually be opposite ends of a continuum (Hojat, Fields, & Gonnella, 2003a; Hojat et al., 2004).

The JSPE was also used to study empathy in 56 female nurses and 42 female physicians in the internal medicine residency program at one hospital. The former group was employees and the latter group was students. Although the JSPE was designed for residents and practicing physicians (Hojat et al., 2002c), the researchers wanted to continue exploring empathy among other health professionals. The JSPE developers have reported its psychometric properties (Hojat et al., 2001a; Hojat et al., 2001b). Convergent validity, discriminate validity and construct validity were determined (Hojat et al., 2002b). The JSPE is designed around an operational measure of empathy defined as "a *cognitive* (as opposed to affective) attribute that involves *understanding* of the inner experiences of the patient, combined with a capacity to *communicate* this understanding to the patient" (Hojat et al., 2002b, p. 4). The three italicized terms emphasize their significance in the construct of empathy in patient care (Hojat et al., 2003b; Hojat et al., 2002a). Although the findings are not generalizable due to the limited sample size and setting, the findings suggest moderate differences between nurses and physicians on a few items of the JSPE. Although medicine views empathy as a cognitive attribute and nursing views empathy as an affective attribute, the researchers believe that the JSPE is a reliable research tool to assess empathy among health professionals, including nurses.

## *Emerging Affective Domain Initiatives and Technology*

The literature review led to emerging trends of importance to future nurse scholars considering educational research study of the affective domain. Although no nursing studies were found related to the trends, it is evident that the trends are in process primarily in the education, medicine and business fields. These research trends are national in scope and some involve technology built to recognize and enhance affective responses.

In non-health care fields, there is a national effort to intentionally study the relationship between cognitive and affective learning. Most teachers have been socialized to value cognitive learning and to ignore or marginalize affective — that is, the emotional component — of teaching and learning. As a result, the Carnegie Foundation and the American Association for Higher Education supported Oxford College of Emory University in assuming a leadership position, along with four other institutions: Agnes Scott College, Kennesaw State University of Georgia, Community College of Philadelphia, and Wright State University School of Medicine. This group established the Cognitive-Affective Learning Initiative (Owen-Smith, 2004) and is working together to focus on specific methods to create campus environments that strengthen the connection between affective and cognitive domains. Activities include assessing campuses' methods of facilitating connections between the heart and mind (i.e., service learning, reflection-centered and problem-based classes, etc.), intentionally provoking and evoking ways to raise sociopolitical consciousness and problematize courses so as to create disorienting moments that contribute to enduring learning, and working to create campus climates that will intentionally focus on the affective domain as a critical and necessary aspect of the learning process. They view this project as returning to the work initiated years ago by the great educational philosophers who believed that the intellect rests in the mind and the heart. Within this project, the first issue of its *Journal of Cognitive Affective Learning* was initiated fall 2004. The journal is a peer-reviewed, open-access journal devoted to advancing the understanding of the connection between the cognitive and affective in teaching and learning.

New learning technologies have emerged that are automating learning designed for the affective domain (Adkins, 2004). These affective learning technologies are beyond the research phase and are rapidly proliferating. Spurred by workforce selection and retention, workplace ethics, customer analytics and public safety and national security, there is an effort to meet the need for affective alignment to work positions. Studies have documented large percentages of workforce disengagement with their work. New affective-based personality assessments are being used routinely in precandidate employment screening. These are not personality tests but are new forms of assessment to map a candidate's personality profile. The psychometrics of these instruments is reported to be defensible in court. The best known personality assessment taxonomy is the Big Five, which identifies five primary subcategories of the affective domain: extraversion, emotional stability, agreeableness, conscientiousness, and openness to experience. A person's score on these assessments is used to determine his or her appropriateness for particular jobs.

Ethics training is proliferating due to corporate scandals, compliance mandates and legal risks. There is an e-learning product line called Legal Compliance and Ethics Center that contains conventional courses on ethics. The company claims a research link between ethics training and quality of products. Other companies such as SimuLearn, WILL Interactive, Kaplan, and Insight Experience are bringing affective learning products to the market that encourage ethical behavior via simulation, which is the current method (of instruction) of choice. The products generate experiences for workers and, as the simulation unfolds, the technology measures beliefs and emotional state of mind. The best known e-learning product dealing with the affective domain is SimuLearn's Virtual Leader. It uses complex artificial intelligence routines to control the behavior of virtual characters, who have a large repertoire of verbal responses. The product uses a library of over 200 body gestures and facial responses designed to elicit behavior from the real participants.

A worker's emotional state will often influence behavior. One product, PeopleView, claims to boost employee performance through improved emotional intelligence. Usually people can determine the emotional status of a person face-to-face; a new technology can gauge a person's emotional status by analyzing his or her voice or text-based conversations. Utopy, Inc. produced emotion detection software called SpeechMiner, designed primarily for call centers. In real time, it enables an agent to visually see when a customer is resisting a sale or when a customer's anger begins to escalate. It also allows a manager to monitor the ongoing emotional flow of several agents at one time and can ensure that agents are properly reading all disclosures without misrepresentations. Other similar products can defuse customer anger or frustration and mitigate performance problems and fill skills gaps as they arise. These are studied in business and training situations.

The Semantic Web, conceived by the innovator of the World Wide Web, is an extension of the current Web, in which information is given well-defined meaning, better enabling computers and people to work in cooperation. It is an infrastructure that enables software and machines to reason about information on the Web. Also, it is focused on creating the next generation of knowledge management tools using the latest technologies. Semantic Web is already being used by government agencies for gathering intelligence and homeland security risks. It allows agencies not only to learn about the belief systems of people, but also to learn the intentions of various groups and people.

Not only are new affective learning technologies being marketed, but they are promoted as XML objects that can be integrated with enterprise applications. There are components that measure the affective state of an individual and components that attempt to modify that person's state of mind. There are products working on a standard to frame and embed contextual human characteristics, including cultural, social, kinesic, psychological and intentional features within conveyed information. The closest working XML standard that combines all three of Bloom's Taxonomy domains is the new Medical Markup Language already being used in medical training products in Germany. These integrated technologies are rare, but it is now possible to develop a learning strategy that delivers remediation to all three learning domains simultaneously.

Another national initiative is funded by the National Science Foundation. Through the Massachusetts' Institute of Technology's Media Lab, a Learning Companion (LC) is being designed to mitigate belief systems that undermine learning accomplishments of children. The LC is viewed as an effective companion that attempts to alleviate frustration and self-doubt in young learners. Initially, LC establishes a relationship with the child, then attempts to ascertain the cognitive state of the child and interacts with the child depending on that cognitive state. The complexities are enormous; this is a formalized analytical model that describes the dynamics of emotional states during model-based learning experiences. All of these products indicate a growing trend to simulate and alter human affective response in various contexts, including the learning environment.

## CONCLUSIONS

Why is affective learning important to nurse educators and learners? The affective research findings support the following conclusions:

1.  Learner anxiety that is a detriment to learning can be lowered.
2.  Learner failure and learner resistance can be reduced.
3.  A supportive community of caring learners can be developed to facilitate learning and retention.
4.  Education is moving from teacher-centered to learner-centered.
5.  The learner's self-confidence can be increased.
6.  Knowledge attainment and retention are enhanced through the affective domain.
7.  Attitudes can be fostered that enhance nursing practice effectiveness and ultimately patient health outcomes.
8.  Affective learning fosters the highest development of professional values, professional responses such as caring and empathy, and professional identity.

The most striking database findings were the difficulty in retrieving information from existing electronic databases and the constant change in search descriptors used to describe the affective domain. These descriptor changes appear to represent societal, educational, and research trends. Also, diverse and overlapping use of affective terms made it difficult to weave a comprehensive overview and interrelationship of the research findings.

Considering the recent efforts to revise and address nursing's professional values, a corresponding emerging effort by nurse educators has been initiated to study the promotion of values in educational settings. The affective domain of nursing, such as professional values, attitudes, caring and compassion, underpins nurses' practice and, as such, deserves priority attention in the nursing curriculum. The link to patient outcomes is an emerging area being explored; for example, incivility in the workplace has been linked to poor health and safety outcomes.

Findings demonstrate the struggles of authors and disciplines to describe, operationalize, research and articulate this complex domain. All articles acknowledged the overlap in domains. However, attempts to study the affective domain continue.

Studies of related disciplines depict some usable research methodologies and findings to guide the development of affective teaching and learning in nursing education. An emerging body of affective domain research is present in the nursing education literature. Incorporating affective learning may facilitate student retention of knowledge while also developing professional values. Also, interdisciplinary and multi-site affective learning research is rare.

Research findings are fragmented and isolated from one another. Little effort has been dedicated to consolidating results and relating them in a meaningful fashion; thus, the development of the science of nursing education regarding affective domain teaching and learning has been difficult to advance. Also, there is limited research concerning the affective domain teaching and learning in different nursing program types and in relation to different nursing student characteristics, such as gender, age, and ethnicity.

Measurement tools used to describe and assess affective learning were usually author-developed and rarely replicated in other published studies. Most instruments lacked the extensive rigor that can be achieved through validity and reliability measures.

Cognitive processes are completed through affective learning. If so, nurse educators could mediate affect when the students attend class or interact with the teacher through technology to facilitate learner knowledge attainment and retention.

Education research exists on affect concepts; some, such as caring and empathy, are more developed than others. Incivility incidents in nursing education have been documented and further study would benefit nurse educators as they cope with immediate incidents and their aftermath. Fostering civility and other professional values while learning needs further research attention.

There is limited affective educational research that is built upon educational theories. A lack of identification of key aspects of the affective domain in nursing exists. Though some tools to measure affective domain learning have been constructed and tested, many are not based on nor grounded in theory.

Beliefs, values, and attitudes are reported as affective learning but may, in fact, be the end product of affective learning (Maier-Lorentz, 1999; Martin et al., 2000; Rodriguez et al., 1996; Snider, 2001). End products or outcomes of affective learning are posited because all authors describe some cognitive or consciousness processing of affect to achieve these outcomes (L. Taylor, personal communication, October 22, 2004).

Sample sizes in affective domain learning studies typically have been small and frequently limited to one course within a nursing program or one specific teaching intervention. Most studies used pre-post-designs within a course rather than a longitudinal design that may be more appropriate in measuring affective outcomes, since such outcomes often take a significant length of time to develop. Several studies were reported where more than one site or several groups were used for comparison results, but these were few in number. Few studies of strategies to foster affective learning development were reported, and none were found relating affective domain maturity to effectiveness in clinical practice.

Considerable research about caring, values and ethics has been reported, and most of this research had a theoretical base that specified affective learning as a primary concern. However, theoretical frameworks used in the studies were varied, and only a few publications, such as those focused on caring, described development of theories about the affective concepts studied (e.g., Alligood, 1992). Research on some topics seemed to fall in and out of favor (e.g., "values clarification" was a dominant theme in early studies, with a change to "ethical principles" as a related dominant concept evident in recent studies); this leads to difficulty in developing and following professional values research.

The complexities in defining caring in nursing may contribute to differing caring beliefs and attitudes in nursing education. As Brown (2005) found, an appreciable number of nursing faculty, while valuing the importance of caring as an affective objective, do not believe that caring can be taught in a classroom or that it can be measured. If an expectation of students, and, ultimately, of professional nurses is that they practice as caring people (Boykin & Schoenhofer, 2001), then it becomes imperative that nurse educators design learning transactions that facilitate movement of caring attitudes, values, and beliefs from one environment to another.

Finally, a lengthy delay occurs from the time of publication to entry of the publication in relevant electronic databases. Also, search descriptors need to be broadened to contain terms and concepts that have been in the literature for over a decade. Authors and those maintaining electronic databases need to be aware of this basic problem, which hampers the retrieval and interconnectedness of findings for furthering the science of nursing education in the affective domain.

## RECOMMENDATIONS

Serious development of educational research that corresponds to the profession's affective values, attitudes and behaviors needs to be embraced. All affective domain aspects of nursing need to be identified, promoted, and developed with accompanying teaching-learning strategies, measurement tools, and program (all types) outcome indicators. Such an effort has the potential to improve quality care efforts of national importance.

Since major nursing organizations have recently revised and clarified the profession's values, the nurse educator interested in affective learning has a golden opportunity to be on the cutting edge of exploring and strengthening teaching and learning of values. "Core values" have been explicitly described (AACN, 2008) for baccalaureate programs; wide gaps of similar discourse in other program types exist. All nursing programs incorporate the ANA *Code of Ethics* (2001) as a nursing practice document; however, it has yet to be fully studied in our teaching, learning and program outcomes.

Strong nurse educator development in the affective domain is needed within the discipline. Based on the review of the domains of learning and the national expectations of teachers, especially at the postsecondary level, nurse educator preparation needs depth and breadth to incorporate specific and overlapping aspects of the affective learning domain.

For teachers, effectiveness is directly related to affective and interpersonal aspects of teaching-learning. Affective characteristics are supported in Chickering and Gamson's (1987) Inventory of Effective Faculty Behaviors. Also, common teacher behaviors that may cause negative student affect interfere with student motivation and stymie learning. These behaviors can be altered with minor shifts in their approach to student learning and satisfaction. Affect is not a troublesome extra to be dealt with in the classroom. Affect parallels intelligence in learning.

Nursing is a highly regulated field. The additive curriculum and the national nursing educator shortage leave little time for nurse educators to explore strategies that develop nursing students as affective learners. Pressure is felt at all levels within nursing programs to foster graduates' success on the national licensure exam, a computerized testing format that measures content application using the cognitive domain, and to quickly produce graduates for the workforce (Joynt & Kimball, 2008). Thoughtful examination of curricula to ensure development in all learning domains and teachers with the abilities to foster all domains are critical to meeting societal needs.

The development of appropriate evaluation instruments to assess learner progress toward attainment of affective competences is needed. Specifying classroom and clinical learning strategies would assist students in achieving affective learning outcomes. Outcome measures, specific to nursing practice success, should be developed for the affective domain. As affective recognition technology increases in employment settings, nursing educator research on its use by nursing students from all programs should be developed.

Affective domain learning occurs within the curriculum with or without planning (Beane, 1990) and assessing. The effectiveness of nursing education and ultimately nursing practice could be increased with dedicated studies and resources to explore this topic. Theory building in the affective domain would be a logical step for nurse educators to pursue.

Clarifying and defining affective competencies would benefit nursing education and practice. Supporting competency development around affective domain expectations as conceived by related disciplines and nurse researchers would enhance planning, teaching and assessing learning.

Nursing education research in the affective domain should not be completed in isolation within educational institutions. The research supports the need to study learning using a tri-model framework that is academic, professional organization and practice based. A challenge will be to translate the practice setting expectations into language and learner changes that are relevant to an educational environment.

Valuing of the research in nursing education is imperative both within and outside the discipline of nursing. Equally important is the funding of nursing education research studies. Following the current practice model of nursing research, identifying priority areas of nursing education research (revised by the NLN in 2008) and then conducting the research at multiple educational sites and in multiple stages seems to be a worthy undertaking of a discipline claiming to teach critical thinkers with professional values.

As nurse educators gain knowledge and expertise researching the affective domain, results could help student nurses who then become graduate nurses as they teach patients, because educator (or teacher) is one of the major roles of nurses in practice. Teaching strategies, tested in academe, may have implication for practice. Incorporating affective learning knowledge could improve the recall of patients seeking to understand the management of their illnesses. For example, patients with low literacy levels may be able to understand health information conveyed in a storying format rather than traditional teaching materials such as providing pamphlets, Internet information, and other handouts.

Gaps exist in research of professional values such as "altruism" and "professional boundaries." Nurse educators need to address these in studies of teaching-learning strategies and evaluation measures.

Integration at the conceptual level and more theory-driven studies are encouraged for theory development and more systematic investigation of affective teaching and learning. The use of phenomenology, a model for understanding learner development in the affective domain, may prove useful in this area of study.

Existing formative and summative evaluations in nursing curricula emphasize knowledge and thinking attainment, not the development of nurses; the latter arguably consists of affective development. Affect is difficult to measure in a cause-and-effect manner. Affect is not a visible construct, but study of it would require a written format through the use of phenomenology, which examines phenomena that cannot be easily measured. Creating a description and framework of nursing education through phenomenology and hermeneutics would provide nurse educators the opportunity to examine affective domain maturation of the learner and create teaching strategies that enhance learner development rather than concentrating solely on content retention and application.

The need for affective competencies is evident; however, there is a scarcity of affective research in nursing education for numerous reasons, including a lack of clarity as to what the concept "affective" means to nursing and learning in nursing programs. However, this scarcity is not limited to nursing and an interdisciplinary study approach is nonexistent.

Non-nursing disciplines have published more studies and for a longer period of time on the topic of affective learning. There is a need to determine the relevance of these studies, particularly from behavioral neuroscience, to nursing education and clinical situations.

The affective component of learning in nursing education takes time to develop within the learner. Consequently, affective learning expectations would supposedly be more prominent in curricula as nurses advance in their education. The studies support that there is a positive correlation between education and the development of affective competencies. However, affective studies focusing on graduate nursing education are needed to expand the existing literature base.

Nurse educators are encouraged to incorporate aspects of the affective domain into their educational research. Although complex, and challenging, the public desires and deserves nurses with well-developed professional values and other affective components such as caring. At no other time have we had the number of nurse educator researchers, the collective knowledge and abilities, the capacity to network and collaborate, and the combined energies to markedly change nursing education and ultimately nurse practice.

## References

Adkins, S. S. (2004). Beneath the tip of the iceberg: Technology plumbs the affective learning domain. *American Society for Training and Development. [Online]*. Available: http://www.learningcircuits.org/2004/feb2004/adkins.htm.

Akin, G., & Palmer, I. (2000). Putting metaphors to work for change in organizations. *Organizational Dynamics, 28(3)*, 67-77.

Alligood, M. R. (1992). Empathy: The importance of recognizing two types. *Journal of Psychosocial Nursing and Mental Health Services*, 30(3), 14-17.

Alpers, R., & Zoucha, R. (1996). Comparison of cultural competence and cultural confidence of senior nursing students in a private southern university. *Journal of Cultural Diversity, 3(1)*, 9-15.

Altun, I. (2002). Burnout and nurses' personal and professional values. *Nursing Ethics*, 9, 269-278.

Amada, G. (1994). *Coping with the disruptive college student: A practical model.* Asheville, NC: College Administration Publishers.

American Academy of Nursing (1998). *Nursing research position statement.* Washington, D.C.: Author.

American Association of Colleges of Nursing (1998). *The essentials of baccalaureate education for professional nursing practice.* Washington, D.C.: Author.

American Association of Colleges of Nursing. (2008). *Draft 3: The essentials of baccalaureate education for professional nursing practice.* Washington, DC: Author.

American Nurses Association. (2001). *Code of ethics for nurses with interpretive statements.* Silver Spring, MD: Author.

American Nurses Association. (2002). *Code for conduct.* Kansas City, MO: ANA Press.

Andersen, J. F. (1979). Teacher immediacy as a predictor of teaching effectiveness. In D. Nimmo (Ed.), *Communication yearbook 3* (pp. 543-559). New Brunswick, NJ: Transaction Books.

Anderson, A. K., & Phelps, E. K. (2002). Is the human amygdala critical for the subjective experience of emotion? Evidence of intact dispositional affect in patients with amygdala lesions. *Journal of Cognitive Neuroscience,* 14, 709-720.

Arangie-Harrell, P. A. R. (1998). Moral development among college nursing students: Cognitive and affective influences (Doctoral dissertation, University of Memphis). Dissertation Abstracts International, 59, 09A.

Astin, A. W. (1977). Four critical years: Effects of college on beliefs, attitudes, and knowledge. San Francisco: Jossey-Bass.

Astin, J. (1997). Stress reduction through mindfulness meditation: Effects on psychological symptomology, sense of control, and spiritual experience. Psychotherapy and Psychosomatics, 66, 97-106.

Asuncion-Lande, N.C. (1975). A program guide for a re-entry/transition seminar-workshop. (ERIC Document Reproduction Service No. ED 344557)

Atkins, M. W., & Steitz, J. A. (2000). The assessment of empathy: An evaluation of the interpersonal reactivity index. [Online]. Available: http://www.uu.edu/union/academ/tep/research/atkins.htm.

Baillie, L. (1996). A phenomenological study of the nature of empathy. Journal of Advanced Nursing, 24, 1300-1308.

Ballou, K. A. (1998). A concept analysis of autonomy. Journal of Professional Nursing, 14, 102-110.

Bandura, A. (1997). Self-efficacy: The exercise of control. New York: W.H. Freeman.

Banyard, V. (1994). Survival on the streets: Coping strategies of mothers who are homeless (Doctoral dissertation, University of Michigan). Dissertation Abstracts International, 55, 3578B. (UMI No. AAG95-00883).

Banyard, V. L., & Graham-Bermann, S. A. (1995). Building an empowerment policy paradigm: Self-reported strengths of homeless mothers. American Journal of Orthopsychiatry, 65, 479-491.

Barrett-Lennard, G. T. (1993). The phases and focus of empathy. British Journal of Medical Psychology, 66, 3-14.

Bartol, G. M., & Richardson, L. (1998). Using literature to create cultural competence. Journal of Nursing Scholarship, 30(1), 75-79.

Batson, C. D. (1991). The altruism question: Toward a social-psychological answer. Hillsdale, NJ: Erlbaum.

Beal, J. A., Lynch, M. M., & Moore, P. S. (1989). Communicating nursing research: Another look at the use of poster sessions in undergraduate programs. *Nurse Educator,* 14(1), 8-10.

Beane, J. A. (1990). *Affect in the curriculum: Toward democracy, dignity, and diversity.* New York: Teachers College Press.

Bechara, A., Damasio, H., & Damasio, A. R. (2000). Emotion, decision-making and the orbitofrontal cortex. *Cerebral Cortex,* 10, 295-307. [Online]. Available: http://www.cercor. oupjournals.org/cgi/content/full/10/3/295#top.

Beck, C. T. (1986). Strategies for teaching nursing research: Small group games for teaching nursing research. *Western Journal of Nursing Research,* 8, 233-238.

Beck, C. T. (2000). The experience of choosing nursing as a career. *Journal of Nursing Education,* 39, 320-322.

Beck, C. T. (2001). Caring within nursing education: A metasynthesis. *Journal of Nursing Education,* 40, 101-109.

Beck, D., Hackett, M. B., Srivastava, R., McKim, E., & Rockwell, B. (1997). Perceived level and sources of stress in baccalaureate nursing students. *Journal of Nursing Education,* 36, 180-186.

Beddoe, A. E., & Murphy, S.,O. (2004). Does mindfulness decrease stress and foster empathy among nursing students? *Journal of Nursing Education,* 43, 305-312.

Bednash, G., Fagin, C., & Mezey, M. (2003). Geriatric content in nursing programs: A wake-up call. [Guest editorial]. *Nursing Outlook,* 51, 149-150.

Belenky, M., Clinchy, B., Goldberger, N., & Tarule, J. (1986). *Women's ways of knowing: The development of self, voice, and mind.* New York: Basic Books.

Bem, S. L. (1974). The measurement of psychological androgyny. *Journal of Consulting and Clinical Psychology,* 42, 155-162.

Benner, P. (1984). *From novice to expert: Excellence and power in clinical nursing practice.* Menlo Park, CA: Addison-Wesley.

Benner, P. (1999). Claiming the worth and wisdom of clinical practice. *Nursing and Health Care Perspectives,* 20, 312-319.

Benner, P., & Wrubel, J. (1989). *The primacy of caring: Stress and coping in health and illness.* Menlo Park, CA: Addison-Wesley.

Bennett, J. A. (1995). Methodological notes on empathy: Further considerations. *Advances in Nursing Science,* 18(1), 28-50.

Bennett, M. J. (1986). A developmental approach to training for intercultural sensitivity. *International Journal of Intercultural Relations,* 10(2), 179-196.

Bevis, O. E., & Watson, J. (1989). *Toward a caring curriculum: A new pedagogy for nursing.* New York: National League for Nursing.

Biestek, F. (1957). *The casework relationship.* Chicago: Loyola University Press.

Bilinski, H. (2002). The mentored journal. *Nurse Educator,* 27, 37-41.

Bixler, G., & Bixler, R. (1945). The professional status of nursing. *American Journal of Nursing,* 45, 730-735.

Bloom, B. S. (Ed.). (1956). *Taxonomy of educational objectives: The classification of educational goals, Handbook I: Cognitive domain.* New York: McKay.

Bolen, J. S. (1996). *Close to the bone: Life-threatening illness and the search for meaning.* New York:Simon & Schuster.

Boughn, S. (1995). An instrument for measuring autonomy-related attitudes and behaviors in women nursing students. *Journal of Nursing Education,* 34, 106-113.

Boughn, S. & Lentini, A. (1999). Why do women choose nursing? *Journal of Nursing Education,* 38, 156-161.

Boykin, A., & Schoenhofer, S. (2001). *Nursing as caring: A model for transforming practice.* Boston: Jones & Bartlett.

Brooker, R., & MacDonald, D. (1999). Did we hear you? Issues of student voice in a curricular innovation. *Journal of Curriculum Studies,* 31(1), 83-97.

Brown, L. P. (2005). Caring in nursing curriculum design: A quantitative study of attitudes, beliefs, and practices of associate degree nursing faculty (Doctoral dissertation, Capella University) *Dissertation Abstracts International,* 66, 08A.

Brubaker, C. L. (2005). An instrument to measure ethical caring in clinical encounters between student nurses and patients (Doctoral dissertation, Illinois State University). *Dissertation Abstracts International,* 66, 11B.

Bruner, J. (1963). *On knowing.* Cambridge, MA: Belknap Press.

Bucher, L. (1991). Evaluating the affective domain: Consider a Likert scale. *Journal of Nursing Staff Development,* 7, 234-238.

Buckenham, M. A. (1988). Student nurse perception of the staff nurse role. *Journal of Advanced Nursing,* 13, 662-670.

Burbank, P. M., Dowling-Castronovo, A., Crowther, M. R., & Capezuti, E. A. (2006). Improving knowledge and attitudes toward older adults through innovative educational strategies. *Journal of Professional Nursing,* 22(2), 91-97.

Cahill, L., Babinsky, R., Markowitsch, H. H., & McGaugh, J. L. (1995). The amygdala and emotional memory. *Nature,* 377, 295-296.

Campinha-Bacote, J., & Padgett, J. J. (1995). Cultural competence: A critical factor in nursing research. *Journal of Cultural Diversity,* 2(1), 31-34.

Campinha-Bacote, J. (1999). A model and instrument for addressing cultural competence in health care. *Journal of Nursing Education,* 38, 203-207.

Capper, C. A. (1993). *School administration in a pluralistic society.* Albany, NY: State University of New York Press.

Carper, B. A. (1978). Fundamental patterns of knowing in nursing. *Advances in Nursing Science,* 1(1), 13-23.

Cassells, J. M., & Redman, B. K. (1989). Preparing students to be moral agents in clinical nursing practice. *Nursing Clinics of North America,* 24, 463-473.

Cassidy, V. R. (1991). Ethical responsibilities in nursing: Research findings and issues. *Journal of Professional Nursing,* 7(2), 112-118.

Chickering, A. (1969). *Education and identity.* San Francisco: Jossey-Bass.

Chickering, A. W., & Gamson, Z. F. (1987). Seven principles for good practice in undergraduate education. *American Association for Higher Education Bulletin,* 39(7), 3-7.

Chinn, P. L., & Kramer, M. K. (1999). *Theory and nursing: Integrated knowledge development* (4th ed.). St. Louis, MO: Mosby.

Chrisman, N. (1998). Faculty infrastructure for cultural competency education. *Journal of Nursing Education,* 37, 45-47.

Clark, C. M. (in press a). Faculty and student assessment and experience with incivility in nursing education: A national perspective. *Journal of Nursing Education.*

Clark, C. M. (in press b). The dance of incivility in nursing education as described by nursing faculty and students. *Advances in Nursing Science.*

Clark, C. M. (2006). Incivility in nursing education: Student perceptions of uncivil faculty behavior in the academic environment (Doctoral dissertation, University of Idaho). *Dissertation Abstracts International.* AAT 3220867.

Clark, C. M. (2008). Student perspectives on incivility in nursing education: An application of the concept of rankism. *Nursing Outlook,* 56(1), 4-8.

Clark, C. M, & Springer, P. J. (2007a). Incivility in nursing education: A descriptive study of definitions and prevalence. *Journal of Nursing Education,* 46(1), 7-14.

Clark, C.M., & Springer, P. J. (2007b). Thoughts on incivility: Student and faculty perceptions of uncivil behavior in nursing education. *Nursing Education Perspectives,* 28(2), 93-97.

Clarke, A. (1999). Changing attitudes through persuasive communication. *Nursing Standard,* 13(30), 14-20.

Coates, C. (1997). The Caring Efficacy Scale: Nurses' self-reports of caring in practice settings. *Advanced Practice Nursing Quarterly,* 3(1), 53-59.

Colesante, R., & Biggs, D. (1999). Teaching about tolerance with stories and arguments. *Journal of Moral Education,* 28, 185-199.

Comstock, J., Rowell, E., & Bowers, J. W. (1995). Food for thought: Teacher nonverbal immediacy, student learning and curvilinearity. *Communication Education,* 44, 251-266.

Congress, E., & Lyons, B. (1992). Ethnic differences in health beliefs: Implications for social workers in health care settings. *Social Work in Health Care,* 17(3), 81-96.

Cook, P. R., & Cullen, J. A. (2003). Caring as an imperative for nursing education. *Nursing Education Perspectives,* 24(4), 192-197.

Cook, T. H., Gilmer, M. J., & Bess, C. J. (2003). Beginning students' definitions of nursing: An inductive framework of professional identity. *Journal of Nursing Education,* 42, 311-317.

Cowles, K. V., Strickland, D., & Rodgers, B. L. (2001). Collaboration for teaching innovation: Writing across the curriculum in a school of nursing. Journal of Nursing Education, 40, 363-367.

Cress, C. M., & Ikeda, E. K. (2003). Distress under duress: The relationship between campus climate and depression in Asian American college students. NAPSA Journal, 40(2), 74-97.

Cullen, J. A. (1994). Determining affective workplace competencies for associate degree nurses (Doctoral dissertation, University of South Carolina). Dissertation Abstracts International, 55, 11A.

Cutcliffe, J. R., & Cassedy, P. (1999). The development of empathy in students on a short, skills based counseling course: A pilot study. Nurse Education Today, 19, 250-257.

Davidhizar, R. E., & McBride, A. (1985). How nursing students explain their success and failure in clinical experiences. Journal of Nursing Education, 24, 284-290.

Davis, M. H. (1983). The effects of dispositional empathy on emotional reactions and helping: A multidimensional approach. Journal of Personality, 51, 167-184.

Dean, P. G. (1986). Strategies for teaching nursing research: Participant observation. Western Journal of Nursing Research, 8, 378-382.

Dearman, C. N. (2003). Using clinical scenarios in nursing education. Annual Review of Nursing Education, 1, 341-355.

DeLashmutt, M. B. (2000). Spiritual needs of mothers raising children while homeless (Doctoral dissertation, George Mason University). Dissertation Abstracts International, 61, 03B. (UMI No. AA19964758)

DeLashmutt, M. B. (2007). Students' experience of nursing presence with poor mothers. Journal of Obstetric, Gynecologic and Neonatal Nursing, 36(2), 183-189.

DeLashmutt, M. B., & Rankin, E. (2005). A different kind of clinical experience: Poverty up close and personal. Nurse Educator, 30(4), 143-149.

DeLashmutt, M. B., & Rankin, E. (2006). Finding spirituality and nursing presence: The student's challenge. Journal of Holistic Nursing, 24, 282-288.

Diaz, E., & De la Casa, G. (2002). Latent inhibition in human affective learning. Emotion 2(3), 242-250.

Diekelmann, N., & Ironside, P. M. (1998). Preserving writing in doctoral education: Exploring the concernful practices of schooling, learning, and teaching. _Journal of Advanced Nursing,_ 28, 1347-1355.

Dierckx de Casterle, B., Janssen, P. J., & Grypdonck, M. (1996). The relationship between education and ethical behavior of nursing students. _Western Journal of Nursing Research,_ 18, 330-350.

Donovan, N. (2002). Providing a home care clinical experience that benefits clients, students, and agencies. _Home Healthcare Nurse,_ 20, 443-448.

du Toit, D. D. (1995). A sociological analysis of the extent and influence of professional socialization on the development of a nursing identity among nursing students at two universities in Brisbane, Australia. _Journal of Advanced Nursing,_ 21, 164-171.

Duchscher, J. E. B. (2001). Peer learning: A clinical teaching strategy to promote active learning. _Nurse Educator,_ 26(2), 59-60.

Duckett, L., Rowan-Boyer, M., Ryden, M. B., Crisham, P., Savik, K., & Rest, J. R. (1992). Challenging misperceptions about nurses' moral reasoning. _Nursing Research,_ 41, 324-331.

Duggleby, W. (1998). Improving undergraduate nursing research education: The effectiveness of collecting and analyzing oral histories. _Journal of Nursing Education,_ 37, 247-252.

Dzurec, L., Allchin, L., & Engler, A. (2007). First-year nursing students' accounts of reasons for student depression. _Journal of Nursing Education,_ 46, 545-551.

Eifried, S. (2003). Bearing witness to suffering: The lived experience of nursing students. _Journal of Nursing Education,_ 42(2), 59-67.

Eisner, E.W. (1997). The promise and perils of alternative forms of data representation. _Educational Researcher,_ 26(6), 4-10.

Emblem, J. (1992). Religion and spirituality defined according to current use in nursing literature. _Journal of Professional Nursing,_ 8, 41-47.

Emrich, K., Thompson, T., & Moore, G. (2003). Positive attitude: An essential element for effective care of people with mental illnesses. _Journal of Psychosocial Nursing,_ 41(5), 18-25.

Esters, I. G., Cooker, P. G., & Ittenbach, R. (1998). Effects of a unit of instruction in mental health on rural adolescents' conceptions of mental illness and attitudes about seeking help. Adolescence, 33, 469-476.

Evans, B. C., & Bendel, R. (2004). Cognitive and ethical maturity in baccalaureate nursing students: Did a class using narrative pedagogy make a difference? Nursing Education Perspectives, 25(4), 188-195.

Evans, B. C., & Severtsen, B. M. (2001) Storytelling as cultural assessment. Nursing and Health Care Perspectives, 22(4), 180-183.

Evans, G. W., Wilt, D. L. Alligood, M. R., & O'Neil, M. (1998). Empathy: A study of two types. Issues in Mental Health Nursing, 19, 453-461.

Everhart, D. E., & Demaree, H. A. (2003). Low alpha power (7.5-9.5 Hz) changes during positive and negative affective learning. Cognitive, Affective, & Behavioral Neuroscience, 3(1), 39-45.

Everhart, D. E., Demaree, H. A., & Wuensch, K. L. (2003). Healthy high-hostiles evidence low alpha power (7.5-9.5 Hz) changes during negative affective learning. Brain and Cognition, 52, 334-342.

Ewell, P. T. (1987). Establishing a campus-based assessment program. In D. F. Halpern (Ed.), Student outcomes assessment: What institutions stand to gain. New Directions for Higher Education, 59, 9-24.

Facione, P., Facione, N., & Giancarlo, C. (1998). CCTDI test manual. Millbrae, CA: California Academic Press.

Fagerberg, I., & Ekman, S. (1998). Swedish nursing students' transition into nursing during education. Western Journal of Nursing Research, 20, 602-620.

Fagermoen, M. S. (1997). Professional identity: Values embedded in meaningful nursing practice. Journal of Advanced Nursing, 25, 434-441.

Fahrenwald, N. L. (2003). Teaching social justice. Nurse Educator, 28, 222-226.

Fahrenwald, N. L., Bassett, S. D., Tschetter, L., Carson, P. P., White, L., & Winterboer, V. J. (2005). Teaching core nursing values. Journal of Professional Nursing, 21(1), 46-51.

Fandetti, D., & Goldmeier, J. (1988). Social workers as culture mediators in health care settings. Health and Social Work, 13(3), 171-179

Feeley, E. M. (1991). Campus wellness vacation: A creative clinical experience with the elderly. Nurse Educator, 16(1), 16-21.

Feldman, K. A., & Newcomb, T. M. (1969). The impact of college on students. Vol. 1. San Francisco: Jossey-Bass.

Felton, G. M., & Parsons, M. A. (1987). The impact of nursing education on ethical/ moral decision making. Journal of Nursing Research, 26(1), 7-11.

Festa, J. V. S. (1987). The effect of telling experiential and fantasy stories on learning a psychomotor nursing skill (Doctoral dissertation, Adelphi University). Dissertation Abstracts International, 40, 03B.

Forsyth, G. L. (1980). Analysis of the concept of empathy: Illustration of one approach. Advances in Nursing Science, 2(2), 33-42.

Fosbinder, D., & Vos, H. (1989). Setting standards and evaluating nursing performance with a single tool. Journal of Nursing Administration, 19(10), 23-30.

Fowler, M. (2008). Guide to the Code of Ethics for Nurses: Interpretation and application for nursing education and professional development. Silver Spring, MD: American Nurses Association.

Frankl, V. (1946). ...trotzdem Ja zum Leben sagen: Ein Psychologe erlebt das Konzentrationslager [...saying yes in spite of everything: A psychologist experiences the concentration camp]. Man's search for meaning (2000, 4th ed.). (I. Lasch, Trans., n.d.). Boston: Beacon Press.

Frymier, A. B. (1994). A model of immediacy in the classroom. Communication Quarterly, 42, 433-144.

Frymier, A. B., & Thompson, C. A. (1995). Using student reports to measure immediacy: Is it a valid methodology? Communication Research Reports, 12, 85-93.

Gardner, K. (1992). The historical conflict between caring and professionalization: A dilemma for nursing. In D. Gaut (Ed.), The presence of caring in nursing (pp. 241-255). New York: National League for Nursing.

Gaul, A. L. (1989). Ethics content in baccalaureate degree curricula: Clarifying the issues. Nursing Clinics of North America, 24, 475-483.

Gething, L., Fethney, J., McKee, K., Goff, M., Churchward, M., & Matthews, S. (2002a). Knowledge, stereotyping and attitudes towards self-ageing. Australian Journal on Ageing, 21, 64-79.

Gething, L., Fethney, J., McKee, K., Goff, M., Churchward, M., & Matthews, S. (2002b). Knowledge, stereotyping and attitudes towards self-ageing. *Clinical Nurse Specialist*, 5, 165-168.

Gilligan, C. (1982). *In a different voice: Psychological theory and women's development.* Cambridge, MA: Harvard University Press.

Glen, S. (1998). The key to quality nursing care: Toward a model of personal and professional development. *Nursing Ethics*, 5, 95-102.

Gormley, K. J. (1996). Altruism: A framework for caring and providing care. *International Journal of Nursing Studies*, 33, 581-588.

Gregory, M. (2004). Pedagogical disjunctions, or, if I say I want my students to be mainly learning X, why do I think mostly about teaching Y? *Journal of Cognitive Affective Learning*, 1, 2-10.

Griffith, J. W., & Bakanauskas, A. J. (1983). Student-instructor relationships in nursing education. *Journal of Nursing Education*, 22, 104-107.

Grinnell, S. K. (1989). Post conference reflections: Autonomy and independence for health professionals? *Journal of Allied Health*, 18(1), 115-121.

Grossman, S., & Wheeler, K. (1999). Integrating multidimensional stress management into a baccalaureate nursing curriculum. *Nursing Connections*, 12, 23-28.

Gudykunst, W. B., & Hammer, M. R. (1983). Dimensions of intercultural effectiveness: Culture specific or culture general? *International Journal of Intercultural Relations*, 8, 1-10.

Gudykunst, W. B., & Kim, Y. Y. (1984). *Communication with strangers: An approach to intercultural communication.* Reading, MA: Addison-Wesley.

Haight, B. K., & Olson, M. (1989). Teaching home health aides the use of life review. *Journal of Nursing Staff Development*, 5(1), 11-16.

Halldorsdottir, S. (1990). The essential structure of a caring and uncaring encounter with a teacher: The perspective of the nursing student. In M. Leininger & J. Watson (Eds.), *The caring imperative in education* (pp. 95-108). New York: National League for Nursing.

Halloran, L. (1996). Promoting research consumerism in BSN students. *Western Journal of Nursing Research*, 18, 108-110.

Halter, M. J. (2004). Stigma and help seeking related to depression: A study of nursing students. _Journal of Psychosocial Nursing, 42(2),_ 42-51.

Hamm, A. O., & Vaitl, D. (1996). Affective learning: Awareness and aversion. _Psychophysiology, 33,_ 698-710.

Hamm, A. O., Weike, A. I., Schupp, H. T., Treig, T., Dressel, A., & Kessler, C. (2003). Affective blindsight: Intact fear conditioning to a visual cue in a cortically blind patient. _Brain, 126,_ 267-275.

Hanna, K. R. (1997). Self-paced mastery learning in adult learners: A descriptive study of a nursing curriculum (Doctoral dissertation, University of California, Santa Barbara). _Dissertation Abstracts International, 58,_ 07A.

Hanson, L. E., & Smith, M. J. (1996). Nursing students' perspectives: Experience of caring and not-so-caring interactions with faculty. _Journal of Nursing Education, 35,_ 105-112.

Hanson, M. F. (2001). Classroom incivility: Management practices in large lecture courses (Doctoral dissertation, South Dakota State University). _Dissertation Abstracts International, 61,_ 2618.

Harrison, L. L., & Novak, D. (1988). Evaluation of a gerontological nursing continuing education programme: Effect on nurses' knowledge and attitudes and on patients' perceptions and satisfaction. _Journal of Advanced Nursing, 13,_ 684-692.

Harrison, L. L., Lowery, B., & Bailey, P. (1991). Changes in nursing students' knowledge about and attitudes toward research following an undergraduate research course. _Journal of Advanced Nursing, 16,_ 807-812.

Harrison, M. D. (1999). Writing and being: The transformational power of storytelling reported through narrative based evaluation (Doctoral dissertation, Arizona State University). _Dissertation Abstracts International, 39,_ 06.

Harrow, A. J. (1972). _Taxonomy of the psychomotor domain: A guide for developing behavioral objectives._ New York: McKay

Heaman, D. (1995). The quieting response (QR): A modality for reduction of psychophysiologic stress in nursing students. _Journal of Nursing Education, 34,_ 5-10.

Heinrich, K. T. (1992). The intimate dialogue: Journal writing by students. _Nurse Educator, 17(6),_ 17-20.

Heinrich, K. T., & Neese, M. R. (2004). Assessing the ineffable: A creative challenge for nurse educators and students. Annual Review of Nursing Education, 2, 71-88.

Heinrich, K. T., & Witt, B. (1998). Serendipity: A focus group turned hermeneutic evaluation. Nurse Educator, 23(4), 40-44.

Heinrich, K. T., Bona, G., McKelvey, M., & Solernou, S. (2001, September). Is scholarly identity development an outcome of a transformative learning environment? Initiating a research-based curriculum. Paper presented at the NLN Education Summit. Anaheim, CA.

Heinrich, K. T., Chiffer, D., McKelvey, M. M., & Zraunig, M. (2002, June). Assessing the ineffable: An alchemy of science, art and synchronicity. Paper presented at the American Association for Health Education conference. Boston, MA.

Herth, K. (1996). Hope from the perspective of homeless families. Journal of Advanced Nursing, 24, 743-753.

Hodges, H. F. (1996). Journal writing as a model of thinking for RN-BSN students: A leveled approach to learning to listen to self and others. Journal of Nursing Education, 35, 137-141.

Hoffman, S. B., Brand, F. R., Beatty, P. G., & Hamill, L. A. (1985). Geratrix: A role-playing game. The Gerontologist, 25(6), 568-572.

Hofmeyer, A. (2002). Using text as data and writing as the method of inquiry and discovery. Nursing Inquiry, 9, 215-217.

Hojat, M., Mangione, S., Gonnella, J. S., Nasca, T. J., Veloski, J. J., & Kane, G. (2001a). Empathy in medical education and patient care. Academic Medicine, 76, 669.

Hojat, M., Mangione, S., Nasca, T. J., Cohen, M. J. M., Gonnella, J. S., & Erdmann, J.B. et al. (2001b). The Jefferson Scale of Physician Empathy: Development and preliminary psychometric data. Educational and Psychological Measurement, 61, 349-365.

Hojat, M., Gonnella, J. S., Mangione, S., Nasca, T. J., Veloski, J. J., & Erdmann, J.B. et al. (2002a). Empathy in medical students as related to academic performance, clinical competence and gender. Medical Education, 36, 522-527.

Hojat, M., Gonnella, J. S., Nasca, T. J., Mangione, S., Veloski, J. J., & Magee, M. (2002b). The Jefferson Scale of Physician Empathy: Further psychometric data and differences by gender and specialty at the item level. Academic Medicine, 77(Supplement), S58-S60.

Hojat, M., Gonnella, J. S., Nasca, T. J., Mangione, S., Vergare, M., & Magee, M. (2002c). Physician empathy: Definition, components, measurement, and relationship to gender and specialty. American Journal of Psychiatry, 159, 1563-1569.

Hojat, M., Fields, S. K., & Gonnella, J. S. (2003a). Empathy: An NP/MD comparison. The Nurse Practitioner, 28, 45-47.

Hojat, M., Gonnella, J. S., Mangione, S., Nasca, T. J., & Magee, M. (2003b). Physician empathy in medical education and practice: Experience with the Jefferson Scale of Physician Empathy. Seminars in Integrative Medicine, 1, 25-41.

Hojat, M., Mangione, S., Nasca, T. J., Rattner, S., Erdmann, J. B., Gonnella, J.S. et al. (2004). An empirical study of decline in empathy in medical school. Medical Education, 38, 934-941.

Holland, K. (1999). A journey to becoming: The student nurse in transition. Journal of Advanced Nursing, 29, 229-236.

Hoopes, D. S., & Ventura, P. (1979). Intercultural sourcebook: Cross-cultural training methodologies. LaGrange Park, IL: Intercultural Network.

Jackson, C., Yorker, B., & Mitchem, P. (1996). Teaching cultural diversity in a virtual classroom. Journal of Child and Adolescent Psychiatric Mental Health Nursing, 9(4), 40-42.

Jacobs, B. B. (2001). Respect for human dignity: A central phenomenon to philosophically unite nursing theory and practice through consilience of knowledge. Advances in Nursing Science, 24, 17-35.

Jeffreys, M. R., & Smodlaka, I. (1999). Construct validation of the transcultural self-efficacy tool. Journal of Nursing Education, 38, 222-227.

Johnson, J. H., Zerwic, J. J., & Theis, S. L. (1999). Clinical simulation laboratory: An adjunct to clinical teaching. Nurse Educator, 24, 37-41.

Jones, M. C., & Johnston, D. W. (1997). Distress, stress and coping in first-year student nurses. Journal of Advanced Nursing, 26, 475-482.

Joynt, J., & Kimball, B. (2008). Blowing open the bottleneck: Designing new approaches to increase nurse education capacity [White paper]. Arlington, VA: Nursing Education Capacity Summit.

Kabat-Zinn, J. (1990). *Full catastrophe living: Using the wisdom of your body and mind to face stress.* New York: Delacorte.

Kahn, E., Lass, S. L., Hurtley, R., & Kornreich, H. K. (1981). Affective learning in medical education. *Journal of Medical Education,* 56, 646-652.

Katims, I. (1995). The contrary ideals of individualism and nursing value of care. *Scholarly Inquiry for Nursing Practice,* 9, 231-240.

Kealey, D. J., & Ruben, B. D. (1983). Cross-cultural personnel selection criteria, issues and methods. In D. Landis & R. Brislin (Eds.), *Handbook for intercultural training: Vol. 1. Issues in theory and design.* New York: Pergamon.

Keddy, K. (2002, November). *Socio-spatial characteristics of nursing activities: A poststructuralist feminist research framework.* Paper presented at the Twelfth Annual International Conference on Critical and Feminist Perspectives in Nursing. Portland, ME.

Kelley, D. H., & Gorman, J. (1988). Effects of immediacy on recall of information. *Communication Education,* 37, 198-207.

Kelly, G. (1963). *A theory of personality.* New York: Norton.

Kemp, E. (1999). Metaphor as a tool for evaluation. *Assessment and Evaluation in Higher Education,* 24, 81-90.

Kendrick, P. (2000). Comparing the effects of stress and relationship style on student and practicing nurse anesthetists. *American Association of Nurse Anesthetists Journal,* 68, 115-122.

Kennedy, M. (2001). Teaching communication skills to medical students: Unexpected attitudes and outcomes. *Teaching in Higher Education*, 6(1), 119-123.

Kessenich, C. R. (1996). Bringing reality to the research classroom. *Journal of Nursing Education,* 35, 187-188.

Kim, Y. Y. (1988). *Communication and cross-cultural adaptation: An integrative theory.* Clevedon, England: Multilingual Matters.

Kimball, B. (1993). Student assessment of career "professionalism": Course profile differences. *Journal of Education for Business,* 1(1), 29-35.

King, E. C. (1984). *Affective education in nursing: A guide to teaching and assessment.* Rockville, MD: Aspen Systems.

Kinsella, T. D., & Verhoef, M. J. (1993). Alberta euthanasia survey: 1. Physicians' opinions about the morality and legalization of active euthanasia. Canadian Medical Association Journal, 148, 1921-1926.

Kirchner, J. H., & Hogan, R. A. (1972). Student values: A longitudinal study. Psychology, 9(3), 36-39.

Kirkpatrick, M. K., Brown, S. T., & Atkins, T. (1998). Using the Internet to integrate cultural diversity and global awareness. Nurse Educator, 23(2), 15-17.

Kirschling, J. M., Fields, J., Imle, M., Mowery, M., Tanner, C. A., Perrin, N. et al. (1995). Evaluating teaching effectiveness. Journal of Nursing Education, 34, 401-410.

Kleehammer, K., Hart, A. L., & Keck, J. F. (1990). Nursing students' perceptions of anxiety-producing situations in the clinical setting. Journal of Nursing Education, 29, 183-187.

Kneipp, S., & Snider, M. J. (2001). Social justice in a market model world. Journal of Professional Nursing, 17, 113.

Knowles, M. C. (1980). The modern practice of adult education: From pedagogy to andragogy. New York: Cambridge, The Adult Education Co.

Kogan, N. (1961). Attitudes toward old people: The development of a scale and an examination of correlates. Journal of Abnormal and Social Psychology, 62, 44-54.

Kohlberg, L. (1972). Development as the aim of education. Harvard Educational Review, 42, 449-496.

Kohls, R., & Ax, E. (1979). Methodologies for trainers: A compendium of learning strategies. Washington, D.C.: Future Life Press.

Kolb, D. A. (1984). Experiential learning: Experience as the source of learning and development. Englewood Cliffs, NJ: Prentice-Hall.

Kosowski, M. M. R. (1995). Clinical learning experiences and professional nurse caring: A critical phenomenological study of female baccalaureate nursing students. Journal of Nursing Education, 34, 235-242.

Kovner, C. T., Mezey, M., & Harrington, C. (2002). Who cares for older adults? Workforce implications of an aging society: Geriatrics needs to join pediatrics as a required element of training the next generation of health care professionals. Health Affairs, 21, 78-89.

Kraiger, K., Ford, J. K., & Salas, E. (1993). Application of cognitive, skill-based, and affective theories of learning outcomes to new methods of training evaluation. *Journal of Applied Psychology, 78*, 311-328.

Kramer, M., & Schmalenberg, C. (1993). Learning from success: Autonomy and empowerment. *Nursing Management, 24(5)*, 58-64.

Krathwohl, D.R., Bloom, B., & Masia, B. (1964). *Taxonomy of educational objectives, Handbook II: Affective domain.* New York: David McKay.

Krechevsky, M., & Stork, J. (2000). Challenging educational assumptions: Lessons from an Italian-American collaboration. *Cambridge Journal of Education, 30(1)*, 57-74.

Krichbaum, K. (1994). Clinical teaching effectiveness described in relation to learning outcomes of baccalaureate nursing. *Journal of Nursing Education, 33*, 306-316.

Kritzer, H., & Phillips, C. A. (1966). Observing group psychotherapy—An affective learning experience. *American Journal of Psychotherapy, 20*, 471-476.

Krueger, P. M., & Irvine, L. (2001). Visualizing the ineffable: Using drawn and written representations to assess students' stereotypes of sociologists. *Sociological Imagination, 38*, 78-92.

Kuhlenschmidt, S. L., & Layne, L. E. (1999). Strategies for dealing with difficult behavior. In S.M. Richardson (Ed.), *Promoting civility: A teaching challenge* (pp. 45-58). San Francisco: Jossey-Bass.

Kushnir, T. (1986). Stress and social facilitation: The effects of the presence of an instructor on student nurses' behaviour. *Journal of Advanced Nursing, 11(1)*, 13-19.

LaMonica, E. L. (1986). *Nursing leadership and management: An experiential approach.* Boston: Jones and Bartlett.

LaMonica, E. L., Wolf, R. M., Madea, A. R., & Oberst, M. T. (1987). Empathy and nursing outcomes. *Scholarly Inquiry for Nursing Practice, 1*, 197-213.

Lamude, K. G., & Chow, L. (1993). Relationship of students' affective learning to teachers' type A scores. *Psychological Reports, 72*, 178.

Laschinger, H. S., Johnson, G., & Kohr, R. (1990). Building undergraduate nursing students' knowledge of the research process in nursing. *Journal of Nursing Education, 29*, 114-117.

Lashley, M. E. (1994). Vulnerability: The call to woundedness. In M. E. Lashley, M. T. Neal, E. T. Slunt, L. M. Berman, & F. H. Hultgren (Eds.), _Being called to care_ (pp. 41-51). Albany: State University of New York Press.

Lawrence, E. J., Shaw, P., Baker, D., Baron-Cohen, S., & David, A. S. (2004). Measuring empathy: Reliability and validity of the Empathy Quotient. _Psychological Medicine,_ 34, 911-919.

Leder, D. (1990). _The absent body._ Chicago: University of Chicago Press.

Leininger, M. M. (1991). The theory of culture care diversity and universality. In M. M. Leininger, _Culture care diversity and universality: A theory of nursing._ (pp. 5-68). New York: National League for Nursing.

Lenburg, C. B. (Ed.). (1995). _Promoting cultural competence in and through nursing education: A critical review and comprehensive plan for action._ Washington, D.C.: American Academy of Nursing.

Letizia, M. (1996). Nursing student and faculty perceptions of clinical post-conference learning environments (Doctoral dissertation, Loyola University of Chicago). _Dissertation Abstracts International,_ 56, 12B.

Letizia, M. (1998). Strategies used in clinical postconference. _Journal of Nursing Education,_ 37, 315-317.

Levenson, R. W., & Ruef, A. M. (1992). Empathy: A physiological substrate. _Journal of Personality and Social Psychology,_ 63, 234-246.

Levinson, W., Roter, D. L., Mullooly, J. P., Dull, V. T., & Frankel, R. M. (1997). Physician-patient communication: The relationship with malpractice claims among primary care physicians and surgeons. _Journal of the American Medical Association,_ 277, 553-559.

Liaschenko, J. (1999). Can justice coexist with the supremacy of personal values in nursing practice? _Western Journal of Nursing Research,_ 21, 35-50.

Lipp, O. V., Neumann, D. L., & Mason, V. (2001). Stimulus competition in affective and relational learning. _Learning and Motivation,_ 32, 306-330.

Lockhart, J. S., & Resick, L. K. (1997). Teaching cultural competence: The value of experiential learning and community resources. _Nurse Educator,_ 22(3), 27-31.

Luparell, S.M. (2003). Critical incidents of incivility by nursing students: How uncivil encounters with students affect nursing faculty (Doctoral dissertation, University of Nebraska). _Dissertation Abstracts International,_ 64, 2128.

Luparell, S. M. (2004). Faculty encounters with uncivil nursing students: An overview. *Journal of Professional Nursing, 20(1)*, 59-67.

Luparell, S. M. (2005). Why and how we should address student incivility in nursing programs. In M. H. Oermann & K. T. Heinrich (Eds.), *Annual review of nursing education: Vol. 3: Strategies for teaching, assessment, and program planning* (pp. 23-36). New York: Springer Publishing.

Luparell, S. M. (2007). The effects of student incivility on nursing faculty. *Journal of Nursing Education, 46(1)*, 15-19.

Macnab, D., Fitzsimmons, G., & Casserly, C. (1985). *Administrator's manual for the life roles inventory values and salience.* Edmonton, Canada: PsiCan Consulting.

Macnab, D., Fitzsimmons, G., & Casserly, C. (1987). Development of the Life Roles inventory-values scale. *Canadian Journal of Counseling, 21*, 86-98.

Magnussen, L. (1998). Women's choices: An historical perspective of nursing as a career choice. *Journal of Professional Nursing, 14*, 175-183.

Mahat, G. (1996). Stress and coping: First-year Nepalese nursing students in clinical settings. *Journal of Nursing Education, 35*, 163-169.

Maheux, B., & Beland, F. (1986). Students' perceptions of values emphasized in three medical schools. *Journal of Medical Education, 61*, 308-316.

Maier-Lorentz, M. M. (1999). Writing objectives and evaluating learning in the affective domain. *Journal for Nurses in Staff Development, 15(4)*, 167-171.

Maki, P. (2002). Using multiple assessment methods to explore student learning and development inside and outside the classroom. [Online]. Available: http://www.naspa.org/NetResults/ (document available only to members).

Mallory, C., Konradi, D., Campbell, S., & Redding, D. (2003). Identifying the ideal qualities of a new graduate. *Nurse Educator, 28(3)*, 104-106.

Manderino, M. A., Ganong, L. H., & Darnell, K. F. (1988). Survey of stress management content in baccalaureate nursing curricula. *Journal of Nursing Education, 27*, 321-325.

Manninen, E. (1998). Changes in nursing students' perceptions of nursing as they progress through their education. *Journal of Advanced Nursing, 27*, 390-398.

Marchesani, L. S., & Adams, M. (1992, Winter). Dynamics of diversity in the teaching-learning process: A faculty development model for analysis and action. _New Directions for Teaching and Learning,_ No. 52, 9-20.

Marcus, E. R. (1999). Empathy, humanism, and the professionalization process of medical education. _Academic Medicine,_ 74, 1211-1215.

Margalith, I., Musgrave, C. F., & Goldschmidt, L. (2003). Physician-assisted dying: Are education and religious beliefs related to nursing students' attitudes? _Journal of Nursing Education,_ 42(2), 91-96.

Martin, M. W., Myers, S. A., & Mottet, T. P. (2000). Students' motives for communicating with their instructors and affective and cognitive learning. _Psychological Reports,_ 87, 830-834.

Masters, K. R. (2005). Educational innovation: A student home visiting program for vulnerable, community-dwelling older adults. _Journal of Nursing Education,_ 44(4), 185-186.

May, W. T., & Ilardi, R. L. (1970). Change and stability of values in collegiate nursing students. _Nursing Research,_ 19, 359-362.

Mayberg, H. S., Liotti, M., Brannan, S. K., McGinnis, X., Mahurin, R. K., Jerabek, P.A. et al. (1999). Reciprocal limbic-cortical function and negative mood: Converging PET findings in depression and normal sadness. _American Journal of Psychiatry,_ 156, 676-682.

Mayo, K. (2000). Social responsibility in nursing education. _Journal of Holistic Nursing,_ 14(1), 24-43.

McAllister, G., & Irvine, J. J. (2002). The role of empathy in teaching culturally diverse students: A qualitative study of teachers' beliefs. _Journal of Teacher Education,_ 53, 433-443.

McAllister, M., & Osborne, Y. (1997). Peer review: A strategy to enhance cooperative student learning. _Nurse Educator,_ 22(1), 40-44.

McCausland, L. L. (2002). A precepted perioperative elective for baccalaureate nursing students. _Association of Operating Room Nurses,_ 76, 1032-1039.

Mehrabian, A. (1969). Significance of posture and position in the communication of attitude and status relationships. _Psychological Bulletin,_ 71, 359-372.

Meisenhelder, J. B. (1987). Anxiety: A block to clinical learning. _Nurse Educator,_ 12(6), 27-30.

Meisenhelder, J. B. (2006). An example of personal knowledge: Spirituality. In L. C. Andrist, P. K. Nichols, & K. A. Wolf (Eds.), _A history of nursing ideas_ (pp. 151-155). Boston: Jones and Bartlett.

Mentkowski, M. (1991). _Designing a national assessment system assessing abilities that connect education and work._ Milwaukee, WI: Alverno College. (ERIC Document Reproduction Service No. ED 340 759)

Meraviglia, M. (1999). Critical analysis of spirituality and its empirical indicators: Prayer and meaning in life. _Journal of Holistic Nursing,_ 17, 18-33.

Mezey, M., & Fulmer, T. (2002). The future history of gerontological nursing. _Journals of Gerontology. Series A: Biological Sciences and Medical Sciences,_ 57A, M438-M441.

Miller, B., Haber, J., & Bryne, M. (1990). The experience of caring in the teaching-learning process of nursing education. In M. Leininger & J. Watson (Eds.), _The caring imperative in education_ (pp. 125-135). New York: National League for Nursing.

Miller, K., Stiff, J., & Ellis, B. H. (1988). Communication and empathy as precursors to burnout among human service workers. _Communication Monographs,_ 55, 250-265.

Miller, S. I., & Morgan, R. R. (2000). Establishing credibility of alternative forms of data representation. _Educational Studies._ 31, 119-131.

Moloney, M. M. (1992). _Professionalization of nursing: Current issues and trends._ Philadelphia: Lippincott.

Moore, W. (1988). _The measure of intellectual development: An instrument manual._ Olympia, WA: Center for the Study of Intellectual Development.

Morris, J. S., Ohman, A., & Dolan, R. J. (1998). Conscious and unconscious emotional learning in the human amygdala. _Nature,_ 393, 467-470.

Morse, J. M., Bottorff, J., Anderson, G., O'Brien, B., & Solberg, S. (1992). Beyond empathy: Expanding expressions of caring. _Journal of Advanced Nursing,_ 17, 809-821.

Morse, J.M., Solberg, S.M., Neander, W.L., Bottorff, J.L. & Johnson, J.L. (1990). Concepts of caring and caring as a concept. _Advances in Nursing Science,_ 13(1), 1-14.

Motowidlo, S. J., Packard, J. S., & Manning, M. R. (1986). Occupational stress: Its causes and consequences for job performance. _Journal of Applied Psychology, 71,_ 618-629.

Motwani, J., Hodge, J., & Crampton, S. (1995). Managing diversity in the health care industry. _Health Care Supervisor, 13(3),_ 16-24.

Murray, M. G., & Steffen, J. J. (1999). Attitude of case managers toward people with serious mental illness. _Community Mental Health Journal, 35,_ 505-514.

Myers, S. A. (2002). Perceived aggressive instructor communication and student state, motivation, learning, and satisfaction. _Communication Reports, 15(2),_ 113-122.

National Council of State Boards of Nursing (Producer). (1997). _Crossing the line: A nurse's guide to the importance of appropriate professional boundaries._ [Video]. (Available from producer, 111 East Wacker Drive, Suite 2900, Chicago, IL 60601-4277).

National League for Nursing. (2008). Priorities for research in nursing education. [Online]. Available: http://www.nln.org/research/priorities.htm.

National League for Nursing Accrediting Commission. (2005). _Accreditation manual and interpretive guidelines by program type for postsecondary and higher degree programs in nursing._ New York: Author.

Neidich, B. (1990). A method to facilitate student interest in research: Chart review. _Journal of Nursing Education, 29,_ 139-140.

Neidt, C. O., & Hedlund, D. E. (1969). Longitudinal relationships between cognitive and affective learning outcomes. _Journal of Educational Research, 37(3),_ 56-60.

Nelms, T. P., Jones, J. M., & Gray, D. P. (1993). Role modeling: A method for teaching caring in nursing education. _Journal of Nursing Education, 32,_ 18-23.

Nightingale, F. (1980). _Notes on nursing: What it is and what it is not_ (Originally published in 1859). New York: Churchill Livingstone.

Noddings, N. (1984). _Caring: A feminine approach to ethics and moral education._ Berkeley, CA: University of California Press.

Noddings, N. (1992). _The challenge to care in schools: An alternative approach to education._ New York: Teachers College Press.

Noddings, N. (1995). Teaching themes of care. _Phi Delta Kappan, 76(9),_ 675-679.

Noddings, N. (2002). *Educating moral people: A caring alternative to character education.* New York: Teachers College Press.

Oermann, M. E., & Heinrich, K. T. (Eds.). (2003-2007). *Annual review of nursing education, Volumes. 1-5.* New York: Springer Publishing.

Ohlen, J., & Segesten, K. (1998). The professional identity of the nurse: Concept analysis and development. *Journal of Advanced Nursing,* 28, 720-727.

Olson, J. K. (1995). Relationships between nurse-expressed empathy, patient-perceived empathy and patient distress. *Image,* 27, 317-322.

Omdahl, B. L., & O'Donnell, C. (1999). Emotional contagion, empathic concern and communicative responsiveness as variables affecting nurses' stress and occupational commitment. *Journal of Advanced Nursing,* 29, 1351-1359.

Oswald, P. A. (2002). The interactive effects of affective demeanor, cognitive processes and perspective-taking focus on helping behavior. *Journal of Social Psychology,* 142, 120-132.

Owen-Smith, P. (2004, Fall). What is cognitive-affective learning (CAL)? *Journal of Cognitive Affective Learning,* 1, 11.

Oz, F. (2001). Impact of training on empathic communication skills and tendency of nurses. *Clinical Excellence for Nurse Practitioners,* 5, 44-51.

Paige, R. M., & Martin, J. N. (1983). Ethical issues and ethics in cross-cultural training. In D. Landis & R. W. Brislin (Eds.), *Handbook of intercultural training, Vol. 1: Issues in theory and design* (pp. 36-60). New York: Pergamon.

Palmore, E. B. (1998). *The facts on aging quiz: A handbook of uses and results* (2nd ed.). New York: Springer Publishing.

Pascarella, E. T. (1985). Students' affective development within the college environment. *Journal of Higher Education,* 56, 640-663.

Pascarella, E. T., & Terenzini, P. (1991). *How college affects students: Findings and insights from twenty years of research.* San Francisco: Jossey-Bass.

Perry, W. (1970). *Forms of intellectual and ethical development in the college years.* New York: Holt, Rinehart & Winston.

Perry, W. (1981). Cognitive and ethical growth: The making of meaning. In A. Chickering (Ed.), *The modern American college* (pp. 76-116). San Francisco: Jossey-Bass.

Pond, E. F., & Bradshaw, M. J. (1996). Attitudes of nursing students towards research: A participatory exercise. *Journal of Nursing Education,* 35, 182-185.

Pope-Davis, D. B., Eliason, M. J., & Ottavi, T. M. (1994). Are nursing students multiculturally competent? An exploratory investigation. *Journal of Nursing Education,* 33, 31-33.

Puentes, W. J. (1995). Effects of a reminiscence learning experience on registered nurses' attitudes toward and empathy with older adults (Doctoral dissertation, Widener University, Chester, PA).

Puentes, W. J., & Cayer, C.A. (2001). Research briefs: Effects of a modified version of Feeley's campus wellness vacation on baccalaureate registered nurse students' knowledge of and attitudes toward older adults. *Journal of Nursing Education,* 40(2), 86-89.

Pugsley, K. E., & Clayton, L. H. (2003). Research brief – Traditional lecture of experiential learning: Changing student attitudes. *Journal of Nursing Education,* 42, 520-525.

Pullen, R. L., Murray, P. H., & McGee, K. S. (2001). Care groups: A model to mentor novice nursing students. *Nurse Educator,* 26, 283-288.

Pusch, M. D. (Ed.). (1981). *Multicultural education: A cross-cultural training approach.* Chicago: Intercultural Press.

Raya, A. (1990). Can knowledge be prompted and values ignored? Implications for nursing education. *Journal of Advanced Nursing,* 15, 504-509.

Redelmeier, D. A., Molin, J. P., & Tibshirani, R. J. (1995). A randomized trial of compassionate care for the homeless in an emergency department. *Lancet,* 345, 1131-1134.

Regan, R. (2000). The effect of gaming on the empathic communication of associate degree nursing students (Doctoral dissertation, Widener University). *Dissertation Abstracts International,* 61, 02B.

Reilly, D. E. (Ed.). (1978). *Teaching and evaluating the affective domain in nursing programs.* Thorofare, NJ: C.B. Slack.

Reilly, D. E., & Oermann, M. H. (1992). *Clinical teaching in nursing education.* New York: National League for Nursing.

Reutter, L., Field, P. A., Campbell, I. E., & Day, R. (1997). Socialization into nursing: Nursing students as learners. *Journal of Nursing Education,* 36, 149-155.

Rew, L. (1996). Affirming cultural diversity: A pathways model for nursing faculty. *Journal of Nursing Education,* 35(7), 310-314.

Rew, L., Becker, H., Cookston, J., Khosropour, S., & Martinez, S. (2003). Measuring cultural awareness in nursing students. *Journal of Nursing Education,* 42(6), 249-257.

Reynolds, W. J., & Presly, A. S. (1988). A study of empathy in student nurses. *Nurse Education Today,* 8, 123-160.

Richmond, V. P., & McCroskey, J. C. (Eds.), (1992). *Power in the classroom: Communication, control, and concern.* Hillsdale, NJ: Erlbaum.

Ritchie, M. A. (2003). Faculty and student dialogue through journal writing. *Journal for Specialists in Pediatric Nursing,* 8(1), 5.

Rodriguez, J. I., Plax, T. G., & Kearney, P. (1996). Clarifying the relationship between teacher nonverbal immediacy and student cognitive learning: Affective learning as the central causal mediator. *Communication Education,* 45, 293-305.

Rosenfeld, P., Bottrell, M., Fulmer, T., & Mezey, M. (1999). Gerontological nursing content in baccalaureate nursing programs: Findings from a national survey. *Journal of Professional Nursing,* 15, 84-94.

Rosenkranz, J. A., Moore, H., & Grace, A. A. (2003). The prefrontal cortex regulates lateral amygdala neuronal plasticity and responses to previously conditioned stimuli. *Journal of Neuroscience,* 23(35), 11054-11064.

Ross, J. M., & Stanley, I. M. (1985). A system of affective learning behaviors of medical education. *Family Practice—An International Journal,* 2(4), 213-218.

Roth, B. (2001). Mindfulness-based stress reduction at the Yale School of Nursing. *Yale Journal of Biology and Medicine,* 74, 249-258.

Rushton, J. P. (1980). *Altruism, socialization, and society.* Englewood Cliffs, NJ: Prentice-Hall.

Russo, T., & Benson, S. (2005). Learning with invisible others: Perceptions of online presence and their relationship to cognitive and affective learning. Educational Technology & Society, 8(1), 54-62.

Ryan, A. A., & McKenna, H. P. (1994). A comparative study of the attitudes of nursing and medical students to aspects of patient care and the nurse's role in organizing that care. Journal of Advanced Nursing, 19, 114-123.

Rychalak, J. F. (1975). Affective assessment, intelligence, social class, and racial learning style. Journal of Personality and Social Psychology, 32, 989-995.

Saarmann, L, Freitas, L., Rapps, J, & Riegel, B. (1992). The relationship of education to critical thinking ability and values among nurses: Socialization into professional nursing. Journal of Professional Nursing, 8(1), 26-34.

Sadler, J. (1997). Defining caring in professional nursing: A triangulated study. International Journal for Human Caring, 1(3), 12-21.

Sadler, J. (2003). A pilot study to measure the caring efficacy of baccalaureate nursing students. Nursing Education Perspectives, 24(6), 295-299.

Saltzberg, C. W. (2002). Nursing students' uncertainty experiences and epistemological perspectives (Doctoral dissertation, Cornell University). Dissertation Abstracts International, 62, 12A.

Sanders, J. A., & Wiseman, R. L. (1990). The effects of verbal and nonverbal teacher immediacy on perceived cognitive, affective, and behavioral learning in the multicultural classroom. Communication Education, 39, 341-353.

Sanford, R. (2000). Caring through relation and dialogue: A nursing perspective for patient education. Advances in Nursing Science, 22(3), 1-15.

Sax, L. J., Bryant, A. N., & Gilmartin, S. K. (2002, November). A longitudinal investigation of emotional health among first-year students: Comparisons of men and women. Paper presented at the annual meeting of the Association for the Study of Higher Education, Sacramento, CA.

Schlapman, N. (1989). Creative teaching strategies. Nurse Educator, 14(5), 6.

Schmitz, B., Paul, S. P., & Greenberg, J. D. (1992, Spring). Creating multicultural classrooms: An experience derived faculty development program. New Directions for Teaching and Learning, No. 49, 75-87.

Schön, D. A. (1987). *Educating the reflective practitioner.* San Francisco: Jossey-Bass.

Schön, D. A. (Ed.). (1991). *The reflective turn: Case studies in and on educational practice.* New York: Teachers College Press.

Schutzenhofer, K. K. (1987). The measurement of professional autonomy. *Journal of Professional Nursing, 3,* 278-283.

Schutzenhofer, K. K. (1988). The problem of professional autonomy in nursing. *Health Care for Women International, 9,* 93-106.

Schutzenhofer, K. K., & Musser, D. B. (1994). Nurse characteristics and professional autonomy. *Image, 26,* 201-205.

Sciortino, R. (1970). Allport-Vernon-Lindzey study of values: I. Factor structure for a combined sample of male and female college students. *Psychological Reports, 27,* 955-958.

Severtsen, B. M., & Evans, B. C. (2000). Education for caring practice. *Nursing and Health Care Perspectives, 21,* 172-177.

Shapiro, J., Morrison, E. H., & Boker, J. R. (2004). Teaching empathy to first-year medical students: Evaluation of an elective literature and medicine course. *Education for Health, 17(1),* 73-84.

Shapiro, S. L., Schwartz, G. E., & Bonner, G. (1998). Effects of mindfulness-based stress reduction on medical and premedical students. *Journal of Behavioral Medicine, 21,* 581-599.

Sheffler, S. J. (1995). Do clinical experiences affect nursing students' attitudes toward the elderly? *Journal of Nursing Education, 34(7),* 312-316.

Shor, I. (1992). *Empowering education: Critical teaching for social change.* Chicago: University of Chicago Press.

Simpson, E. (1972). *The classification of educational objectives in the psychomotor domain (Vol. 3).* Washington, DC: Gryphon House.

Simpson, J. R., Ongur, D., Akbudak, E., Conturo, T. E., Ollinger, J. M., Snyder, A.Z. et al. (2000). The emotional modulation of cognitive processing: An MRI study. *Journal of Cognitive Neuroscience, 12(2),* 157-170.

Sims, S. L., & Swenson, M. M. (2001). Preparing teachers and students for narrative learning. _Journal of Scholarship of Teaching and Learning,_ 1(2), 24-37. [Online]. Available: http://www.iupui.edu/~josotl/VOL_1/NO_2/sims_vol_1_no_2.htm.

Slimmer, L. W. (1992). Effect of writing across the curriculum techniques on students' affective and cognitive learning about nursing research. _Journal of Nursing Education,_ 31, 75-78.

Smith, M. J. (2000). A reflective teaching-learning process to enhance personal knowing. _Nursing and Health Care Perspectives,_ 21, 130-132.

Snider, S. (2001). Cognitive and affective learning outcomes resulting from the use of behavioral objectives in teaching poetry. _Journal of Educational Research,_ 333-338.

Sodowsky, G. R., Taffe, R. C., Gutkin, T. B., & Wise, S. L. (1994). Development of the multicultural counseling inventory: A self-report measure of multicultural competencies. _Journal of Counseling Psychology,_ 41, 137-148.

Solomon, L. C., Bisconti, A. S., & Ochsner, N. L. (1977). _College as a training ground for jobs._ New York: Praeger.

Sorbye, L. W., Sorbye, S., & Sorbye, S. W. (1995). Nursing students' attitudes towards assisted suicide and euthanasia: A study from four different schools of nursing. _Scandinavian Journal of Caring Science,_ 9, 119-122.

Southall, V. H. (2002). Nursing home buddies: A unique service learning opportunity. _Nurse Educator,_ 27(3), 101-102.

Spouse, J. (2000). An impossible dream? Images of nursing held by pre-registration students and their effect on sustaining motivation to become nurses. _Journal of Advanced Nursing,_ 32, 730-739.

Stancato, F. A., & Hamachek, A. L. (1990). The interactive nature and reciprocal effects of cognitive and affective learning. _Education,_ 111(1), 77-82.

Starr-Glass, D. (2002). Metaphor and totem: Exploring and evaluating prior experiential learning. _Assessment and Evaluation in Higher Education,_ 27, 221-231.

Super, D. E. (1957). _The psychology of careers._ New York: Harper.

Super, D. E. (1970). _Work Values Inventory._ Boston: Houghton Mifflin.

Super, D. E. (1973). The Work Values Inventory. In D.G. Zytowski (Ed.), _Contemporary approaches to interest measurement_ (pp. 189-205). Minneapolis: University of Minnesota Press.

Super, D. E., & Sverko, B. (Eds.). (1995). Life roles, values, and careers: International findings of the Work Importance Study. San Francisco: Jossey-Bass.

Swenson, I., & Kleinbaum, A. (1984). Attitudes toward research among undergraduate nursing students. Journal of Nursing Education, 23, 380-386.

Sword, W., Reutter, L., Meagher-Stewart, D., & Rideout, E. (2004). Baccalaureate nursing students' attitudes toward poverty: Implications for nursing curricula. Journal of Nursing Education, 43, 13-19.

Sywester, R. (1994). How emotions affect learning. Educational Leadership, 52(2), 211-215.

Tanner, C. A. (1990). Caring as a value in nursing education. Nursing Outlook, 38(2), 70-72.

Thorpe, K., & Loo, R. (2003). The values profile of nursing undergraduate students: Implications for education and professional development. Journal of Nursing Education, 42, 83-90.

Thrasher, S., & Mowbray, C. (1995). A strengths perspective: An ethnographic study of homeless women with children. Health & Social Work, 20, 93-101.

Tiberius, R. G., & Flak, E. (1999). Incivility in dyadic teaching and learning. New Directions for Teaching and Learning, No. 77, 3-12.

Tompkins, E. S. (1992). Nurse/client values congruence. Western Journal of Nursing Research, 14, 225-236.

Tompson, G. H., & Dass, P. (2000). Improving students' self-efficacy in strategies management: The relative impact of cases. Simulation and Gaming, 31(1), 22-42.

Treharne, G. (1990). Attitudes toward the care of elderly people: Are they getting better? Journal of Advanced Nursing, 15, 777-781.

Ulloth, J. K. (2002). The benefits of humor in nursing education. Journal of Nursing Education, 41, 476-481.

Ulloth, J. K. (2003). A qualitative view of humor in nursing classrooms. Journal of Nursing Education, 42, 125-131.

Valiga, T. (1983). Cognitive development: A critical component of baccalaureate nursing education. Image, 15(4), 115-119.

Vogler, D. E. (1991). Performance instruction: Planning, delivering, evaluating. Eden Prairie, MN: Instructional Performance Systems.

Wade, G. H. (1999). Professional nurse autonomy: Concept analysis and application to nursing education. *Journal of Advanced Nursing, 30,* 310-318.

Wade, G. H. (2004). A model of the attitudinal component of professional nurse autonomy. *Journal of Nursing Education, 43,* 116-124.

Wagner, A. L. (1998). A study of baccalaureate nursing students' reflection on their caring practice through creating and sharing story, poetry, and art (Doctoral dissertation, University of Massachusetts Lowell). *Dissertation Abstracts International, 59,* 08B.

Warda, M. R. (1997). *Development of a measure of culturally competent care.* Unpublished doctoral dissertation, University of California at San Francisco.

Watson, J. (1988a). *Nursing: Human science and human care.* New York: National League for Nursing.

Watson, J. (1988b). Human caring as moral context for nursing education. *Nursing & Health Care, 9(8),* 423-425.

Watson, J. (1990). Caring knowledge and informed passion. *Advances in Nursing Science, 13(1),* 15-24.

Watson, R., Deary, I. J., & Lea, A. (1999). A longitudinal study into the perceptions of caring and nursing among student nurses. *Journal of Advanced Nursing, 29,* 1228-1237.

Webb, S. S., Price, S. A., & Coeling, H. V. E. (1996). Valuing authority/responsibility relationships. *Journal of Nursing Administration, 26(2),* 28-33.

Weiss, G. L. (1996). Attitudes of college students about physician-assisted suicide: The influence of life experiences, religiosity, and belief in autonomy. *Death Studies, 20,* 587-599.

Wheeler, K., Barrett, E. A. M., & Lahey, E. M. (1996). A study of empathy as a nursing care outcome measure. *International Journal of Psychiatric Nursing Research, 3,* 281-289.

Williams, C. A. (1989). Empathy and burnout in male and female helping professions. *Research in Nursing & Health, 12,* 169-179.

Williams, K. A., Kolar, M. M., Roger, B. E., & Pearson, J. C. (2001). Evaluation of a wellness-based mindfulness stress reduction intervention: A controlled trial. *American Journal of Health Promotion, 15,* 422-432.

Williams, R.A., Lusk, S.L., & Kline, N.W. (1986). Knowledge of aging and cognitive syles in baccalaureate nursing students. *The Gerontologist, 26,* 545-550.

Wiseman, T. (1996). A concept analysis of empathy. _Journal of Advanced Nursing, 23_, 1162-1167.

Wolf, T. M., Balson, P. M., Faucett, J. M., & Randall, H. M. (1989). A retrospective study of attitude change during medical education. _Medical Education, 23_, 19-23.

Wolff, A., & Rideout, E. (2001). The faculty role in problem-based learning. In E. Rideout (Ed.), _Transforming nursing education through problem-based learning._ Sudbury, MA: Jones and Bartlett.

Wood, W. (2000). Attitude change: Persuasion and social influence. _Annual Review of Psychology, 51_, 539-570.

Wood, W., Christensen, P. N., Hebl, M. R., & Rothgerber, H. (1997). Conformity to sex-typed norms, affect, and the self-concept. _Journal of Personality and Social Psychology, 73_, 523-535.

Woods, J. H. (1993). Affective learning: One door to critical thinking. _Holistic Nursing Practice, 7(3)_, 67-70.

Woodward, V. M. (1997). Professional caring: A contradiction in terms? _Journal of Advanced Nursing, 26(5)_, 999-1004.

Young, A., Volker, D., Rieger, P. T., & Thorpe, D. M. (1993). Oncology nurses' attitudes regarding voluntary, physician-assisted dying for competent, terminally ill patients. _Oncology Nursing Forum, 20_, 445-451.

Young, J. R. (2003). Prozac campus: More students seek counseling and take psychiatric medication. _Chronicle of Higher Education, 49(23)_, A37-A38.

Young, L. E., Bruce, A., Turner, L., & Linden, W. (2001). Student nurse health promotion: Evaluation of a mindfulness-based stress reduction (MBSR) intervention. _Canadian Nurse, 97(6)_, 23-26.

Yuker, H. E., Block, J. R., & Campbell, J. (1966). _The measurement of attitudes toward disabled persons._ Albertson, NY: Human Resources Center.

Zimmerman, B. J., & Phillips, C. Y. (2000). Affective learning: Stimulus to critical thinking and caring practice. _Journal of Nursing Education, 39_, 422-425.

Zrinyi, M., & Balogh, Z. (2004). Student nurse attitudes towards homeless clients: A challenge for education and practice. _Nursing Ethics, 11(4)_, 334-348.

# 7

## CHAPTER 7
### ONGOING DEVELOPMENT OF THE
### SCIENCE OF NURSING EDUCATION

*Theresa M. Valiga, EdD, RN, FAAN*

"How many experiences life offers us everyday. We let them
pass, but a deep thinker [a scholar] gathers them up and
makes his treasure of them."

**Sertillanges**

Developing the science of nursing education is a journey that involves many individuals and many activities. It is a never-ending task that incorporates the continual asking of questions and the ongoing search for understanding. But it is a journey worth taking, since the outcome of science-building efforts will be the identification and implementation of best practices in teaching the discipline of nursing. The use of such best practices results in the preparation of graduates who are most capable of providing safe, quality care to patients, families and communities; can manage the uncertainty and ambiguity that characterizes the health care arena; and will provide leadership that changes the practice of nursing.

As noted in earlier chapters and depicted in the NLN's Science of Nursing Education Model (see Figure 1.1), the ongoing development of the science of nursing education will require the efforts of faculty, educational administrators, students, graduate students in teacher preparation programs, clinical partners, and colleagues in other disciplines. This is not a task that is the responsibility of only a handful of nursing education scholars, though such individuals are expected to provide the leadership needed to guide and sustain the science-building effort.

## SCIENCE-BUILDING RESPONSIBILITIES

### Faculty Members

As they engage in classroom, laboratory and clinical teaching, advise students, create policies, design curriculum plans, and collaborate with colleagues from other disciplines, faculty must employ a critical mind and questioning spirit. Every faculty member can contribute to the development of the science of nursing education by searching for evidence to support the teaching strategies and evaluation methods to be used in their courses and talking with colleagues about gaps in our knowledge when such evidence is not found.

Faculty also need to reflect on their teaching practices and document — in a systematic way — the impact of those practices on students. Did a new classroom strategy challenge students to ask higher-order questions? Did students report that a course assignment made them "really think" and "pull it all together"? Did staff members in an affiliating clinical agency comment more positively on students' abilities to make decisions in complex situations when the nature of student clinical experiences was more flexible and student-driven than "routine" and teacher-driven? By documenting the outcomes of innovative teaching practices, any faculty member can generate questions to be pursued through rigorous research.

### Pedagogical Scholars

The National League for Nursing (NLN) has contributed significantly to the development of the science of nursing education by outlining and continually refining *Priorities for*

*Research in Nursing Education* (NLN, 2008). Such priorities direct investigators in the kinds of questions they need to study ... those that help educators create reform through innovations, evaluate reform through the conduct of evaluation research, and lead evidence-based reform through building the science. These pedagogical scholars then need to design and conduct systematic inquiries that are rigorous and stand up to the scrutiny of the scientific community.

Such studies need to be designed within frameworks that are relevant for nursing education, and pedagogical scholars need to take responsibility for helping to build those frameworks. As noted in previous chapters, many of the studies conducted in nursing education today lack an organizing framework. Often, each study uses a different framework, which makes it difficult to draw comparisons between them. Thus, building frameworks that can be used to conceptualize and study significant nursing education questions is a step that needs attention if we are to build a science of nursing education.

Nursing education scholars also must provide leadership to the nursing education community in coming to some common understanding about how terms are defined, so that the findings from one study can be synthesized with those of another investigation. For example, there have been many studies done about nursing students' critical thinking abilities, but each study defines that core term differently, which challenges scholars who try to draw conclusions about trends in the findings.

Once rigorous studies have been completed, scholars then need to disseminate the findings of their research and open up their work for critique and their findings for further testing and application. Such dissemination can occur through presentations and dialogue, both of which are helpful; but in order to build a science, they must be published and integrated into databases so that others can find them when conducting searches. Thus, the building of databases — particularly those that are unique to nursing education — is another significant component of building the science of nursing education to which pedagogical scholars can contribute.

### Graduate Students

Students enrolled in teacher preparation programs at the master's or doctoral level also have a responsibility to contribute to the development of the science of nursing education. Like faculty, they need to employ a critical mind and questioning spirit as they pursue their studies, read the educational literature, develop creative projects, participate in practicum experiences, observe master teachers, attend education-focused conferences, and complete course assignments. But such students can make other significant contributions to this effort as well.

Graduate students can be challenged to conduct scholarly analyses of concepts that are central to nursing education. For example, the nursing education community would benefit from a deeper conceptual understanding of the changing nature of relationships between students and teachers, what it means to live with or make decisions in uncertainty and ambiguity, the impact of learning style, the nature of effective doctoral dissertation advisement, making clinical assignments, or any number of other elements of the educational experience. The conduct and publication of such scholarly concept analyses help graduate students develop their scholarly skills, but they also help both students and faculty better understand and know how to most positively influence the teaching/learning enterprise.

Graduate students also can be called upon to conduct comprehensive syntheses of research on specific educational topics (e.g., the use of concept mapping, the development of students as leaders) so that the evidence for such topics is readily accessible to faculty and pedagogical scholars. As they review the literature to do this work, graduate students would be critiquing extant research and identifying gaps in knowledge of teaching the practice of nursing, both of which are needed components of building a science.

### Undergraduate Students

Oftentimes, we underestimate undergraduate or pre-licensure students in terms of their scholarliness or their ability to help us better understand what it means to learn a practice. All students should be expected to employ a critical mind and questioning spirit as they proceed through their educational program, and such a "spirit" should not only be tolerated by faculty, it should be encouraged, expected and rewarded.

Students also participate as subjects in research projects being conducted by pedagogical scholars, which is another way they can contribute to developing the science. However, we can learn even more from students and engage them in the process more deeply if we spent time talking with them after a research project is completed. Faculty could make explicit to students why they are studying various approaches to teaching or new evaluation methods. They could help students reflect on what the experience of being a study subject was like for them. And they could show students how the findings from that study (or others) will be used to enhance the educational experience for other learners.

### Educational Administrators

Finally, those in administrative positions have a responsibility to create environments that support and encourage science-building efforts. When faculty propose using new teaching/ learning strategies or evaluation methods based on what they have read in the literature, deans/directors are in a position to encourage such innovation and provide resources to develop new approaches.

Deans/Directors can also encourage faculty to use criteria for peer review and faculty performance evaluations that promote the scholarship of teaching (Boyer, 1990), recognize and reward contributions to building the science of nursing education, and acknowledge the expertise of pedagogical scholars. As leaders of our educational programs, administrators can be expected to challenge faculty to continually question their teaching practices, the evaluation methods used, the design of the curriculum, the effectiveness of student learning experiences, and other aspects of the educational environment ... all in an effort to achieve excellence in nursing education and help build the science that underlies that area of practice.

### Summary

It is clear that the responsibility for building the science of nursing education cannot be left to a handful of pedagogical scholars alone. There are too many questions to be asked and studied, too many activities that need to be undertaken (see Figure 1.1) to build a science, and too many missed opportunities if all faculty, students, and educational administrators do not participate.

Each faculty member or group of faculty may benefit from extended discussions about the science-building model (see Figure 1.1) and how they can embrace it as a guide to day-to-day implementation of their role as educators. Such efforts could lead to a school "carving out a niche" related to some element of building the science of nursing education and providing leadership within the nursing education community in a specific area. But as such activities are implemented, there are a number of issues that need to be addressed.

## Significant Areas in Need of Study in Nursing Education

It is clear from the discussions in the preceding chapters that, while many studies have been conducted in nursing education, the foundation for building a science remains weak. Chapter authors and others have noted that "there is a lack of replication of studies ... few nurse educators have extended their work ... [and] one time studies dominate" (Oermann, 1990, p. 24). In addition, they conclude that most studies are descriptive or evaluative in nature, few have been guided by a theoretical framework, sample sizes tend to be small, and measurement instruments tend to be researcher-developed, used only in one study, and not necessarily valid or reliable. Finally, this review shows that many studies are conducted in a single school and often with homogeneous populations, which limits the generalizability of findings.

Nurse educators should not be discouraged by such a state of affairs, however. The science of nursing *practice* has been developing for more than 30 years, and the powerful impact of such efforts has been evident only recently. During those 30 years, significant funding has been available to support clinical investigations, programs have been designed to train nurse scientists, and schools of nursing have created research centers to help evolving scholars design studies, write proposals, and pursue programs of research. Nursing education can learn a great deal from the profession's efforts to build the science of nursing practice and use those insights to build the science of nursing education more expeditiously.

In order to build that science, then, pedagogical scholars must conduct large-scale, multi-site studies that are developed within relevant frameworks, use valid and reliable instruments, replicate and extend the work of other scholars, and take into consideration the diversity of students, faculty and the communities served by our schools of nursing. We also must address questions of significance. Following are a number of questions that faculty, pedagogical scholars, and students might consider as we join together on the journey to build the science of nursing education:

- What is the impact on the quality of education when schools are mandated to increase their enrollments to meet nursing practice shortages in a given area?

- How is teaching graduate students similar to and different from teaching pre-licensure students?

- What does it cost to develop and deliver a nursing program that is described as excellent?

- What is the effect on student learning when many different faculty "take turns" teaching a course as opposed to when one faculty member has responsibility for a course?

- How can the diversity of a school's student population be "exploited" to enhance the learning of all students?

- What are the most effective ways to help new faculty develop their knowledge and skills in each of the NLN's nurse educator competencies (NLN, 2005)?

- What is the impact on the type/level/complexity of questions posed by students when faculty "think out loud" and make visible to students how they manage complex situations?

- Which elements of the NLN's Excellence Model (NLN, 2006) have the greatest potential for moving a school of nursing from "good to great" (Collins, 2001)?

- What factors in the learning environment most influence students' excitement about learning and their taking responsibility for their own learning?

- How does the use of technology affect the learning process?

- What are the unplanned/unexpected outcomes of the educational experience, as reported by students?

- What learning experiences are most powerful in helping students clarify and internalize a set of values that are congruent with professional expectations?

- How do the teaching and learning climates at schools that focus on evidence-based teaching practices compare with the teaching and learning climates at schools that do not have such a focus?

Each of the preceding chapters outlines more specific questions that need to be studied as the nursing education community advances with building our science. In addition, the "What if ..." or "Why not ..." questions raised by nurse educators in relation to their teaching and student learning serve as fodder for areas of scholarly reflection and investigation.

## CONCLUSION

The questions to ask about nursing education are limitless at this point in our development as a science, but if we are to build that science systematically, deliberately and efficiently, we must be asking significant questions, conducting rigorous investigations of those questions, disseminating the findings of those investigations broadly, and applying those findings in our everyday teaching practices. In addition, each of us must join in the journey and contribute in some way.

With such concerted effort, the science of nursing education will evolve, continually be refined, and provide faculty with the evidence base needed to make sound decisions about curriculum design, teaching strategies, and evaluation methods. Our students deserve nothing less than excellence in education, and engaging in evidence-based nursing education can help us achieve that goal.

## REFERENCES

Boyer, E. L. (1990). *Scholarship reconsidered: Priorities of the professoriate.* New York: John Wiley & Sons.

Collins, J. (2001). *Good to great: Why some companies make the leap ... and others don't.* New York: Collins Business Publishers.

National League for Nursing. (2005). *Core competencies of nurse educators with task statements.* [Online]. Available http://www.nln.org/facultydevelopment/pdf/corecompetencies.pdf.

National League for Nursing. (2006). *Excellence in nursing education model.* New York: Author.

National League for Nursing. (2008). *Priorities for research in nursing education.* [Online]. Available: http://www.nln.org/research/priorities.htm.

Oermann, M. H. (1990). Research on teaching methods. In Clayton, G. M. & Baj, P. A. (Eds.). *Review of research in nursing education* (Volume III). New York: National League for Nursing.

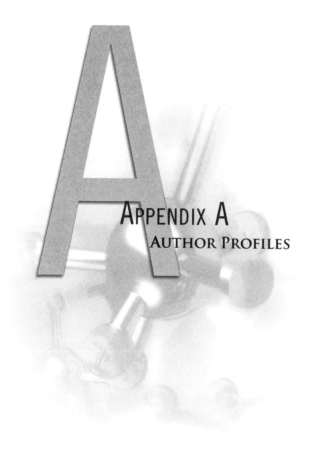

# Appendix A
## Author Profiles

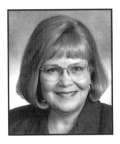

# CATHLEEN M. SHULTZ, PhD, RN, CNE, FAAN

*Professor and Dean of Nursing, Harding University (Searcy, AR)*
*NLN President-Elect 2007-2009; President 2009-2011*
*NLN Task Group on Teaching-Learning Paradigms Chair (2001-2006)*

Dr. Shultz is professor and dean of nursing at Harding University in Arkansas. She received a diploma in nursing from East Liverpool City Hospital (Ohio), a BSN from the University of South Carolina, a master's in nursing from Emory University (Atlanta, GA) and a doctorate from Vanderbilt University (Nashville, TN). A nurse educator for 30+ years, she has taught and learned from excellent nursing students (over 2000+) and a cadre of quality, caring colleagues. She has taught diploma, baccalaureate, master's and doctoral students and served three prior positions in hospital staff development. Her interests are curriculum design, innovations in teaching-learning, mentoring, professional values and evaluation of learning. Having twice received Harding University's Outstanding Teacher Award, she maintains an active teaching practice. She is a past treasurer of the NLN (2005-2007) and past chair-elect of the NLN's Measurement and Evaluation Advisory Council (2004-2005). With international experience in nursing education, she has been privileged to consult with numerous nursing programs for curriculum, faculty development and accreditation needs. Along with NLN colleagues, she was among the founders of the Academy of Nursing Education. She earned the CNE in 2006 and is a Fellow of the American Academy of Nursing.

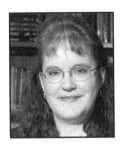

# NELL ARD, PhD, RNC, CNS, CNE

*Director of Nursing for Collin County Community College District*
*(McKinney, TX)*

Dr. Ard has been in nursing education for 20 years and has taught at the diploma, associate, baccalaureate, and master's degree levels. She has served NLN in several capacities: a member of the Task Group on Teaching/Learning, a member of a Task Group on Test Security, and consultant for the Centers of Excellence program. She is currently serving as an Ambassador and a Nominations Committee member, and she recently completed a 3-year term as chair of the Task Group on Clinical Nursing Education. She has presented several times at the NLN Summit. She graduated from Harding University (BSN), West Texas State University (MSN), and University of Texas Health Science Center at San Antonio (PhD in clinical nursing research). Dr. Ard has numerous publications and awards. She was recently honored by her nursing colleagues and students with the funding of a nursing scholarship named for her. She earned NLN's Certification in Nursing Education in 2006.

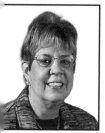

## RUTH SERIS GRESLEY, PhD, RN, CNE

***Professor of Nursing and Dean of the School of Human Services, Concordia University (Mequon, WI)***

Dr. Gresley is professor of nursing and dean of the School of Human Services at Concordia University in Wisconsin. She began her nursing career with a diploma in nursing from Barnes Hospital School of Nursing in St. Louis, MO. She earned her BSN at Washington University and her MSN and PhD in higher education from St. Louis University. She began her teaching career at Southern Illinois University at Edwardsville where she learned teaching, curriculum building and leadership skills. She came to Concordia in 1996 to launch the MSN program and has since developed the nurse educator track. She served two terms as Wisconsin League for Nursing President, and served on the Wisconsin Nursing Redesign Consortium Leadership Council. She is currently on the Northeast Area Health Education Center Board of Directors. Her early research focused on identifying the quality of family member caregiving. Her current research is a qualitative study of teaching/learning strategies for building clinical skills in nurse educator master's students. She is an NLN Certified Nurse Educator.

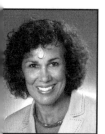

## PAMELA R. JEFFRIES, DNS, RN, FAAN, ANEF

***Associate Professor of Nursing and Associate Dean for Undergraduate Programs, Indiana University (Indianapolis, IN)***
***Project Director for NLN/Laerdal Simulation Projects***

Dr. Jeffries is an associate professor and associate dean for undergraduate programs at Indiana University School of Nursing. Her research and scholarship of teaching are focused on learning outcomes, instructional design, new pedagogies, innovative teaching strategies, and incorporating the use of technology and simulated learning. She has been awarded several grants to support her research and has received several teaching awards, including the NLN Lucile Petry Leone Award for nursing education, the prestigious Elizabeth Russell Belford Award for teaching excellence given by Sigma Theta Tau International, and numerous outstanding faculty awards presented by the graduating nursing classes at Indiana University School of Nursing. She has many publications and a career of scholarly research.

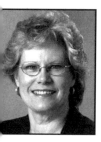

## GAIL C. KOST, MSN, RN, CNE

***Clinical Lecturer of Nursing, Department of Adult Health, Indiana University School of Nursing (Indianapolis, IN)***

Ms. Kost received a BSN from the University of Indianapolis and an MSN from the University of Pennsylvania. She received the Indy Star Salute to Nurses (2007) and was named Nurse Educator of the Year. She is an NLN Certified Nurse Educator.

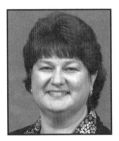

# Sheila Cox Sullivan, PhD, RN, CNE

*At the time of writing: Associate Professor and Associate Dean of Nursing, Harding University (Searcy, AR)*
*Current position: Associate Chief for Research, Central Arkansas Veterans Healthcare System (Little Rock, AR)*

Dr. Sullivan completed her basic nursing education at Harding University in Searcy, AR. She received her master's degree in critical care nursing from the University of Virginia and her PhD from the University of Arkansas for Medical Sciences in Little Rock. After working in critical care for over a decade, Dr. Sullivan worked as a supplemental staff educator and case manager. She began her nurse educator role at Virginia Tricollege Nursing Program, based in Abingdon, VA, an associate degree program serving the southwestern portion of Virginia. She then joined the faculty at her alma mater, Harding University, teaching baccalaureate students in critical care nursing, research, leadership and management, and nursing interventions courses. In January 2007, Dr. Sullivan became an NLN Certified Nurse Educator. While at Harding, graduating classes chose Dr. Sullivan to speak at the pinning exercises on three occasions, and she was named to Who's Who in America's Teachers four times. In January 2008, she accepted a position as the associate chief for research at the Central Arkansas Veterans Healthcare System. Dr. Sullivan recently served on the NLN's Clinical Nursing Education Task Group and has made numerous presentations and publications. She received several research and leadership awards and has held offices in the Arkansas Nurses Association. She was an NLN Ambassador.

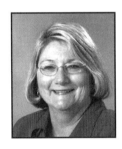

# Vema Sweitzer, MSN, RN, CNE

*Visiting Lecturer in Nursing, Department of Adult Health, Indiana University School of Nursing (Indianapolis, IN)*

Ms. Sweitzer graduated with a BSN from the University of Florida and received her master's in nursing from Emory University in Atlanta, GA. She is an NLN Certified Nurse Educator.

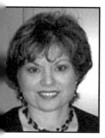

## CESARINA (CES) THOMPSON, PHD, RN

***Assistant to the Dean of the School of Health and Human Services
Former Chairperson and Professor of Nursing, Southern Connecticut
State University (New Haven, CT)***

Dr. Thompson recently assumed the role of assistant to the dean for the School of Health and Human Services at Southern Connecticut State University (SCSU). Prior to this appointment, she served as chairperson of the school's Department of Nursing for 13 years. Dr. Thompson has more than 20 years of experience as a nurse educator and has taught students at the associate, baccalaureate, and master's level. She taught the nurse educator courses in SCSU's MSN-Nurse Educator program and secured external funding to financially support MSN nurse educator students and convert some of the courses to online to enhance accessibility. Dr. Thompson's scholarly activities have focused on teaching effectiveness, evaluation and assessment. She has authored a number of articles and book chapters related to nursing education and has conducted research on teaching effectiveness and measuring program outcomes. Active in several professional organizations at the state and national levels, Dr. Thompson has also served on multiple task groups for the NLN including Teaching/Learning Paradigms and the Critical Thinking Think Tank, which developed a discipline-specific critical thinking definition and guidelines for critical thinking measurement instruments; the NLN's critical thinking test was based on this group's work.

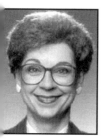

## THERESA M. (TERRY) VALIGA, EDD, RN, FAAN

***At the time of writing: Chief Program Officer, National League for
Nursing (New York, NY)
Current position: Director, Institute for Educational Excellence, Duke
University School of Nursing (Durham, NC)***

Dr. Valiga received both a master's and a doctorate in nursing education from Teachers College, Columbia University in New York. Prior to her appointment at the National League for Nursing, she held faculty and administrative positions in five different universities over a 26-year period and had the good fortune to teach hundreds of exceptional students and work with many outstanding faculty colleagues. In her role as chief program officer, Dr. Valiga collaborated with many talented NLN members to develop a number of NLN initiatives, including the Centers of Excellence program, the Academy of Nursing Education, position statements, the Hallmarks of Excellence in Nursing Education, the Excellence in Nursing Education Model, and several publications. She has received several prestigious awards for excellence in nursing education, presented on education topics at national and international conferences, published widely on issues related to nursing education, and consulted with nursing faculty groups in the United States, Canada, Japan, and China on curriculum development, program evaluation, innovations in teaching, and the faculty role. She also is an expert in the area of leadership and has co-authored a book (now in its third edition) on this complex phenomenon. After nine years with the NLN, Dr. Valiga joined Duke University's School of Nursing in July 2008 to create and lead their new Institute for Educational Excellence.

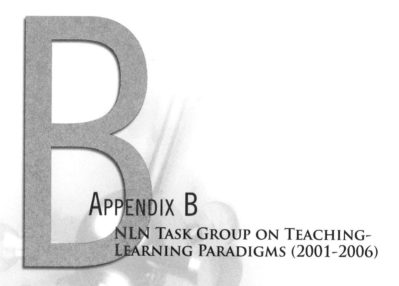

# Appendix B
## NLN Task Group on Teaching-Learning Paradigms (2001-2006)

## THE NLN TASK GROUP ON TEACHING-LEARNING PARADIGMS (2001-2006)

**Cathleen M. Shultz, PhD, RN, CNE, FAAN (Chair)**
*Dean and Professor*
*Harding University College of Nursing*
*Searcy, Arkansas*

**Nell Ard, PhD, RNC, CNS, CNE**
*Director of Nursing*
*Collin County Community College District*
*McKinney, Texas*

**Darlene Nebel Cantu, MSN, RNC (2001-2003)**
*Chief Nursing Officer*
*Baptist Health System*
*San Antonio, Texas*

**Ruth Seris Gresley, PhD, RN, CNE**
*Professor of Nursing*
*Dean, School of Human Sciences*
*Concordia University*
*Mequon, Wisconsin*

**Pamela R. Jeffries, DNS, RN, FAAN, ANEF**
*Associate Professor of Nursing*
*Associate Dean for Undergraduate Programs*
*Indiana University School of Nursing*
*Indianapolis, Indiana*

**Sheila Cox Sullivan, PhD, RN, CNE**
*Associate Chief for Research*
*Central Arkansas Veterans Healthcare System*
*Little Rock, Arkansas*
*(Note: Work was completed while Associate Professor*
*Harding University College of Nursing*
*Searcy, Arkansas)*

**Cesarina "Ces" Thompson, PhD, RN**
*Assistant to the Dean, School of Health and Human Services*
*Former Chairperson, Department of Nursing, and Professor of Nursing*
*Southern Connecticut State University*
*New Haven, Connecticut*

**Joyce Newman Giger, EdD, RN, CS, FAAN (2001-2002)**
*Professor, Graduate Studies*
*University of Alabama at Birmingham School of Nursing*
*Birmingham, Alabama*

**Martha M. Scheckel, PhD, RN**
*Assistant Professor of Nursing*
*Winona State University*
*Winona, Minnesota*
*(Note: Work was completed while a doctoral student intern with the NLN)*

**Theresa M. "Terry" Valiga, EdD, RN, FAAN**
*Director of the Institute for Educational Excellence*
*Duke University School of Nursing*
*Durham, North Carolina*
*(Note: Work was completed while Chief Program Officer*
*National League for Nursing*
*New York, New York)*

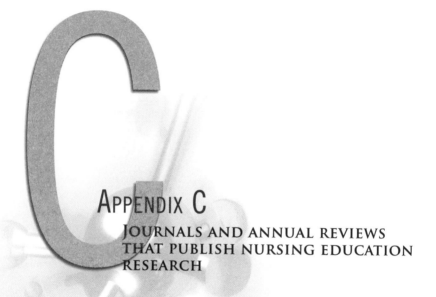

# Appendix C
## Journals and annual reviews that publish nursing education research

| Journal | Publisher |
|---|---|
| *Annual Review of Nursing Education* | Springer Publishing |
| *International Journal of Nursing Education Scholarship* | Berkeley Electronic Press |
| *Journal of Nursing Education* | Slack |
| *Journal of Nursing Scholarship* | Blackwell Publishing |
| *Journal of Professional Nursing* | Elsevier |
| *Nurse Education in Practice* | Elsevier |
| *Nurse Educator* | Lippincott Williams & Wilkins |
| *Nursing Education Perspectives* | National League for Nursing |

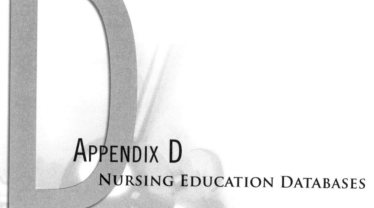

# APPENDIX D
## NURSING EDUCATION DATABASES

*Janet M. Phillips, PhDc, RN*
*Associate Instructor*
*Indiana University School of Nurssing*

| Database/URL* | Description |
|---|---|
| **Books@Ovid**<br>http://www.ovid.com/site/index.jsp | Provides key medical, nursing, and pharmacy e-texts from a variety of publishers. |
| **CDSR**<br>http://www.cochrane.org/reviews/ | Cochrane Database of Systematic Reviews. Provides full text of the regularly updated systematic reviews of the results of health care. The database is prepared by The Cochrane Collaboration. |
| **CINAHL**<br>http://www.ebscohost.com/cinahl/ | Cumulative Index of Nursing and Allied Health Literature. Covers the nursing and allied health literature from 1982 to the present. |
| **Education Full Text**<br>http://www.hwwilson.com/databases/educat.htm | Comprehensive coverage of an international range of periodicals, monographs and yearbooks. Full text of articles from hundreds of journals. |
| **EMBASE**<br>http://www.ovid.com/site/products/ovidguide/embase.htm | Excerpta Medicus Database Guide, produced by Elsevier, is a major biomedical and pharmaceutical database indexing over 3,500 international journals. There is selective coverage for nursing, dentistry, veterinary medicine, psychology, and alternative medicine. |
| **ERIC**<br>http://www.eric.ed.gov/ | Educational Resources Information Center database is sponsored by the U.S. Department of Education to provide extensive access to education-related literature, with access to up to 14,000 documents and over 20,000 journal articles per year |
| **HAPI**<br>http://www.ovid.com/site/catalog/DataBase/866.jsp | Health and Psychosocial Instruments. Provides a variety of valid and reliable measurement instruments for health fields |
| **Health Source**<br>http://www.ebscohost.com/titleLists.php?topicID=380&tabForward=titleLists http://www.hwwilson.com/databases/educat.htm | Nursing/Academic Edition available through EBSCOhost WebDatabases. Provides nearly 550 scholarly full-text journals focusing on many medical disciplines. |
| **Journals@Ovid**<br>http://www.ovid.com/site/index.jsp | Journals at Ovid Full Text. Provides hundreds of full text scientific, technical, and medical journals with graphics from over 82 publishers and societies. |
| **MEDLINE®**<br>http://www.ncbi.nlm.nih.gov/sites/entrez | MEDLINE® is the United States National Library of Medicine's (NLM®) premier bibliographic database, providing information from nursing, medicine, dentistry, veterinary medicine, allied health, and pre-clinical sciences from 1950 to the present month. |

| Database/URL* | Description |
|---|---|
| **MEDLINE® Daily Update**<br>http://medlineplus.gov/ | MEDLINE® database, which is updated daily. |
| **Ovid HealthStar**<br>http://www.ovid.com/site/index.jsp | Contains citations to the published literature on health services, technology, administration, and research. Focus is on both clinical and nonclinical aspects of health care delivery. |
| **PDC**<br>http://www.ebscohost.com/thisTopic.php?topicID=123&marketID=1 | Professional Development Collection. Provides a highly specialized collection of electronic information for professional educators from children's health and development to pedagogical theory and practice. Offered by EBSCO. |
| **PQDT**<br>http://www.proquest.com/products_pq/descriptions/pqdt.shtml | ProQuest Dissertations and Theses. Provides a comprehensive database of doctoral dissertations and master's theses. |
| **Professional Collection**<br>http://www.gale.cengage.com/servlet/ItemDetailServlet?region=9&imprint=000&titleCode=IACSBC&cf=n&type=4&id=174860 | A selection of more than 300 full-text journals for educators, with coverage for any professional educator in arts and humanities, child and adolescent psychology and development, drug and alcohol abuse, health/nutrition/fitness, learning disabilities, literature, science and technology, social sciences and sports/athletic training. Offered through Gale Information Search Engine. |
| **PsycINFO**<br>http://www.apa.org/psycinfo | Provides access to international literature in psychology and related disciplines such as psychiatry, education, business, medicine, nursing, pharmacology, law, linguistics, and social work. |
| **PubMed**<br>http://www.ncbi.nlm.nih.gov/pubmed/ | List of abstracts developed in conjunction with publishers of biomedical literature as a search tool for accessing literature citations and linking to full-text journals at websites of participating publishers. |
| **TRC**<br>http://web.ebscohost.com/ehost/search?vid=1&hid=102&sid=51a72957-843f-4e91-bdaa-3868017ec17e%40sessionmgr102 | Teacher Reference Center. Provides indexing and abstracts for over 280 of the most popular teacher and administrator trade journals to assist professional educators. |

# Appendix E

## Summary of Major Categories of Krathwohl, Bloom, & Masia's Affective Domain Taxonomy

*Cathleen M. Shultz, PhD, RN, CNE, FAAN*

| Description of the Major Categories in the Affective Domain | Illustrative General Instructional Objectives | Illustrative Verbs for Stating Specific Learning Outcomes |
|---|---|---|
| 1. **Receiving.** Receiving refers to the student's willingness to attend to particular phenomena or stimuli (classroom activities, textbook, music, etc.). From a teaching standpoint, it is concerned with getting, holding, and directing the student's attention. Learning outcomes in this area range from the simple awareness that a thing exists to selective attention on the part of the learner. Receiving represents the lowest level of learning outcomes in the affective domain. | • Listens attentively<br>• Shows awareness of the importance of learning<br>• Shows sensitivity to human needs and social problems<br>• Accepts differences of race and culture<br>• Attends closely to classroom activities | Asks, chooses, describes, follows, gives, holds, identifies, locates, names, points to, replies, selects, uses |
| 2. **Responding.** Responding refers to active participation on the part of the student. At this level, he or she not only attends to a particular phenomenon, but also reacts to it in some way. Learning outcomes in this area may emphasize acquiescence in responding (reads assigned material), willingness to respond (voluntarily reads beyond assignment), or satisfaction in responding (reads for pleasure or enjoyment). The higher levels of this category include those instructional objectives that are commonly classified under "interest"; that is, those that stress the seeking out and enjoyment of particular activities. | • Completes assigned homework<br>• Obeys school rules<br>• Participates in class discussion<br>• Completes laboratory work<br>• Volunteers for special tasks<br>• Shows interest in subject<br>• Enjoys helping others | Answers, assists, complies, conforms, discusses, greets, helps, labels, performs, practices, presents, reads, recites, reports, selects, tells, writes |

| Description of the Major Categories in the Affective Domain | Illustrative General Instructional Objectives | Illustrative Verbs for Stating Specific Learning Outcomes |
|---|---|---|
| 3. **Valuing.** Valuing is concerned with the worth or value a student attaches to a particular object, phenomenon, or behavior. This ranges in degree from the simpler acceptance of a value (desires to improve group skills) to the more complex level of commitment (assumes responsibility for the effective functioning of the group). Valuing is based on the internalization of a set of specified values, and clues to these values are expressed in the student's overt behavior. Learning outcomes in this area are concerned with behavior that is consistent and stable enough to make the value clearly identifiable. Instructional objectives that are commonly classified under "attitudes" and "appreciation" would fall into this category. | • Demonstrates belief in the democratic process<br><br>• Appreciates good literature (art or music)<br><br>• Appreciates the role of science (or other subjects) in everyday life<br><br>• Shows concern for the welfare of others<br><br>• Demonstrates problem solving attitude<br><br>• Demonstrates commitment to social improvement | Completes, describes, differentiates, displays, explains, follows, forms, initiates, invites, joins, justifies, proposes, reads, reports, selects, shares, studies, works |
| 4. **Organization.** Organization is concerned with bringing together different values, resolving conflicts between them, and beginning the building of an internally consistent value system. Thus, the emphasis is on comparing, relating, and synthesizing values. Learning outcomes may be concerned with the conceptualization of a value (recognizes the responsibility of each individual for improving human relations) or with the organization of a value system (develops a vocational plan that satisfies his or her need for both economic security and social service). Instructional objectives relating to the development of a philosophy of life would fall into this category. | • Recognizes the need for balance between freedom and responsibility in a democracy<br><br>• Recognizes the role of systematic planning in solving problems<br><br>• Accepts responsibility for his or her own behavior<br><br>• Understands and accepts his or her own strengths and limitations<br><br>• Formulates life plan in harmony with his or her abilities, interests, and beliefs | Adheres, alters, arranges, combines, compares, completes, contrasts, defends, explains, generalizes, identifies, integrates, modifies, orders, organizes, prepares, relates, synthesizes |

| Description of the Major Categories in the Affective Domain | Illustrative General Instructional Objectives | Illustrative Verbs for Stating Specific Learning Outcomes |
|---|---|---|
| 5. **Characterization by a Value or Value Complex.** At this level of the affective domain the individual has a value system that has controlled his or her behavior for a sufficiently long time for him or her to have developed a characteristic "life-style." Thus, the behavior is pervasive, consistent, and predictable. Learning outcomes at this level cover a broad range of activities, but the major emphasis is on the fact that the behavior is typical or characteristic of the student. Instructional objectives that are concerned with the student's general patterns of adjustment (personal, social, emotional) or response would be appropriate here. | • Demonstrates self-reliance working Independently<br><br>• Practices cooperation in group activities<br><br>• Uses objective approach in problem solving<br><br>• Demonstrates industry, punctuality, and self-discipline<br><br>• Maintains good health habits<br><br>• Displays safety consciousness | Acts, discriminates, displays, influences, listens, modifies, performs, practices, proposes, qualifies, questions, revises, serves, solves, uses, verifies |

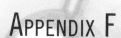

# Appendix F

### Latin American Scientific Contribution to New Teaching/Learning/Evaluation Paradigms to Advance Nursing Education: A Progress Review of the Portuguese and Spanish Literature

Collaborators:

Maria da Gloria Miotto Wright, PhD, RN
*Inter-American Commission on Drug Abuse Control (CICAD)*
*Organization of American States (OAS)*

Federal University of Santa Catarina, Brazi
Maria Itayra Coelho de Souza Padilha, PhD, RN
Kenya Schmitz Reibnitz, Doctoral Student
Joel Rolim Mancia, Graduate Student

University of Nuevo Leon, Monterrey, México
Silvia Espinoza Ortega, MNSc

## BACKGROUND

Scientific nursing publication in Latin America is strongly linked to the production of graduate nursing educational programs, the organization of national conferences, workshops and seminars, and individual initiatives by nursing faculty. In Latin America, graduate nursing education started in the 1970s, with Brazil being the leader by opening the first graduate program (master's in the 70s and doctoral programs in the 80s) (Almeida et al., 2003). Other countries began their general graduate education in the late 80s and early 90s (Wright & Alarcon, 1999). As a result, graduate programs became an important tool to advance nursing training and education, and, in turn, increase scientific knowledge, specialized journals, and other nursing-related publication.

This report portraits a preliminary progress result of seven Latin American countries: Argentina, Brazil, Chile, Costa Rica, Colombia, Cuba, and Mexico. It covers ten years of scientific publications in nursing journals, as well as other areas related to nursing education.

The International Coordinator of the Nursing Schools Project on Demand Reduction for Latin America of the Inter-American Drug Abuse Control Commission (CICAD) was the liaison from the NLN's Nursing Education Research, Technology, and Information Management Advisory Council who worked with The Task Group on Teaching-Learning Paradigms, along with faculty and graduate students from the Nursing Department of the Federal University of Santa Catarina, Brazil, and the Nursing Faculty of University of Nuevo Leon, Mexico. They reviewed the literature of Portuguese and Spanish nursing journals to identify the Latin American scientific contribution of nursing education on the subject of "New Teaching and Learning Evaluation Paradigms, Theories, and Methods of Nursing Education."

## FINDINGS

The Latin American nurses published a total of 209 articles on nursing education between 1994 and 2004. There were a total of 180 articles in Portuguese and 29 in Spanish.

The articles in Portuguese were published in 10 journals: nine in nursing-related journals, and one outside the nursing field. Three articles were published in English. The majority of Brazilian nursing journals (seven in total) are based in the South and Southeast regions of the country, while the other three originate from Brazil's Northeast and Midwest regions. Some of the themes and emphasis of these Portuguese-language articles about nursing education are as follows (Padilha, Reibnitz, & Mancia, 2003):

- Autonomy and Nurse Emancipation Process
- Case Studies Model as a Teaching Strategy
- Communication and Nursing Education
- Competence and Performance of Nursing Faculty

- Constructivism as a Methodological Strategy
- Continuing Education
- Critical Thinking and Nursing Education
- Critical-Holistic Paradigm and Model
- Critical-Reflective Approach for Capacity-Building Nursing Programs
- Curriculum Development from a Dialectic Perspective
- Development of Educational Software for Pediatrics
- Distance Educational Technology
- Distance Nursing Education and Problem-Raising Methodology
- Educating Toward Autonomy
- Educational Health Process in the Group Dimension
- Emancipator Nursing Educational Experiences
- Ethnography and Pedagogical Practice
- Evaluation Following a Constructive Perspective
- Evaluation of the Teaching-Learning Process
- Evaluation Process – Emphasis on Novelties
- Evaluation Process and Integrated Curriculum
- Faculty and Clinical Nursing Partnerships
- Health Education
- Humanized and Participatory Evaluation Process
- Information and Education Strategies
- Initiatives in the Innovation of Teaching Nursing in Latin America
- Innovation and Teaching-Learning Process at the Graduate Level
- Institutional Nursing Learning Analysis
- International Health and Nursing Education
- Learners, Educators, and New Esthetic Values
- Learning Negotiating
- New Methodologies for Nursing Education at the Technical, Undergraduate, and Graduate Levels
- New Pedagogical Proposal for Nursing Education
- Nursing Care Plan
- Nursing Curriculum in an Integrated Model
- Nursing Network
- Nursing Political-Pedagogic Approach
- Nursing Process and Problem-Raising Pedagogy
- Nursing Teaching and Research
- Participant-Research and Didactic-Pedagogical Education
- Path for Teaching-Learning and Research
- Paulo Freire's Educational Model Applied to Nursing Education and Practice

- Pedagogical Capacity-Building for Nurses
- Pedagogical Transformation in Nursing Education
- Playing Social Roles as a Teaching-Learning Strategy
- Political-Pedagogical Project Focused on the Culture of Care
- Political-Pedagogy Project for Undergraduate Nursing Courses
- Problem-Solving in a Teaching-Learning Process
- Public Health Nursing and Pedagogical and Agricultural Advice in Rural Communities
- Quality of Teaching and Evaluation Model
- Reflection about Theoretical-Practical Nursing Education
- Research as an Educational Experience
- Rethinking Nursing Education
- Rituals of Power in Formal Nursing Education
- Sharing and Curriculum Evaluation
- Software for Teaching Basic Needs
- Specialized Education in the Areas of Gerontology, Administration, Women's Health, Psychiatry, Children and Adolescents, Surgery, Home Health, and Community Health
- Strategies for Multiprofessional and Multidisciplinary Integration in Health
- Structure of Nursing Curricula
- Supervision and Nursing Education
- Support Technician in a Nursing Assistance Project
- Teachers Practice a New Concept of Quality in Nursing Education
- Teaching of Nursing and Pedagogic Trends
- Teaching Strategies and Learning Process
- The Interdisciplinary Approach in Nursing Education
- Theater as an Alternative for Health Education
- Theory Support for the Creative Teaching Process

The articles in Spanish were published in 19 nursing journals from six Latin American countries: Argentina (7), Mexico (4), Colombia (4), Chile (2), Costa Rica (1), and Cuba (1). Some of the themes and emphasis in this literature are as follows (Espinoza, 2003):

- Bio-Ethics in Nursing
- Computers and Nursing Education
- Curriculum Development
- Evaluation of Distance Education Programs
- Evaluation Process
- Gerontology and Nursing Education

- Human Resources Development
- Innovation and Teaching Models
- National State of Nursing Research
- Nursing Care
- Nursing Degrees via Internet
- Research and Nursing Education
- Research Skills
- Self-Education Strategies
- Teaching-Learning Process
- Time and Theoretical-Practice Exams
- Use of Research Results in Clinical Practice

The themes and emphasis classification of nursing articles in the Portuguese and Spanish languages, according to the NLN *Priorities for Research in Nursing Education*, are shown in Table F.1. This compilation is the first attempt to use the NLN research priorities to examine literature from outside the United States to identify trends and their corresponding implications. The NLN research priorities (in 2001, when this analysis was completed) are as follows:

I.  Competencies for nursing graduates for practice in the 21st century;

II.  Accountability links between educational programs and health outcomes;

III.  Infusion of technologies into concepts, structure, and process of nursing education;

IV.  Resource accountability models for educating the nursing workforce;

V.  Educator competencies for changing the social, health care, and educational worlds; and

VI.  Research-based paradigms, strategies and evaluation models for nursing education.

The articles in Portuguese and Spanish were distributed across all priority areas. The data indicate that the articles in Portuguese fell more frequently under priorities I, V, and VI, and less frequently under priorities II, III, and IV. As for the Spanish articles, they fell more frequently under priorities III and VI, and less frequently under priorities I, II, IV, and V.

## ANALYSIS

By analyzing the data, we concluded that Latin American nursing journals regarding the project's main theme were more common in Brazil than in the other Latin countries. This conclusion points out, in some respect, the impact that graduate nursing programs have had in advancing the scientific and technological aspects of nursing education and the nursing profession in Brazil. In contrast, Spanish-speaking nurses have only recently begun to receive the benefits of graduate nursing education.

In analyzing the most frequent themes regarding nursing journals in Portuguese related to priorities I, V, and VI in Table F.1, we realized the importance Brazilian nurses give to issues such as international health, the relationship between political and pedagogical approaches to education, critical thinking, dialectic perspective, interdisciplinary, emancipation, negotiation, and autonomy aspects in the preparation of nurses for the 21st century. Hence, the importance of preparing educators with competencies and goals toward the autonomy, understanding power within nursing education, communication, and supervision aspects. In addition, Brazilian nurses value the development of new paradigms for education, test innovative didactic-pedagogy methodologies, use the evaluation process to improve nursing education and curriculum development, and value the importance of using research as a tool to advance nursing education.

The analysis of less frequent themes in nursing journals in Portuguese related to priorities II, III, and IV in Table F.1 shows that the accountability between educational programs and health outcomes, as well as the importance of educating the nurse workforce, is a new area of study for nurses in Brazil. However, the infusion of technologies within nursing education has become a reality among Brazilian nurses. They have developed distance education programs and specific software as new initiatives to advance the field of nursing.

The analysis of the most common themes regarding nursing journals in Spanish related to priorities III and VI in Table F.1 indicates the importance Spanish-speaking nurses give to the infusion of technology in nursing education, and to research as a tool to advance the same. However, priorities I, II, IV, and V are still new research areas for most nurses in Spanish-speaking Latin America.

## CONCLUSION

The search initiated with this project is only the first step in understanding more about the trends regarding nursing education and its research implications toward advancing science and technology for the nursing profession in Latin America.

It is evident that nursing education and research in Brazil is more advanced than in the above-mentioned Latin American countries, and it is the contribution of graduate nursing programs that facilitate this process. Spanish-speaking nurses in Latin America, therefore, need to advance their education at the graduate level to demonstrate their contribution to the development of science and technology, both within the nursing community and outside of it.

The research priorities for nursing education developed by NLN indicates six new areas of study for nurses in Latin America. Brazil is the only country that has advanced in these areas of study to some extent. Latin American nurse researchers should conduct a more profound analysis of the factors determining and conditioning this situation. Another aspect that needs to be addressed in this study is the fact that the NLN priorities were developed for nursing education in the United States. Consequently, when they are applied to research studies elsewhere, we must consider the trends and realities of nursing education in other countries, especially because their political, economic, social, cultural, and technological realities are very different than those faced by the United States.

The analysis and conclusions of this report demonstrate the importance and necessity of working toward integration and collaboration of nurses around the world, and especially those in Latin America.

## REFERENCES

Almeida, M.C. P. et al. (2003). The doctoral programs in Latin America: The case study of Brazil. In _The new nursing doctoral programs and their contribution to demand reduction in Latin America: Challenges and perspectives._ Washington, D.C.: Inter-American Drug Abuse Control Commission/CICAD. Washington, D.C.: Author. (Title translated to English; the original title is in Spanish.)

Espinoza, S.O. (2003). _Nursing education – Trends of knowledge in Latin America. Technical Report._ Brasilia, Brazil: Ministry of Health. (Title translated to English; the original title is in Spanish.)

Padilha, M.I.C.Z,; Reibnitz, K.S., & Mancia, J.R. (2003). _Nursing education – Trends of knowledge in Brazil._ Technical Report. Brasilia, Brazil: Ministry of Health. (Title translated to English; the original title is in Spanish.)

Wright, M.G.M., & Alarcon, N.G. (1999). Critical-holistic analysis of graduate nursing education programs in Latin America. In _Nursing in the Americas. Scientific Publication # 571._ Washington, D.C.: Pan American Health Organization/World Health Organization: Author. (Title translated to English; the original title is in Spanish.)

**Table F.1.** Classification of Themes and Emphasis of Nursing Articles in Portuguese and Spanish Related to the NLN's Priorities for Research in Nursing Education

| NLN Priorities for Research in Nursing Education | Themes & Emphasis of Nursing Articles in Portuguese | Themes & Emphasis of Nursing Articles in Spanish |
|---|---|---|
| I. Competencies of Nursing Graduates for Practice in the 21st Century | Autonomy and Nurse Emancipation Process<br>Constructivism as a Methodological Strategy<br>Critical Thinking and Nursing Education<br>Curriculum Development from a Dialectic Perspective<br>Emancipator Nursing Educational Experiences<br>International Health and Nursing Education<br>Learning Negotiation<br>Nursing Political-Pedagogic Approach<br>Political-Pedagogical Project Focused on the Culture of Care<br>Political-Pedagogy Project for Undergraduate Nursing Courses<br>Rethinking Nursing Education<br>Strategies for Multiprofessional and Multidisciplinary Integration in Health<br>The Interdisciplinary Approach in Nursing Education | Bio-Ethics in Nursing |
| II. Accountability Links between Educational Programs and Health Outcomes | Faculty and Clinical Nursing Partnerships<br>Nursing Network | Use of Research Results in Clinical Practice |
| III. Infusion of Technology into Concepts, Structure, and Processes of Nursing Education | Developing Educational Software for Pediatrics<br>Distance Education Technology<br>Distance Nursing Education and Problem-Raising Methodology<br>Information and Education Strategies<br>Initiatives in the Innovation of Teaching Nursing in Latin America<br>Software for Teaching Basic Needs | Computers and Nursing Education<br>Evaluation of Distance Education Programs<br>Nursing Degrees via Internet |
| IV. Resource Accountability Models of Educating the Nursing Workforce | Institutional Nursing Learning Analysis<br>Nursing Care Plan<br>Support Technician in a Nursing Assistance Project | Human Resources Development |

**Table F.1. Classification of Themes and Emphasis of Nursing Articles in Portuguese and Spanish Related to the NLN's Priorities for Research in Nursing Education (continued)**

| NLN Priorities for Research in Nursing Education | Themes & Emphasis of Nursing Articles in Portuguese | Themes & Emphasis of Nursing Articles in Spanish |
|---|---|---|
| V. Educator Competencies for Changing Social, Health Care and Educational Worlds | Communication and Nursing Education<br>Competence and Performance of Nursing Faculty<br>Educating toward Autonomy<br>Learners, Educators and the New Esthetic Model<br>Pedagogical Capacity-Building for Nurses<br>Rituals of Power in Formal Nursing Education<br>Supervision and Nursing Education<br>Teachers Practice a New Concept of Quality in Nursing Education<br>Teaching Strategies and Learning Process | Nursing Care |
| VI. Research-Based Paradigms, Strategies and Evaluation Models for Nursing Education | Case Studies Model as a Teaching Strategy<br>Continuing Education<br>Critical-Holistic Paradigm<br>Critical-Reflective Approach for Capacity-Building Nursing Programs<br>Educational Health Process in the Group Dimension<br>Ethnography and Pedagogical Practice<br>Evaluation Following a Constructive Perspective<br>Evaluation of Teaching-Learning Process<br>Evaluation Process – Emphasis on Novelties<br>Evaluation Process and Integrated Curriculum<br>Health Education<br>Humanized and Participatory Evaluation Process<br>Innovation and Teaching-Learning Process at the Graduate Level<br>New Methodologies for Nursing Education at the Technical, Undergraduate, and Graduate Levels<br>New Pedagogical Proposal for Nursing Education<br>Nursing Curriculum in an Integrated Model<br>Nursing Process and Problem-Raising Pedagogy<br>Nursing Teaching and Research<br>Participant-Research and Didactic-Pedagogical Education<br>*(continued)* | Curriculum Development<br>Evaluation Process<br>Gerontology and Nursing Education<br>Innovation and Teaching Learning Process<br>National State of Nursing Research<br>Research and Nursing Education<br>Research Skills<br>Self-Education Strategies<br>Teaching-Learning Process<br>Time and Theoretical-Practice Exams |

| Table F.1. Classification of Themes and Emphasis of Nursing Articles in Portuguese and Spanish Related to the NLN's Priorities for Research in Nursing Education (continued) | | |
|---|---|---|
| NLN Priorities for Research in Nursing Education | Themes & Emphasis of Nursing Articles in Portuguese | Themes & Emphasis of Nursing Articles in Spanish |
| VI. Research-Based Paradigms, Strategies and Evaluation Models for Nursing Education (continued) | Path for Teaching-Learning and Research | |
| | Paulo Freire's Educational Model Applied to Nursing Education and Practice | |
| | Pedagogical Transformation in Nursing Education | |
| | Playing Social Roles as a Teaching-Learning Strategy | |
| | Problem-Solving in a Teaching-Learning Process | |
| | Public Health Nursing and Pedagogical and Agricultural Advice in Rural Communities | |
| | Quality of Teaching and Evaluation Model | |
| | Reflection about Theoretical-Practical Nursing Education | |
| | Research as an Educational Experience | |
| | Sharing and Curriculum Evaluation | |
| | Specialized Education in the Areas of Gerontology, Administration, Women's Health, Psychiatry, Children and Adolescents, Surgery, Home Health, and Community Health | |
| | Structure of Nursing Curricula | |